Researching the Autism Spectrum

Contemporary Perspectives

This selection of contemporary studies provides up-to-date perspectives from leading investigators who are at the cutting edge of research into Autism Spectrum Disorders. The book allows readers to grasp new approaches to understanding the autism spectrum. Key areas of theory and research are covered, from classification and diagnosis, genetics, neurology and biochemistry, to socio-cognitive, developmental and educational perspectives, essential to a broader understanding of the autism spectrum. In addition, it introduces new emphases on MEG, epilepsy and memory. In highlighting both biomedical and psychological perspectives, this book reflects the multi-level focus of contemporary thinking about autism. By addressing key unanswered questions, *Researching the Autism Spectrum* acts as a guidepost for future research and provides an authoritative and multi-disciplinary perspective.

ILONA ROTH is Senior Lecturer in Psychology in the Department of Life Sciences at the Open University. Her textbooks and media materials have a wide audience in and beyond the OU. Her research focuses on alterations of cognitive and socio-cognitive functioning in Autism Spectrum Disorders and dementia. Key recent publications focus on imagination and on the autism spectrum.

PAYAM REZAIE is Reader in Neuropathology in the Department of Life Sciences at the Open University. His research interests and expertise lie in clinical and experimental neuropathology and in developmental neurobiology. He is leading a programme of research into the neuropathology of autism supported by Autism Speaks and the Autism Tissue Program (USA).

Researching the Autism Spectrum

Contemporary Perspectives

Edited by

ILONA ROTH

The Open University

PAYAM REZAIE

The Open University

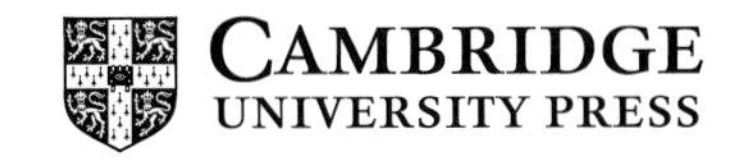

CAMBRIDGE UNIVERSITY PRESS
Cambridge, New York, Melbourne, Madrid, Cape Town, Singapore,
São Paulo, Delhi, Dubai, Tokyo, Mexico City

Cambridge University Press
The Edinburgh Building, Cambridge CB2 8RU, UK

Published in the United States of America by Cambridge University Press, New York

www.cambridge.org
Information on this title: www.cambridge.org/9780521518963

First published 2011

Printed in the United Kingdom at the University Press, Cambridge

A catalogue record for this publication is available from the British Library

Library of Congress Cataloguing in Publication data
Researching the autism spectrum : contemporary perspectives / [edited by]
Ilona Roth, Payam Rezaie.
p. cm.
Includes index.
ISBN 978-0-521-51896-3 (hardback)
1. Autism spectrum disorders. I. Roth, Ilona. II. Rezaie, Payam.
RC553.A88R48 2011
616.85′882 – dc22 2010038766

ISBN 978-0-521-51896-3 Hardback
ISBN 978-0-521-73686-2 Paperback

Contents

The colour plates are to be found between 208 and 209.

Preface

There is widespread concern about the apparently growing prevalence of autism, although this increase may be due, in large part, to factors such as changes in diagnostic criteria and ascertainment practices. Public and scientific interest in the causes and fundamental nature of autism has never been stronger. Research in this field has grown exponentially in the last twenty years, with significant financial support in this area provided by Governments, Research Councils and private charities. Studies spanning a whole range of disciplines share the goals of elucidating the core phenomena and underlying aetiology, thereby informing therapeutic interventions, as well as offering valuable insights into normal functioning. Research by individuals and groups in the UK has played a leading role in addressing key unanswered questions about autism, including its causes and psychological substrates, the underlying brain mechanisms, and the most effective ways to work with and support people with autism and their families.

A major conference which we were privileged to organise in 2007, entitled: 'Autism Research UK: from diagnosis to intervention' hosted by the Open University and sponsored by the Medical Research Council, Wellcome Trust, Autism Speaks and a number of other organisations, provided an effective backdrop to this book. At this first national meeting of this scope, internationally renowned speakers and chairpersons convened with representatives from the Medical Research Council, the Wellcome Trust, Economic and Social Research Council, National Autistic Society and Autism Speaks for two days of discussion and debate aimed at elucidating ways forward in understanding the autism spectrum and helping affected individuals and their families. A series of themed scientific sessions charted the way UK-based investigations have shaped and developed our understanding of the autism spectrum over recent years. This provided a strong rationale for an edited volume which would present a selection of 'cutting edge' contributions to theory and practice in this important, rapidly moving field.

This book, encompassing three main sections, presents an authoritative and multi-disciplinary perspective on autism from leading UK-based investigators who are active at the forefront of research in this field. A selection of key areas of research and theory covering classification and diagnosis, genetics, neurology and biochemistry, through to socio-cognitive, developmental and educational perspectives, including new emphases (MEG, autism and epilepsy, memory in autism) are highlighted, and provide the fundamental basis for a broader understanding of the autism spectrum. We are confident that this collection of works will serve as a balanced, authoritative and contemporary reference that will inform current understanding of the science of autism and act as a guidepost for research over the next few years. We expect that this book will appeal to, and inform a wide readership from clinical and academic professionals, to educators, healthcare providers, and policy makers. It will also be of interest to the substantial and growing body of parents and family members of those who are affected by autism.

We are deeply indebted to our colleagues and especially to the authors and contributors for their encouragement, their support and their commitment. We hope that you will find the contents stimulating and informative.

Ilona Roth
Payam Rezaie

Foreword

The editors of this volume, Ilona Roth and Payam Rezaie, have assembled a valuable collection of chapters providing an excellent overview of a wide range of areas relevant to autism research. The book tackles the challenge of early detection; the complex biology of autism, including genetics (from linkage, to association, to CNVs), the autistic brain (from the perspectives of MRI, DTI, MEG, neuroanatomy and epilepsy) and molecular aspects of autism (from serotonin to oxytocin); the complex psychology of autism (from cognitive models, language, memory and executive function); and the challenge of education in autism.

Autism research is currently enjoying considerable growth, with hundreds of researchers joining in the hunt to understand this important set of conditions. This book showcases some of the best autism scientists in the UK who are contributing to this international effort. The editors are to be congratulated on pulling this collection together, since this will inspire a new generation of autism scientists among contemporary students. The hope is that an anthology of this kind will be produced every few years, so we can track this fast-changing field. This multi-disciplinary book nicely illustrates how autism is a multi-level phenomenon that will need integration across levels. This book exemplifies how each level must be represented and contributes to the bigger picture.

Simon Baron-Cohen
Professor of Developmental Psychopathology
Director of the Autism Research Centre
University of Cambridge

Contributors

Professor Anthony Bailey, IMH Chair in Child and Adolescent Psychiatry, UBC Institute of Mental Health, University of British Columbia, Canada

Professor Jill Boucher, Autism Research Group, Department of Psychology, School of Social Sciences, City University London

Professor Dermot Bowler, Autism Research Group, Department of Psychology, School of Social Sciences, City University London

Dr Sven Braeutigam, Oxford Centre for Human Brain Activity (OHBA), University Department of Psychiatry, Medical Sciences Division, Oxford University

Professor Ann Le Couteur, Professor of Child and Adolescent Psychiatry, Institute of Health and Society, Newcastle University

Dr Sebastian Gaigg, Autism Research Group, Department of Psychology, School of Social Sciences, City University London

Professor Christopher Gillberg, Professor of Child Psychiatry, Institute of Neuroscience and Physiology, Child and Adolescent Psychiatry, Queen Silvia's Hospital for Children and Adolescents, University of Göteborg (Gothenburg), Sweden

Dr Ofer Golan, Senior Lecturer, Head of the Child Clinical Program, Bar-Ilan University, Ramat-Gan, Israel

Dr Jessica Hobson, Behavioural and Brain Science Unit, University College London Institute of Child Health, London

Professor R. Peter Hobson, Professor of Developmental Psychopathology, Behavioural and Brain Science Unit, University College London Institute of Child Health, London

Dr Richard Holt, Wellcome Trust Centre for Human Genetics, University of Oxford

Dr Ayla Humphrey, Consultant Clinical Psychologist, Autism Research Centre and Developmental Psychiatry Section, University of Cambridge

Professor Eve C. Johnstone, Professor of Psychiatry, Centre for Clinical Brain Sciences, University Department of Psychiatry, Royal Edinburgh Hospital, Edinburgh

Professor Rita Jordan, Emeritus Professor, School of Education, University of Birmingham

Dr Sophie Lind, Autism Research Group, Department of Psychology, School of Social Sciences, City University London

Professor Anthony P. Monaco, Professor of Human Genetics, Head of Neurogenetics Laboratory, Wellcome Trust Centre for Human Genetics, University of Oxford

Dr Elizabeta B. Mukaetova-Ladinska, Clinical Senior Lecturer and Consultant in Old Age Psychiatry, Institute for Ageing and Health, Newcastle University

Professor Brian Neville, Emeritus Professor of Paediatric Neurology, Neurosciences Unit, The Wolfson Centre, University College London Institute of Child Health, London

Dr Alistair Pagnamenta, Wellcome Trust Centre for Human Genetics, University of Oxford

Dr Elizabeth Pellicano, Senior Lecturer in Autism Education, Centre for Research in Autism and Education, Department of Psychology and Human Development, Institute of Education, University of London

Professor Elaine Perry, Professor of Neurochemical Pathology, Institute for Ageing and Health, Newcastle University

Dr Sara Sopena, Medical Research Council Cognition and Brain Sciences Unit, Cambridge

Dr Inês Girão Meireles de Sousa, Wellcome Trust Centre for Human Genetics, University of Oxford

Dr Michael D. Spencer, Autism Research Centre, University of Cambridge

Dr Andrew C. Stanfield, Centre for Clinical Brain Sciences, University Department of Psychiatry, Royal Edinburgh Hospital, Edinburgh

Professor Stephen J. Swithenby, Professor of Physics, Department of Physics and Astronomy, Faculty of Science, The Open University

Jodie Westwood, Institute for Ageing and Health, Newcastle University

Professor Barbara Wilson, Medical Research Council Cognition and Brain Sciences Unit, Cambridge

Introduction

ILONA ROTH AND PAYAM REZAIE

The term 'Autism Spectrum' currently embraces a cluster of conditions known as Autism Spectrum Disorders or 'ASD', that are characterised by impairments in social functioning, verbal and non-verbal communication, together with repetitive and stereotypical patterns of behaviour and interests. Impairments within each of these 'core' clinical domains can range in severity from mild to profound, and intellectual disability may be present in more severe cases. The classification of ASD broadly includes classic autism (childhood autism; autistic disorder), Asperger syndrome and Pervasive Developmental Disorder Not Otherwise Specified (PDD-NOS) (Levy *et al.* 2009). Classic autism is frequently diagnosed around the age of 3 (and may be diagnosed as early as 2 years of age) (Baird *et al.* 2003; Landa, 2008). Asperger syndrome often presents with more subtle symptoms, and is usually diagnosed later on in childhood (frequently around 11 years of age), and occasionally in adults (Howlin and Asgharian 1999; Toth and King 2008).

While the precise causes of autism remain a mystery, prevalence estimates have risen almost exponentially within the last six decades, making autism a major global concern. Initially considered rare, current estimates suggest that as many as 1% of children under the age of 8 years may have an autism spectrum diagnosis (Baird *et al.* 2006), with boys being diagnosed up to four times more than girls. More than half a million people are thought to be living with autism in the UK alone (National Autistic Society, 2007), and in the US autism is considerably more common today than it was in the 1980s (Yeargin-Allsopp *et al.* 2003).

Terminology relating to the autism spectrum is markedly inconsistent between formal and informal contexts, and between different expert groups. The term 'autism' is often used colloquially as an umbrella term for the entire autism

Researching the Autism Spectrum: Contemporary Perspectives, ed. I. Roth and P. Rezaie. Published by Cambridge University Press.

spectrum, as well as more specifically for the classic or prototypical form of autism spectrum disorder. Some researchers and autism advocates favour the term 'Autism Spectrum Conditions' (ASC), rather than Autism Spectrum Disorders or ASD, one rationale being that the first phrase avoids the connotation of autism as a disorder or disability, and is thus less discriminatory than the second. The terms 'high-functioning' and 'low-functioning' autism reflect a classification employed by many researchers, alongside the diagnostic distinctions, to distinguish those with normal or above normal intellectual abilities from those who are intellectually disabled. The question of whether high-functioning autism and Asperger syndrome denote the same, overlapping or different groups of individuals remains unresolved.

The two major classification systems, DSM-IV (American Psychiatric Association, 2000) and ICD-10 (World Health Organization, 1993), also employ subtly different terms for the sub-groups within the spectrum. The forthcoming version of DSM (DSM-V due to be released in 2013) aims to reduce some of the complexity, and address unreliability in the diagnostic differentiation of sub-groups (American Psychiatric Association, 2010). The Neurodevelopmental Disorders Workgroup have publicised their intention to remove the diagnostic sub-types (autistic disorder, Asperger disorder and PDD-NOS) from the classification, replacing them with a single clinical entity 'Autism Spectrum Disorder', within which individual symptom patterns will be differentiated by a severity score (Swedo, 2008; 2009). Yet, despite its worthy aims, the proposal has stimulated considerable debate, underlining the wide range of views that still prevail in this area. Issues surrounding terminology, classification and diagnosis are discussed further in Chapter 1. In the remainder of this introduction, we will use the terms 'ASD' and 'autism' interchangeably to refer to the spectrum as a whole. In the remaining chapters of this volume we have left authors to adopt the terminology with which they feel most comfortable.

Autism: an evolving concept

Leo Kanner (1943) viewed autism as a syndrome, a specific developmental disorder with a characteristic set of symptoms, likely to have a single underlying cause. Evidence for a different and more nuanced interpretation existed in the contemporary work of Hans Asperger (1944), but it was 40 years before Asperger's work came to wider attention through the work of Lorna Wing (1981). Asperger's work, later translated into English and reprinted by Uta Frith (1991), provided the stimulus for Wing to make two radical proposals: firstly, the notion of autism as a spectrum, rather than a syndrome, and secondly, the idea of Asperger syndrome as a separable sub-type of autism.

The ramifications of these new ideas were profound, including revisions to the diagnostic criteria to include Asperger syndrome as a separate diagnostic entity, diagnosis of many individuals who would not have been recognised as autistic by Kanner, recognition of the complex and possibly incidental relationship between intellectual disability and autism, increasing prevalence estimates and so on.

Three decades on from Wing's pioneering contributions, the concept of the autism spectrum is still evolving: further major changes are being considered with the growing appreciation that the autism spectrum may be best characterised as a continuum rather than as a cluster of sub-types (hence the radical proposals for DSM-V); the concept that autistic traits are graded from those individuals with full expression, to family members with 'shadow traits' constituting the Broader Autism Phenotype, to the existence of some autistic-like characteristics even in the 'neurotypical' population.

The implication of this still moving trajectory is that the characterisation and explanation of autism is far more complex than either Kanner or Asperger could have realised. Despite much progress in research, theory and clinical practice in this field over the last seven decades, autism remains a conundrum, a disorder, or group of disorders, which is compelling and yet elusive, and for which medical remediation (e.g. Coury, 2010) is as yet extremely limited. Moreover the status of autism as a 'disorder' rather than a difference has been contested: there is a substantial diversity of views on whether all forms of autism, and especially Asperger syndrome, require remediation.

What are the reasons for the persisting obscurity surrounding this spectrum or cluster of conditions?

Heterogeneity across the autism spectrum

There is consensus on the substantial variability of autism. The expression and severity of symptoms vary significantly from one affected individual to another, and furthermore, autism may present with or without: (i) full expression of the diagnostic triad of symptoms; (ii) intellectual disability; (iii) marked delay/impairment of language; and (iv) a range of different co-morbid conditions (most notably epilepsy). In addition, autism may affect a solitary member of a family, or occur in multiple family members. From this picture, and from a substantial body of scientific studies, it has become clear that the causal factors involved in autism are likely to be multiple, complex, and quite possibly variable from one individual case and one major symptom group to another, even if different influences can be said to converge towards a 'final common pathway' (Frith *et al.* 1991; Darby and Clark, 1992; Geschwind, 2008). Earlier notions that it might be possible to identify specific biological markers for autism, or even a single gene, as in cystic fibrosis for example, have foundered (see Happé *et al.* 2006; Geschwind, 2008).

Known single gene mutations account for less than 1% of all ASD cases, confirming the aetiological heterogeneity of autism (Geschwind, 2009).

Heterogeneity at both aetiological and behavioural levels has, in turn, led to methodological and interpretative difficulties in research. For instance, in psychological studies, there is limited consensus about the appropriate way of matching experimental and control participants (see for example the Journal of Autism and Developmental Disorders: Special Issue on Research Methodology-Matching, Jacob, 2004), and experimental groups may be heterogeneous in terms of sub-diagnosis and the presence or absence of co-morbid conditions. Experimental studies are also constrained by the difficulty of testing low-functioning individuals, with the result that insights tend to be confined to those at the high-functioning end of the spectrum. Neurobiological research is beset by related methodological difficulties. For instance, in neuropathological and neurochemical studies, samples may be small, clinically heterogeneous, often with co-existing/co-morbid conditions, and difficult to match with suitable controls (Palmen *et al.* 2004; Lam *et al.* 2006; Casanova, 2007). Brain tissue donors may also be at the low-functioning end of the spectrum. These limitations pose difficulties for cross-referencing and integrating psychological and neurobiological findings.

Blind alleys in autism research

As in many clinical fields where there is a pressing need for explanations leading to therapeutic interventions, some superficially appealing hypotheses have attracted undue interest, led nowhere and in the process, substantially undermined the progress of research and clinical practice. In the case of autism an early blind alley was Bruno Bettelheim's hypothesis that the causes of autism lay in emotional detachment and faulty parenting by mothers of those on the autism spectrum (Bettelheim, 1967). This erroneous interpretation of what may in some cases have been genetically mediated 'shadow traits' led to the stigmatisation of several generations of parents, and distress in children from whom they were separated for 'therapeutic' reasons. Bettelheim's theoretical and therapeutic approach to autism, now refuted, resonated strongly with psychoanalytical accounts of child development, which were extremely influential at the time (i.e. during the 1960s and 1970s).

An equally if not more damaging hypothesis put forward by Andrew Wakefield and his collaborators (Wakefield *et al.* 1998), subsequently retracted (Murch *et al.* 2004), identified the MMR vaccine as a possible cause of autism in children. Extensive research in this area, carried out over a number of subsequent years, has provided no evidence linking the MMR vaccine to autism. Such a link is unlikely to exist and cannot be considered a reason for the increase in incidence of autism that has been seen in recent years (see Honda *et al.* 2005). Moreover, while the pattern of inheritance in autism strongly suggests that genetic factors interact with environmental influences to produce susceptibility (Pardo and Eberhart, 2007), the negative publicity that environmental hypotheses have attracted through the work of both Bettelheim and Wakefield has also engendered a greater apparent reluctance amongst researchers to identify significant environmental risk factors.

Neglected topics in autism research

Just as some beguiling avenues of enquiry proved to yield little or no benefit, other potentially important but less seductive topics have been relatively neglected. One of these is the precise relationship of epilepsy to autism. In 1960 one of the first reports linking autism to epilepsy was published (Schain and Yannet, 1960). This was rapidly followed by others (e.g. Gubbay, 1970; Kolvin *et al.* 1971) which indicated that up to one-third of those with autism spectrum diagnoses may have epilepsy, while a review of studies published since 2000 has found that a much higher percentage (up to 60%) have atypical/epileptiform EEG activity (Hughes and Melyn, 2005; Spence and Schneider, 2009). Yet despite the steady accretion of evidence linking epilepsy and autism (see Hughes and Melyn, 2005; Levisohn, 2007; Spence and Schneider, 2009), and further work linking seizures to the sleep disturbances often reported in autism (Malow, 2004), the precise role that seizures play in the aetiology, developmental trajectory and long term outcomes of autism has been sparsely examined. This limitation has impacted further on our understanding of the differentiation of sub-groups within the spectrum. The disproportionate occurrence of epilepsy in those with autism and low IQ, and in females with autism (Amiet *et al.* 2008) highlights yet again the need for caution in generalising about this markedly heterogeneous condition.

There have been important omissions also at the psychological level of enquiry. The major foci of research on the psychology of autism, as well as the target areas for quite a number of interventions, have been the 'triad' of symptoms and characteristics included in the diagnostic criteria for autism. While the precise delineation of these three symptom groups has changed since separate criteria for autism were first included in the DSM-III diagnostic classification in 1980, they still centre upon three main areas of impaired functioning: communication, social interaction, and the rigid and repetitive quality of activities and interests (American Psychiatric Association, 2000; World Health Organisation, 1993). Both Kanner and Asperger documented other difficulties, notably sensory and perceptual problems, atypical memory, and special skills. Pioneering experimental research on memory, sensory and perceptual atypicalities was carried out by Hermelin and O'Connor in the 1960s (Hermelin and O'Connor, 1964; 1970), but due focus on these topics in relatively recent. A recent review by Geschwind (2009) estimates that sensory atypicalities are observed in more than 90% of those with autism spectrum diagnoses. This resonates with the view of many parents and teachers of children on the autism spectrum, as well as individuals themselves, that sensory and perceptual difficulties are of paramount concern (Bogdashina, 2003). However, Rogers and Ozonoff (2005) argue that the evidence that such difficulties are more especially associated with autism than with other developmental disorders is unclear. Consequently, there is understandable reservation among experts about the explanatory status of sensory problems in relation to the autism spectrum, though at least one recent psychological account of autism has proposed atypical modulation of sensory and perceptual processes as a possible key to explanation (Mottron *et al.* 2006).

Other areas comparatively overlooked in research, but highlighted by Geschwind (2009) include the onset and development of motor signs, estimated to affect 60–80% of those on the spectrum, gastrointestinal problems (up to 50% of those on the spectrum) and co-morbid psychiatric diagnoses, in particular the presence of mood/conduct disorders, aggression and ADHD (between 25 and 70% of children on the spectrum). While it may be argued that the relationship of these symptoms to the autism spectrum is non-specific, and therefore their potential as 'core deficits' limited, their frequency of occurrence does emphasise the complex heterogeneity of the spectrum, which explanations need to encompass.

During much of three decades in which psychological theories have abounded, the major focus has been on explaining the deficits: it is only in more recent work that special skills have begun to attract more interest (see for instance Baron-Cohen *et al.* 2002; Happé, 1999). A constraint here has been a lack of clarity about what constitutes a special skill. Prodigious savant talents, as displayed, for instance, by the artist Stephen Wiltshire, are extremely rare, suggesting, once again, that this facet of autism should not be a central focus of explanation. However, according to recent estimates (Howlin *et al.* 2009) a much larger group of individuals on the spectrum (around 30%) have some measure of special skill. This then presents yet another phenomenon which, while not universal, characterises a major subpopulation of the spectrum, meriting consideration in what will be almost certainly (given the heterogeneity of the phenomena) a fractionated account of the whole field.

Finally, at both biological and psychological levels of enquiry, the developmental trajectory of autism, from infancy to adulthood, has been comparatively neglected. Many studies have characterised atypical functioning within a relatively narrow window of time, paying scant attention to the cumulative effects of early biological and psychological deficits in engendering these outcomes. A notable exception to this trend is theoretical work by Hobson (see for instance Hobson 1993; Hobson, 2002) seeking to explain how impaired capacity to engage emotionally and socially with other humans from birth onwards, could fundamentally alter a child's developmental trajectory, resulting in both the cognitive and social deficits seen in autistic conditions. Baron-Cohen (1995) has also offered theoretical proposals for early developmental precursors of later theory of mind deficits. The value of the 'trajectory approach' to developmental disorders is elegantly demonstrated by Thomas *et al.* (2009), while recent studies of the developmental trajectory of behavioural symptoms (Richler *et al.* 2010) and neurobiology (Schumann *et al.* 2010) represent an encouraging shift of emphasis.

Positive trends in biology, psychology and practice

Findings gathered over the last four to five decades have resulted in a substantial contemporary framework of understanding about the causes and key phenomena of autism. From initial sources such as the influential monograph by Bernard Rimland (1964) and the pioneering concordance study by Folstein and Rutter (1977; see also Folstein and Rutter, 1978) came persuasive evidence for biological and genetic factors in the causation of autism. The 1970s and 1980s brought a steady stream of further findings concerning biological aspects of autism. This field has taken significant leaps forward since the 1990s, thanks to revolutionary advances in the fields of brain imaging (Minshew and Keller, 2010; Verhoeven *et al.* 2010) and molecular genetics (Abrahams and Geschwind, 2008; Geschwind, 2008; Weiss, 2009). In relation to the neurobiology of autism there is now little doubt that there are subtle atypicalities in the structure and functioning of the brain and neural pathways in people on the autism spectrum (Amaral *et al.* 2006; DiCicco-Bloom *et al.* 2006; Pardo and Eberhart, 2007). Current opinion views autism as a disorder of functional 'connectivity' between cortical networks (Minshew and Williams, 2007), in which key brain areas involved in verbal and non-verbal communication, social interaction, planning and flexibility, as well as networks that govern emotional responses (including fear and anxiety), facial recognition, and the ability to conceptualise mental states in self and others (theory of mind) are affected to varying degrees. Although a unifying pathology has not been identified, and is perhaps even unlikely to be identified for autism, given the heterogeneity in clinical and behavioural presentation of the spectrum, changes that affect early brain development (evidenced by early brain overgrowth during the post-natal period) are indicated in a significant proportion of children with autism (Courchesne *et al.* 2007). Developmental involvement of the frontal and temporal lobes and the amygdala are strongly implicated (see Geschwind, 2009).

Neurochemical investigations have focused on several transmitter systems in autism, including serotonin, dopamine, noradrenaline, acetylcholine, glutamate, gamma-aminobutyric acid (GABA) and oxytocin (McDougle *et al.* 2005; Lam *et al.* 2006). Overall it has been difficult to draw firm conclusions from these studies mainly due to the limitations highlighted earlier (i.e. heterogeneity of the spectrum, co-morbidities, sample sizes and matching to controls). Although a central role for altered serotonergic function in autism has gained the most empirical evidence, this still requires further investigation and validation. Promising new areas of research include the possibility that oxytocin (the so-called 'social hormone') signalling is perturbed in autism.

Concerning genetic factors, the heritability of autism is now well established. The main focus of interest is in identifying candidate genes and their mode of action on the developmental trajectory in autism (Abrahams and Geschwind, 2008; Geschwind, 2008; Weiss, 2009).

Psychological findings have also played an important role in theory and research on autism from an early stage. Besides offering detailed descriptions of the phenomena of autism, psychological approaches have offered a number of theoretical models seeking to identify the core psychological processes underlying the observed phenomena. A significant breakthrough in the field of theoretical models came with the work of Baron-Cohen, Frith and Leslie (Baron-Cohen *et al.* 1985) initiating two and a half decades of important research on theory of mind deficits in people with autism. An additional impact of this model has been to stimulate the development of a number of rival models, each originally presented as an account of the single 'core deficit' which could explain the full range of symptoms and characteristics in autism. Recently this era of model building has entered a new phase with the realisation that underlying processes proposed within mutually exclusive accounts may in fact constitute parallel factors which operate together to produce the observed pattern of symptoms in autism.

Progress in the field of interventions for autism has been somewhat slower. Some of the most widely used psychological interventions for autism remain those such as the TEACCH framework (Treatment and Education of Autistic and related Communication-handicapped Children) and the behavioural approach pioneered by Ivar Lovaas (Pasco and Roth, 2010). Both originated several decades ago and though reasonably effective in ameliorating certain symptoms of autism, and promoting scope for education, cannot be considered as treatments. Progress in the development of effective pharmacological interventions remains extremely limited. However, some encouraging trends are evident in recent work. For instance, a growing number of interventions seek to address core psychological problems in autism, such as theory of mind or mind-reading deficits (see for example, Golan *et al.* 2010). Moreover, advances in the design and implementation of critical evaluations have greatly enhanced the evidence base for a whole range of treatments, thus limiting the scope for practitioners to make unfounded claims about 'cures' (Pasco and Roth, 2010).

Moving forward – contemporary issues in autism, from diagnosis to development and education

As we have outlined, progress in understanding the autism spectrum combines encouraging progress in some areas with a history of conceptual and methodological difficulties, false trails and puzzling omissions. One important goal of this volume is to redress this uneven and patchy coverage. The selected topics combine contemporary developments in areas widely accepted as fundamental for understanding autism, with new work representing some less widely researched themes and approaches. A recurring theme throughout the volume is the need to develop a suitably nuanced account of autism, fully informed by the heterogeneity and complexity of the phenomena which it presents. All chapters in this compendium are by leading contributors at the forefront in the field of autism theory, research and practice. Their wide-ranging contributions embrace classification and diagnosis, genetics, neurology and biochemistry through to socio-cognitive, developmental and educational perspectives, reflecting the multi-level emphasis of current thinking. This volume aims to promote a broader, more balanced and contemporary understanding of the autism spectrum.

The first section of the book examines classification and diagnosis. In the opening chapter on 'Early assessment and diagnosis of children', Professor Ann Le Couteur from the Institute of Health and Society at Newcastle University first addresses the challenge of dissecting and clarifying the difficult terminology of the autism spectrum, offering an invaluable framework for the volume as a whole. The remainder of this chapter focuses on key aspects of assessment and current diagnostic procedures, including the use of the best estimate clinical diagnosis for clinical and research practice. Difficulties and challenges surrounding diagnosis of childhood autism and ASD are explained and discussed in depth. These are placed in context for the reader with reference to landmark and ongoing studies.

The next section (Chapters 2–6) deals with genetics, neurology and biochemistry. In Chapter 2, 'Unravelling the genetics of autism spectrum disorders', a team of investigators from the Wellcome Trust Centre for Human Genetics at Oxford University led by Professor Anthony Monaco, an integral part of the International Molecular Genetic Study of Autism Consortium (IMGSAC), provide an exceptional insight into this crucial topic. They review and evaluate the extensive body of evidence from linkage and association studies (including genome-wide association), focusing on candidate genes, single gene mutations, epigenetics and copy number variations. They emphasise that the complex aetiology of ASD, which is likely to involve multiple interacting genes and pathways, calls for several different strategies of enquiry, and show how this field of research may move forward, with larger-scale sequencing efforts required to unravel the causal variants involved in ASD.

Dr Michael Spencer at the Cambridge Autism Research Centre and colleagues from the Centre for Clinical Brain Sciences, Royal Edinburgh Hospital Department of Psychiatry consider 'Brain imaging and the neuroanatomical correlates of autism' in Chapter 3. They provide a detailed overview of structural alterations within neural circuits and brain areas involved with social functions, and restricted and repetitive behaviours in autism. Importantly, they discuss key factors that impact on the interpretation of brain imaging studies which, besides the established heterogeneity of the spectrum, include the gender and intellectual ability of individuals, the developmental trajectory of autism, as well as differences in analytical and technical approaches. They conclude that longitudinal studies exploring the developmental trajectory in ASD, and interdisciplinary efforts to combine neuroimaging with genomic techniques, relating these to neuropathological findings, represent a productive route to further important insights into the neurobiology of autism.

In the chapter which follows, 'Magnetoencephalography (MEG) as a tool to investigate the neurophysiology of autism' (Chapter 4), Dr Sven Braeutigam from the Oxford Centre for Human Brain Activity (OHBA) and colleagues introduce this modern functional neuroimaging method, describing its application to investigating dynamic brain activity and neural processing in autism. The technical and analytical approaches are outlined before the authors move on to the 'functional systems', focusing on key aspects of neural processing which may be affected in autism–auditory processing, semantic processing, face processing and theory of mind-associated with activity within the so-called 'mirror neuron' network. An important feature of MEG highlighted in this chapter is the scope it offers to define and further characterise subclinical epilepsy and epileptiform activity (seizures) that may remain otherwise undetected in a significant proportion of individuals on the spectrum. The authors emphasise that while MEG is a relatively new tool, the few studies conducted to date broadly support the notion that autism involves altered cognitive strategies as opposed to cognitive impairments or 'deficits' *per se*. The technique is presented as holding significant promise for advancing understanding of the neural basis of autism.

In the next chapter 'Autism and epilepsy' (Chapter 5), this critically important and often understated relationship is the focus of discussion by Professors Gillberg and Neville, from the University College London Institute of Child Health and the University of Gothenburg in Sweden. They discuss prevalence, gender and differential diagnostic aspects, before examining autistic regression and epilepsy and taking a closer look at the various types of seizures that may be associated/coexist with autism, as well as early-onset epilepsy syndromes. The authors consider investigation and management, emphasising the need for an integrated approach to epilepsy and psychiatric problems, and for neurological investigations to include MRI scanning and biochemical investigation, and discuss the place of EEG in investigating autism and the pathogenesis of autistic regression in epilepsy.

Dr Mukaetova-Ladinska and colleagues from Newcastle University shift the focus to the 'Biochemistry of autism: changes in serotonin, reelin and oxytocin' in Chapter 6. They review the field and present evidence to support the notion that disruption in one or more of these systems, which may be interlinked, is associated with aspects of the clinical phenotype in autism. Currently available pharmacological interventions targeting these systems are evaluated and discussed in the context of these findings. The authors conclude by highlighting some important limitations in these studies and the need for more concerted efforts and validation.

The next section (Chapters 7–12) deals with cognition, development and education. In the opening chapter of this section, 'Psychological models of autism: an overview', Dr Elizabeth Pellicano from the Centre for Research in Autism and Education at the London Institute of Education, sets the scene with an overview of three theoretical accounts of autism which have played a major role in psychological explanation of autism in recent decades (the theory of mind hypothesis, the executive dysfunction hypothesis and the weak central coherence theory). She analyses some of the reasons why the status of these approaches as 'single-deficit' accounts has been challenged, not least that there may be different substrates for the three major symptom groups in autism, leading to the more recent reconfiguration of these proposals within 'multiple-deficit' models. She concludes by stressing the all-important issue of situating explanatory approaches within a developmental context. In relation to cognitive functioning in autism, this chapter uses 'deficit' and associated terminology only where historically appropriate. The author's preference for alternative terms such as 'atypicality' reflects an important and growing trend in the discussion of autism.

In the chapter on 'Cognitive flexibility in autism: a social-developmental account' (Chapter 8), Professor Peter Hobson and Dr Jessica Hobson from the Behavioural and Brain Science Unit at the UCL Institute of Child Health in London offer a theoretical extension of the social-developmental approach to autism. A theory prioritising the impaired capacity of infants later diagnosed with autism to form social and emotional relationships might seem ill-equipped to explain the narrow and repetitive activities and interests that form the third symptom cluster of the triad. However, the authors present an elegant account of how a child's social-developmental endowments could also determine their cognitive capacity for flexible and context-sensitive thinking and engagement with the world. The claim that these may be affected in individuals with autism, leading to specific forms of cognitive restriction and rigidity, provides an interesting counterpoint to the theoretical fractionation of the three symptom clusters, set out in the preceding chapter.

Professor Jill Boucher of the Autism Research Group at the Department of Psychology, City University London, addresses one of the most complex and puzzling patterns of deficit in those on the autism spectrum; in her chapter on 'Language in autism spectrum disorders' (Chapter 9). As she points out, language capacities across the spectrum vary widely across sub-groups and from low- to high-functioning individuals. Among those who have problems with structural language (as opposed to more subtle problems with communication), there is also a range from marked difficulties with grammar, syntax and phonology, to difficulties in processing meaning. Her chapter reviews the possible role of theory of mind and associated impairments, as well as that of co-morbid specific language impairment in generating this complex pattern. She concludes with a hypothesis suggesting a selective but pervasive impairment in the declarative aspects of memory.

In Chapter 10, 'Memory in autism: binding, self and brain', Professor Dermot Bowler and colleagues, also from the Autism Research Group at the Department of Psychology, City University London, continue with the theme of memory difficulties. They provide convincing arguments for the importance of this often-neglected area of impairment in ASD, showing how memory impairment may impact on fundamental aspects of human functioning, including the binding of experience and sense of self, and may also relate closely to known neurosychological atyplicalities.

Dr Ayla Humphrey and colleagues from the Cambridge Autism Research Centre, Developmental Psychiatry Section, and MRC Cognition and Brain Sciences Unit consider the crucial interface between psychological theory and its application in clinical and educational settings in their chapter 'Measuring executive function in children with high-functioning autism spectrum disorders: what is ecologically valid?' (Chapter 11). In so doing, they highlight how the nuanced consideration of differences in symptoms and capacities, which has surfaced repeatedly in this volume, must extend not only to sub-groups, but also to the level of the individual child. Their study suggests that there is in fact no best measure of executive function, and that information from several sources should be considered when evaluating this (and perhaps other neuropsychological functions), in this group of children. Their work provides further important insight into how expectations of parents and teachers of children with ASD influence their views and reporting of a child's abilities and disabilities.

In the concluding chapter, 'Autism Spectrum Disorders in Current Education Provision' (Chapter 12), Professor Rita Jordan of the School of Education at Birmingham University provides a stimulating analysis of the crucial issue of educational provision for children on the spectrum. She examines the evidence base for learning styles in ASD, in particular how psychological characteristics and cognitive style impact on the child's capacity to learn, and on their ability to access key areas of the curriculum. The role of stress and the importance of parental support are further emphasised. The value of different kinds of educational placement, the issue of inclusion, and the need for further research in these and other associated areas are identified in these discussions.

It has been a great privilege and a pleasure to assemble and shape the material in this volume. We hope that readers will enjoy engaging with the content as much as we have enjoyed preparing it.

References

Abrahams, B.S., Geschwind, D.H. (2008). Advances in autism genetics: on the threshold of a new neurobiology. *Nature Reviews Genetics*, **9**: 341–355.

Amaral, D.G., Schumann, C.M., Nordahl, C.W. (2006). Neuroanatomy of autism. *Trends in Neurosciences*, **31**: 137–145.

American Psychiatric Association. (2000). *Diagnostic and Statistical Manual of Mental Disorders 4th edn. Text Revision (DSMIV TR)*. Washington DC: American Psychiatric Association.

American Psychiatric Association. (2010). DSM-5 Development: Disorders usually first diagnosed in infancy, childhood or adolescence. http://www.dsm5.org/ProposedRevisions/Pages/InfancyChildhoodAdolescence.aspx (accessed May 2010).

Amiet, C., Gourfinkel-An, I., Bouzamondo, A., *et al.* (2008). Epilepsy in autism is associated with intellectual disability and gender: evidence from a meta-analysis. *Biological Psychiatry*, **64**: 577–582.

Asperger, H. (1944). Die 'autistichen psychopathen' im kindersalter. *Archive für Psychiatrie und Nervenkrankenheiten*, **117**: 76–136. (Reprinted in Autism and Asperger Syndrome, by U. Frith, editor, 1991, Cambridge UK: Cambridge University Press).

Baird, G., Cass, H., Slonims, V. (2003). Diagnosis of autism. *British Medical Journal*, **327**: 488–493.

Baird, G., Simonoff, E., Pickles, A., *et al.* (2006). Prevalence of disorders of the autism spectrum in a population cohort of children in South Thames: the Special Needs and Autism Project (SNAP). *Lancet*, **368**: 210–215.

Baron-Cohen, S. (1995). *Mindblindness: An Essay on Autism and Theory of Mind*. London: MIT Press.

Baron-Cohen, S., Leslie, A.M., Frith, U. (1985). Does the autistic child have a 'theory of mind'? *Cognition*, **21**: 37–46.

Baron-Cohen, S., Wheelwright, S., Griffin, R., Lawson, J., Hill, J. (2002). The exact mind: empathising and systemising in autism spectrum conditions. In *Handbook of Cognitive Development*. Oxford: Blackwell.

Bettelheim, B. (1967) *The Empty Fortress: Infantile Autism and the Birth of the Self*. New York: Free Press.

Bogdashina, O. (2003). *Sensory Perceptual Issues in Autism: Different Sensory Experiences – Different Perceptual Worlds*. London: Jessica Kingsley.

Casanova, M.F. (2007). The neuropathology of autism. *Brain Pathology*, **17**: 422–433.

Courchesne, E., Pierce, K., Schumann, C.M., *et al.* (2007). Mapping early brain development in autism. *Neuron*, **56**: 399–413.

Coury, D. (2010). Medical treatment of autism spectrum disorders. *Current Opinion in Neurology*, **23**: 131–136.

Darby, J.K., Clark, L. (1992). Autism syndrome as a final common pathway of behavioural expression for many organic disorders. *American Journal of Psychiatry*, **149**: 146–147. Comment on: *American Journal of Psychiatry*, **147**: 1614–1621.

DiCicco-Bloom, E., Lord, C., Zwaigenbaum, L., *et al.* (2006). The developmental neurobiology of autism spectrum disorder. *Journal of Neuroscience*, **26**: 6897–6906.

Frith, U. (1991). *Autism and Asperger syndrome*. Cambridge UK: Cambridge University Press.

Folstein, S., Rutter, M. (1977). Infantile autism: a genetic study of 21 twin pairs. *Journal of Child Psychology and Psychiatry*, **18**: 297–321.

Folstein, S., Rutter, M. (1978). A twin study of individuals with infantile autism. In *Autism: A Reappraisal of Concepts and Treatment*. New York: Plenum Press, pp. 219–242.

Frith, U., Morton, J., Leslie A.M. (1991). The cognitive basis of a biological disorder: Autism. *Trends in Neurosciences*, **14**: 433–438.

Geschwind, D.H. (2008). Autism: many genes, common pathways? *Cell*, **135**: 391–395.

Geschwind, D.H. (2009). Advances in Autism. *Annual Review of Medicine*, **60**: 367–380.

Golan, O., Baron-Cohen, S., Ashwin, E., *et al.* (2010). Enhancing emotion recognition in children with autism spectrum conditions: an intervention using animated vehicles with real emotional faces. *Journal of Autism and Developmental Disorders*, **40**: 269–279.

Gubbay, S.S., Lobascher, M., Kingerlee, P. (1970). A neurological appraisal of autistic children: results of a Western Australian survey. *Developmental Medicine and Child Neurology*, **12**: 422–429.

Happé, F. (1999). Autism: Cognitive deficit or cognitive style? *Trends in Cognitive Sciences*, **3**: 216–222.

Happé, F., Ronald, A., Plomin, A. (2006). Time to give up on a single explanation for autism. *Nature Neuroscience*, **9**: 1218–1220.

Hermelin, B., O'Connor, N. (1964). Effects of sensory input and sensory dominance on severely disturbed, autistic children and on subnormal controls. *British Journal of Psychology*, **55**: 201–206.

Hermelin, B., O'Connor, N. (1970). *Psychological Experiments with Autistic Children*. New York: Pergamon Press.

Hobson, P. (1993). *Autism and the Development of Mind*. Hove: Lawrence Erlbaum Associates.

Hobson, P. (2002). *The Cradle of Thought: Exploring the Origins of Thinking*. London: Macmillan.

Honda, H., Shimizu, Y., Rutter, M. (2005). No effect of MMR withdrawal on the incidence of autism: a total population study. *Journal of Child Psychology and Psychiatry*, **46**: 572–579.

Howlin, P., Asgharian, A. (1999). The diagnosis of autism and Asperger syndrome: findings from a survey of 770 families. *Developmental Medicine and Child Neurology*, **41**: 834–839.

Howlin, P., Goode, S., Hutton, J., Rutter, M. (2009). Savant skills in autism: psychometric approaches and parental reports. *Philosophical Transactions of the Royal Society of London, Series B: Biological Sciences*, **364**: 1359–1367.

Hughes, J.R., Melyn, M. (2005). EEG and seizures in autistic children and adolescents: further findings with therapeutic implications. *Clinical EEG and Neuroscience*, **36**: 15–20.

Jacob, A. (ed.). (2004). *Journal of Autism and Developmental Disorders, Special Issue on Research Methodology – Matching*, **34** (1): 1–92.

Kanner, L. (1943). Autistic disturbances of affective contact. *Nervous Child*, **2**: 217–250.

Kolvin, I., Ounsted, C., Roth, M. (1971). Studies in childhood psychoses. V. Cerebral dysfunction and childhood psychoses. *British Journal of Psychiatry*, **118**: 407–414.

Lam, K.S.L., Aman, M.G., Arnold, L.E. (2006). Neurochemical correlates of autistic disorder: a review of the literature. *Research in Developmental Disabilities*, **27**: 254–289.

Landa, R.J. (2008). Diagnosis of autism spectrum disorders in the first 3 years of life. *Nature Clinical Practice: Neurology*, **4**: 138–147.

Levisohn, P.M. (2007). The autism-epilepsy connection. *Epilepsia*, **48** (S9): 33–35.

Levy, S.E., Mandell, D.S., Schultz, R.T. (2009). Autism. *Lancet*, **374**: 1627–1638.

Malow, B.A. (2004). Sleep disorders, epilepsy and autism. *Mental Retardation and Developmental Disabilities Research Reviews*, **10**: 122–125.

McDougle, C.J., Erickkson, C.A., Stigler, K.A., Posey, D.J. (2005). Neurochemistry in the pathophysiology of autism. *Journal of Clinical Psychiatry*, **66** (S10): 9–18.

Minshew, N.J., Keller, T.A. (2010). The nature of brain dysfunction in autism: functional brain imaging studies. *Current Opinion in Neurology*, **23**: 124–130.

Minshew, N.J., Williams, D.L. (2007). The new neurobiology of autism: cortex, connectivity and neuronal organisation. *Archives of Neurology*, **64**: 945–950.

Mottron, L., Dawson, M., Soulières, I., Hubert, B., Burack, J. (2006). Enhanced perceptual functioning in autism: an update, and eight principles of autistic perception. *Journal of Autism and Developmental Disorders*, **36**: 27–43.

Murch, S.H., Anthony, A., Casson, D., *et al.* (2004) Retraction of an interpretation. *Lancet*, **363**: 750. [Retraction statement made by 10 of the 12 original authors who could be contacted referring to the Early Report 'Ileal-lymphoid-nodular hyperplasia, non-specific colitis, and pervasive developmental disorder in children' published in *The Lancet* in 1998]

National Autistic Society (2007). Statistics: How many people have autistic spectrum disorders? http://www.nas.org.uk/nas/jsp/polopoly.jsp?d=235&a=3527 (accessed May 2010).

Palmen, S.J., van Engeland, H., Hof, P.R., Schmitz, C. (2004). Neuropathological findings in autism. *Brain*, **127**: 2572–2583.

Pardo, C.A., Eberhart, C.G. (2007). The neurobiology of autism. *Brain Pathology*, **17**: 434–447.

Pasco, G., Roth, I. (2010). Perspectives on intervention. In Roth, I. with Barson C., Hoekstra, R., Pasco, G., Whatson, T. *The Autism Spectrum in the 21st Century: Exploring Psychology, Biology and Practice*. London: Jessica Kingsley.

Richler, J., **Huerta, M.**, **Bishop, S.L.**, **Lord, C.** (2010). Developmental trajectories of restricted and repetitive behaviours and interests in children with autism spectrum disorders. *Development and Psychopathology*, **22**: 55–69.

Rimland, B. (1964). *Infantile Autism: The Syndrome and its Implication for a Neural Theory of Behaviour*. New York: Prentice Hall.

Rogers S.J., **Ozonoff, S.** (2005). Annotation: What do we know about sensory dysfunction in autism? A critical review of the empirical evidence. *Journal of Child Psychology and Psychiatry*, **46**: 1255–1268.

Schain, R.J., **Yannet, H.** (1960). Infantile autism. An analysis of 50 cases and a consideration of certain relevant neurophysiologic concepts. *Journal of Pediatrics*, **57**: 560–567.

Schumann, C.M., **Bloss, C.S.**, **Barnes, C.C.**, *et al.* (2010). Longitudinal magnetic resonance imaging study of cortical development through early childhood in autism. *Journal of Neuroscience*, **30**: 4419–4427.

Spence, S.J., **Schneider, M.T.** (2009). The role of epilepsy and epileptiform EEGs in autism spectrum disorders. *Pediatric Research*, **65**: 599–606.

Swedo, S. (2008). Report of the DSM-V Neurodevelopmental Disorders Work Group. American Psychiatric Association. http://www.psych.org/MainMenu/Research/DSMIV/DSMV/DSMRevisionActivities/DSMVWorkGroupReports/NeurodevelopmentalDisordersWorkGroupReport.aspx (accessed October 2010).

Swedo, S. (2009). Report of the DSM-V Neurodevelopmental Disorders Work Group. American Psychiatric Association. http://www.psych.org/MainMenu/Research/DSMIV/DSMV/DSMRevisionActivities/DSM-V-Work-Group-Reports/Neurodevelopmental-Disorders-Work-Group-Report.aspx (accessed October 2010).

Thomas, M.S., **Annaz, D.**, **Ansari, D.**, *et al.* (2009). Using developmental trajectories to understand developmental disorders. *Journal of Speech, Language and Hearing Research*, **52**: 336–358.

Toth, K., **King, B.H.** (2008). Asperger's syndrome: diagnosis and treatment. *American Journal of Psychiatry*, **165**: 958–963.

Verhoeven, J.S., **DeCock, P.**, **Lagae, L.**, **Sunaert, S.** (2010). Neuroimaging of autism. *Neuroradiology*, **52**: 3–14.

Wakefield, A.J., **Murch, S.H.**, **Anthony, A.**, *et al.* (1998). RETRACTED: Ileal-lymphoid-nodular hyperplasia, non-specific colitis, and pervasive developmental disorder in children. *Lancet*, **351**: 637–641.

Weiss, L.A. (2009). Autism genetics: emerging data from genome-wide copy number and single nucleotide polymorphism scans. *Expert Review of Molecular Diagnostics*, **9**: 795–803.

Wing, L. (1981). Asperger's syndrome: a clinical account. *Psychological Medicine*, **11**: 115–129.

World Health Organization (1993). *The ICD-10 Classification of Mental and Behavioural Disorders: Diagnostic Criteria for Research*. Geneva: World Health Organization.

Yeargin-Allsopp, M., **Rice, C.**, **Karapurkar, T.**, *et al.* (2003). Prevalence of autism in a US metropolitan area. *Journal of the American Medical Association*, **289**: 49–55.

PART I CLASSIFICATION AND DIAGNOSIS

1

Early assessment and diagnosis of children

ANN LE COUTEUR

Autism is an organic neurodevelopmental disorder, the prototypical disorder of the group of conditions known as the pervasive developmental disorders. Genetic findings and general population studies indicate that these types of disorders (commonly referred to as Autism Spectrum Disorders (ASD) or more recently Autism Spectrum Conditions (ASC)), probably occur along a broad continuum of severity. This spectrum of presentations include those individuals with a definable disorder and clear evidence of social impairment and incapacity, qualitatively similar behavioural characteristics in other family members (described as the broader autism phenotype), and a range of more subtle social, communicative and repetitive behaviours in the general population. ASD are no longer considered rare, with a replicated reported prevalence of approximately 1 in 100. With increasing public and professional awareness and an emphasis on the importance of both early recognition and access to so-called 'early interventions', there is an expectation of early identification, assessment and diagnosis. This chapter will review the evidence for ASD, the epidemiology and prevalence of these disorders and consider (using the framework of the National Autism Plan for Children) a range of assessment and diagnostic procedures including the use of the best estimate clinical diagnosis for clinical and research practice. Inevitably, the purpose of assessment informs the format and content of the diagnostic process. The chapter will conclude by considering some current diagnostic challenges. Although the focus of this chapter is the diagnosis of ASD in children, there is an increasing awareness that the needs of adults from across the autism spectrum must be recognised. For some individuals this will include access to assessment and

Researching the Autism Spectrum: Contemporary Perspectives, ed. I. Roth and P. Rezaie. Published by Cambridge University Press.

diagnosis during adult life to inform the development of a personalised package of support.

1.1 Definition

Autism Spectrum Disorders are lifelong severe neurodevelopmental disorders with a considerable functional and financial impact on both the individual and their family. In recognition of this broader spectrum of difficulties the terms ASD and ASC have gained wider acceptability over the last twenty years or so (Frith, 1991; Johnson *et al.* 2007; Volkmar *et al.* 2004; Wing, 1978; Wing and Gould, 1979). The terms ASD and ASC have become widely used in lay, clinical and research contexts to include autism, Asperger syndrome, atypical autism and pervasive developmental disorders not otherwise specified (PDD-NOS) (Frith, 1991; Volkmar *et al.* 2004; Wing and Gould, 1979). ASD/ASC is used as a pragmatic category, both for purposes of clinical and research diagnosis and for the identification of special needs in relation to the provision of appropriate support services. Throughout this chapter the term 'Autism Spectrum Disorder' will be used interchangeably to mean autism spectrum disorders/autism spectrum conditions and Pervasive Developmental Disorders (PDD).

Autism is the prototypical disorder of this broad spectrum of disorders. All individuals share a common triad of impairments in social interactions, atypical and often delayed verbal and non-verbal communication together with a repertoire of repetitive and unusual behaviours, interests and play. Studies have shown a wide variation in rates of cognitive impairment. Historically autism was frequently recognised in individuals with severe impairment and learning disability (Rutter, 2005). Estimates suggested learning disabilities (IQ less than 70) affected 70 to 80% of individuals with ASD (Baird *et al.* 2003; Johnson *et al.* 2007). In recent years the inclusion of higher functioning individuals has led to an apparent decrease in the rates of cognitive impairment (Baird *et al.* 2006; Johnson *et al.* 2007). Those higher functioning individuals with autism spectrum disorder may show good verbal skills in contrast to those with autism or PDD-NOS who may perform better in non-verbal measures. However, this 'higher' degree of intelligibility on performance tasks cannot be assumed to reflect their social skills which may be significantly impaired (Carrona *et al.* 2008; Le Couteur, 2003).

Another unique feature of these disorders is the characteristic patchy pattern of deficits and areas of relative strength. Indeed approximately ten percent of individuals with core autism have been shown to possess a skill that is significantly better than would be predicated by their global intellectual ability (Frith, 2003). Howlin (2003) has also reported that adults with high functioning autism can show giftedness in one or more areas of functioning. Frith and her colleagues have proposed that early atypical processing biases may play a role in the development of these so-called splinter skills (Frith, 2003). These skills include perfect pitch, artistic, musical and mathematical ability.

Most authors agree that the spectrum of neurodevelopmental disorders extends beyond ASD to include other specific developmental disorders such as specific language impairment (SLI), specific academic difficulties (such as dyslexia) and other disorders such as attention deficit hyperactivity disorder (ADHD) (Rutter, 2006). Rutter (2006) wrote 'For all these disorders persistence into adult life involves a mixture of the expected and unexpected and substantial challenges remain in the identification of key mediating variables'. These disorders have many features in common including: early onset life long disorders; delay/deviance in maturationally influenced psychological features; a general tendency for impairments to lessen with age; and some degree of accompanying general or specific cognitive impairment. Much of the behavioural symptomology of these disorders shows considerable overlap. These disorders also have in common a genetic liability and marked male preponderance.

One of the first clinical descriptions of Autism was made by Kanner in 1943. He identified an underlying 'innate inability to form the usual biologically provided affective contact with people' (Kanner, 1943). The following year Asperger (1944) reported a number of clinical cases using the term 'autistic psychopathy' and wrote that this 'disturbance results in severe and characteristic difficulties in social integration' (Frith, 1991).

It was not until 1980 that the American Psychiatric Association coined the term pervasive developmental disorders (PDD) highlighting the significant impact on everyday life that these complex neurodevelopmental disorders have across all aspects of functioning. The currently agreed international diagnostic criteria (ICD-10 and DSM IV-TR) define these disorders in relation to particular developmental history profiles and current behavioural characteristics. The subcategories are similar across the two classification systems (American Psychiatric Association, 2000; World Health Organization, 1993) (Table 1.1).

The diagnostic criteria include: qualitative impairments in social interaction; qualitative impairments in social communication; the presence of a repertoire of restricted, repetitive (often non-adaptive) interests, behaviours and activities; together with evidence of delay or deviance in development within the first 3 years of life. There is clear evidence that the diagnosis of autism is valid and can be made reliably from 2 years of age (Charman *et al.* 2004; Lord, 1995; Lord *et al.* 2006; Moore and Goodson, 2003). Studies also show that despite individual variations in presentation and patterns of developmental progress, the diagnosis remains valid at follow-up (up to the age of 9 years) (Baird *et al.* 2006; Lord *et al.* 2006; Volkmar *et al.* 2004). Turner *et al.* (2006) reported that 88% of children who received a diagnosis of autism/autism spectrum disorder at 2 years remained on the autism spectrum at the age of 9 years.

Table 1.1 *International diagnostic sub-categories for Pervasive Developmental Disorders*

Pervasive Developmental Disorders (ICD-10)
(World Health Organization, 1993)

- F84.0 Childhood autism
- F84.1 Atypical autism
- F84.2 Rett's syndrome
- F84.3 Other childhood disintegrative disorder
- F84.4 Overactive disorder associated with mental retardation and stereotyped movements
- F84.5 Asperger syndrome
- F84.9 Pervasive Developmental Disorder, unspecified

Pervasive Developmental Disorders (DSM-IV-TR)
(American Psychiatric Association, 2000)

- Autistic Disorder
- Rett's syndrome
- Childhood Disintegrative Disorder
- Asperger Syndrome
- Pervasive Developmental Disorder Not Otherwise Specified (PDD-NOS)

The nosological validity of the other sub-groups within the pervasive developmental disorder classification is less certain and the use of these diagnoses in early childhood shows more variability and is less reliable (Charman and Baird, 2002; Cox *et al.* 1999; Lord *et al.* 2006; Turner *et al.* 2006).

Taking one specific subcategory, Asperger syndrome (AS), several international clinical and research teams have developed specific sets of diagnostic criteria for Asperger syndrome (Attwood, 2006; Leekam *et al.* 2000; Wing, 1981). These clinical research criteria show areas of both overlap and separation but most include more detailed requirements than the ICD 10/DSM IV-TR descriptions and definitions for Asperger syndrome. Further, a number of studies have highlighted the difficulties replicating the internationally agreed diagnostic criteria (ICD; DSM). This has led to conflicting findings (Gilchrist *et al.* 2001; Howlin, 2003; McConachie *et al.* 2005; McIntosh and Dissanayake, 2004; Szatmari *et al.* 2003). McConachie *et al.* (2005) explored the rates of Asperger syndrome in a cohort of 104 pre-school children recruited in the north-east of England, all of whom had received detailed diagnostic assessments. Only three children met the current ICD-10 criteria. These authors reported that repetitive behaviours seemed to be important for the diagnosis of AS but were more likely to be reported in older children as they enter school age. Several authors have also observed that with age (i.e. into adolescence and adulthood) individuals with an early childhood diagnosis of AS showed similar clinical behavioural characteristics to those with a diagnosis of autism, albeit high functioning autism (Gilchrist *et al.* 2001; Howlin, 2003).

Moving beyond the diagnoses of autism and Asperger syndrome, published reports of both clinical and general population samples identify a spectrum of developmental difficulties and behaviours in individuals presenting with milder clinical traits and evidence of social impairment/incapacity. These types of developmental and functional difficulties meet the internationally agreed diagnostic criteria for atypical autism, Pervasive Developmental Disorder unspecified (ICD-10)/Pervasive Developmental Disorder not otherwise specified (PDD-NOS) (DSM-IV-TR) and would be included within the terminology of Autism Spectrum Disorders. These categories (PDD-NOS) are defined by exclusion (Volkmar, 1998). Volkmar also noted the striking paradox that individuals with PDD-NOS are much less frequently studied but are much more common than other recognised diagnostic Pervasive Developmental Disorder diagnostic categories.

However, the spectrum probably extends even further beyond those individuals with an ASD defined by some degree of impairment in social functioning. Genetic studies of families recruited through individuals with core autism indicate that some affected individuals experience milder variants known as the broader autism phenotype (Bailey *et al.* 1998; Bailey and Parr, 2003; Bolton *et al.* 1994; Le Couteur *et al.* 1996; Parr *et al.* 2006; Pickles *et al.* 2000; Piven *et al.* 1997; Rutter, 2006). Furthermore the study of several other recognised disorders, such as tuberous sclerosis, neuromuscular disorders, Fragile X, cerebral palsy, congenital blindness, congenital rubella and ADHD, has shown autistic-like behavioural characteristics and patterns of development (Brown *et al.* 1997; Chess, 1977; Darke *et al.* 2006; Kerr, 2002; Reiersen *et al.* 2007). The association of known medical conditions is much stronger for the prototypical disorder of autism (childhood autism (ICD-10); autistic disorder (DSM-IV-TR)) than the more broadly defined ASD (Fombonne, 2003).

Finally, several studies using various different measures including study specific self report rating scales and checklists through to ASD screening and diagnostic tools have reported a range of so-called Autism Spectrum Disorder type social-communication and repetitive behavioural traits in general population samples (Constantino and Todd, 2003; Leekam *et al.* 2007; Ronald *et al.* 2006). These findings need replication with valid and reliable measures. However, the conceptual implications of a categorical or continuous dimensional approach to ASD and the implications of a symptom model, factor solution or the continued acceptance of the triad of impairment for defining autism/Autism Spectrum Disorder will significantly influence our future understanding of the aetiology and the investigation of the underpinning constructs of these disorders. Yet it may not be possible to resolve these controversies until there is finally a better understanding of the aetiology of the autism spectrum.

In summary, over recent decades, there have been major changes in both the diagnostic terminology and our conceptual understanding of Autism Spectrum

Disorders across a broad spectrum of presentations from specific diagnoses to so-called dimensional traits in the general population.

1.2 Epidemiology

The most recent UK epidemiological study was conducted by Baird *et al.* (2006) and reported an overall prevalence rate for ASD of approximately 1 in 100 in school aged children (38.9 per 10 000 for autism and 77.2 per 10 000 for other ASD). This study included the direct assessment of a proportion of all the children within the identified study community. These rates are in keeping with other UK and US studies (Chakrabarti and Fombonne, 2005; Newschaffer *et al.* 2007) but in sharp contrast to the reports of the first epidemiological study when autism was defined as a rare disorder with a population prevalence of 4–5 per 10 000 (Lotter, 1966). There are likely to be several factors contributing to this increase. First there is a greater knowledge and awareness about Autism/ASD amongst both the general population and relevant professional groups working with children leading to improved case recognition. Second there is a greater preparedness to extend the diagnostic criteria to include more able individuals rather than to restrict diagnosis to a narrow definition of autism with accompanying significant and severe learning difficulties. Third, there is some evidence to suggest diagnostic substitution for example from learning disabilities to autism/ASD. Finally it is possible that recent studies using systematic standardised screenings of total populations or birth cohorts are likely to have missed fewer children with ASD than in earlier studies (Rutter, 2005). Whether or not these most recently reported prevalence rates for autism/ASD are accurate or an underestimate it is clear that these are common disorders of childhood (Baird *et al.* 2006; Filipek *et al.* 1999). Further a recent report from the Adult Psychiatric Morbidity survey (2007) has indicated that 1% of adults living in the English general population had ASD. The authors highlight that it is the first time that such data have been collected in adults in any country (Brugha *et al.* 2009).

Although the genetic underpinnings of autism/ASD are indisputable (see Chapter 2) there have been a number of hypotheses about possible environmental aetiologies. Some of these hypotheses have received a great deal of media coverage. The published large epidemiological studies have not supported these postulated causal factors (Atladottir *et al.* 2007; Honda *et al.* 2005). If environmental risk factors are relevant they are likely to be operating either in the prenatal period or in the early years of life (Rutter, 2005). New studies of high risk siblings and large scale longitudinal studies may shed light on these controversial areas.

1.3 Assessment and diagnosis

Assessment and diagnosis can be challenging as affected individuals can not only show a wide variation in the degree of both intellectual ability and behavioural severity across the key developmental domains (see above), but their behavioural profiles will inevitably change with age. Any developmental concerns highlighted by parents/carers or identified during routine developmental surveillance require further assessment. However, a lack of concern from parents about their child's early development does not necessarily imply a normal developmental history. Many parents express concerns as early as 15 to 18 months of age and some as early as 11 months (Chawarska *et al.* 2007) but it is often difficult to differentiate clearly when developmental difficulties began (Baird *et al.* 2003). These early symptoms may include: lack of joint attention (Charman *et al.* 1997; Charman, 2003); failure to develop spoken language (McConachie *et al.* 2005); failure to respond to name (Baranek, 2004); and showing decreased imitation of facial expressions, vocal imitations and object-orientated imitation (Bryson *et al.* 2007). Despite these findings the usual age of early pre-school diagnosis in the UK is not before 4 to 5 years of age (Carrona *et al.* 2008; Charman and Baird, 2002, Dumont-Mathieu and Fein, 2005).

At the time of initial presentation in early childhood it can be difficult to determine the significance of behavioural abnormalities with respect to the onset of ASD. For instance there may be uncertainty about the differentiation of developmental impairment/delay from developmental deviance or impaired social reciprocity from social anxiety or withdrawal. The child may have experienced a lack of opportunities to learn to play rather than displaying specific abnormalities in play skills or unusual interests. Other factors such as the presence of sensory deficits and/or the presence of other potentially co-morbid problems such as poor attention, poor concentration and levels of hyperactivity add to the complexity of defining the boundaries of the ASD spectrum. Certainly there are many children, especially at the more intellectually able end of the ASD spectrum, who are unlikely to be identified during the pre-school period. On the other hand there is emerging evidence that early intervention targeted on skills development leads to better outcome (Bryson *et al.* 2003).

Although a number of early general developmental and ASD screening tools have been developed and used in both clinical practice and research, universal use has not been recommended (Bryson *et al.* 2003; Le Couteur, 2003; Robins *et al.* 2001; Rutter 2005; Scottish Intercollegiate Guidelines Network (SIGN), 2007; Stone *et al.* 1999; Swinkels *et al.* 2006). There is a recent optimism regarding the potential for earlier identification and diagnosis of ASD (Johnson *et al.* 2007; see Autism: the

International Journal of Research and Practice, Volume 12, No 5, September 2008, Special Issue on Early Detection).

The age of clinical diagnosis depends on a combination of factors that include parental and professional recognition of presenting concerns, variability of behavioural symptoms and assessment procedures. For example speech delay in pre-school children may activate a referral whereas a child who is high functioning and has adequate language skills may present later with behavioural difficulties or problems with peer relationships as academic and social demands increase. Gilchrist *et al.* (2001), using the Autism Diagnostic Interview (ADI) to obtain retrospective accounts from parents of adolescents with AS, reported that although 70% of parents were aware of some abnormality in their child's behaviour and development before the age of 3, only 35% of those parents sought professional help. In contrast, 92% of parents of young adults with high functioning autism (in the same study) were reportedly aware of problems before the age of 3, and 77% sought help at that early stage. When assessing a particular individual it may be hard to separate the features of ASD, co-morbid condition(s) and any environmental factors; or indeed the diagnosis may include a combination of all three.

1.3.1 Assessment process

> It is equally important to diagnose, and not diagnose, accurately
> (SIGN, 2007)

The purpose of clinical or research assessment in ASD is to make a diagnosis where applicable. The assessment is based on an account of the developmental history, specific individual behavioural assessments and investigations, observation in several settings and the consideration of an appropriate differential diagnosis. The resulting diagnosis should be based on clinical judgement and the expertise of the multi-disciplinary/multi-agency assessments (Levy *et al.* 2009).

Standardised instruments (including diagnostic assessment tools) can enhance or facilitate diagnosis, may not be essential for every clinical assessment, but are required for most published peer reviewed research studies. Diagnostic assessment tools should not be used in isolation and most currently published instruments are less reliable in children under 2 years of age (Charman and Baird, 2002). The multi-disciplinary/multi-agency assessment should also include the identification of the individual's and family's profile of developmental skills and deficits, together with any associated developmental problems and co-morbidities that might impact on the functioning for the individual with ASD and their family.

The **National Autism Plan for Children** (Le Couteur, 2003) and the Scottish Intercollegiate Guidelines Network clinical guideline number 98 (SIGN, 2007)

Table 1.2 *Components for a Multi-agency Assessment*

Multi-agency Assessment (MAA) (NAP-C, 2003)
1. Collate existing information
2. ASD specific developmental history (ADI-R; DISCO; 3di)
3. Observational assessments (incl ADOS)
4. Cognitive assessment
5. Communication assessment
6. Behaviour & mental health assessment
7. Family assessment
8. Physical examination
9. Medical investigations
10. Other investigations (such as Occupational therapy and/or Physiotherapy)

provide a framework for early recognition, assessment and diagnosis and early intervention for young children/children and adolescents respectively. The stages for assessment include:

- Stage 1: **General Developmental Assessment (GDA)** for any child with a possible developmental problem.
- Stage 2: **Multi-agency Assessment (MAA)** including the 'essential' components for a complete ASD diagnostic assessment and differential diagnosis

The components for a multi-agency (MA) assessment are listed in Table 1.2.

1.3.2 ASD-specific developmental history

Standardised instruments, such as the Autism Diagnostic Interview-Revised (ADI-R) (Le Couteur *et al.* 2003; Lord *et al.* 1994), the Diagnostic Interview for Social and Communications Disorders (DISCO) (Leekam *et al.* 2002; Wing *et al.* 2002) and the Developmental Diagnostic and Dimensional Interview (3di) (Skuse *et al.* 2004), provide frameworks for the specific developmental history required for a differential diagnosis of ASD/PDD. Although a criticism of such semi-structured interviews is that they can be time consuming, the detailed developmental history framework may provide relevant information that is not available from assessments of current functioning (Royal College of Psychiatrists (2006) Council Report CR 136).

Autism Diagnostic Interview-Revised (ADI-R) (Le Couteur *et al.* 2003; Lord *et al.* 1994; Rutter *et al.* 2003). The ADI-R is a semi-structured investigator-based interview undertaken with the parents/main caregiver. The format of the interview is designed to provide a framework for a lifetime differential diagnosis of PDD/ASD defined within the internationally accepted diagnostic systems (DSM-IV-TR and ICD-10). The interview emphasises the need to record descriptions of specific behaviours in the three key domains necessary for a diagnosis of autism/ASD (with sections focusing on regression and special skills) and some other relevant clinical behaviours. The interview can be used for individuals of the mental age of 2 years and above. It takes around two to three hours to administer and training is required. The published algorithm provides a threshold for autism/non-autism only. With increasing awareness of the autism spectrum the original authors and a number of other ASD research groups are reanalysing ADI-R datasets to propose new diagnostic algorithm(s) threshold cut-off scores for autism and ASD (Buitelaar *et al.* 1999; Le Couteur *et al.* unpublished data). The interview does not, however, cover the more subtle and milder symptoms of the broader autism phenotype.

The ADI-R format records information about current behaviours (defined as the last three months), lifetime and early childhood ratings. Individual items show high reliability and high diagnostic validity (Rutter *et al.* 2003). However, it is the multiplicity of items across the three domains of enquiry that allows the separation of ASD from general developmental delay/learning disability and other neurodevelopmental disorders (Rutter *et al.* 2003). Further studies by other research groups have reported both good psychometric properties (de Bildt *et al.* 2004; Lecavalier *et al.* 2006) and the usefulness of the ADI-R in research studies (South *et al.* 2005). However, studies have also reported high sensitivity (83–91%) but lower specificity for autism (56–72%) in different age groups and populations. For instance Charman *et al.* (2004) reported that in a sample of 2-year-olds the diagnoses based on ADI-R alone were less stable when the children were followed up at 3 years of age. These findings support the importance of not relying on a single diagnostic measure and that algorithm threshold cut-off scores should not be used as the sole diagnostic criterion (Baird *et al.* 2006; de Bildt *et al.* 2004; Ventola *et al.* 2006). The interview is now available in seventeen languages.

The Diagnostic Interview for Social and Communication Disorders (DISCO) (Leekam *et al.* 2002; Wing *et al.* 2002). The DISCO is a clinical interview schedule based on Wing and Gould's original theoretical proposal that autism is a spectrum of conditions with a particular emphasis on the triad of impairments. It was designed to collect information on development and behaviour for individuals of all ages and levels of ability. The interview evolved from the earlier Handicaps, Behaviours and Skills schedule (HBS) (Wing and Gould, 1978; 1979) and is used to elicit information relevant for the broader autism spectrum, other associated developmental disorders and co-morbid conditions. A set of algorithms and information on developmental skills and atypical behaviours can be derived from the interview but these are not clinical diagnoses (Leekam *et al.* 2002; Wing *et al.* 2002). The semi-structured interview is undertaken with parents/main caregivers. It takes approximately 3 hours to administer and specific training is required. The authors report good to excellent inter-rater reliability on 90% of items. The instrument shows good agreement with the ADI-R. For both the ADI-R and the DISCO, informants (parents/carers) usually report that the experience of taking part in this type of detailed interview is reassuringly thorough and comprehensive.

The Developmental Diagnostic and Dimensional Interview (3di) (Skuse *et al.* 2004). This is a computerised interview assessment procedure that is designed to be administered by a trained interviewer with a parent informant using a laptop computer. A structured computer-generated report is available at the end of the interview, together with algorithms using a dimensional framework of symptom and diagnostic profiles for autism and common non-autistic co-morbidities. The focus is on current functioning. Parents can be sent a pre-interview package of questionnaires to complete. This information can be entered onto the computer and allows an abbreviated face-to-face interview lasting forty-five minutes, compared with ninety minutes for the full interview. The interview was devised to assess autistic traits, social impairment and co-morbidity in children of normal ability and is not recommended for use on pre-school children. The authors report good test inter-rater reliability (Skuse *et al.* 2004).

Vineland Adaptive Behaviour Scale (VABS). An additional structured interview undertaken with the parent/main caregiver that is completed in some studies (clinical and research) immediately after the ASD specific developmental history is the VABS (Sparrow *et al.* 1984). Carter *et al.* (1998) have published supplementary norms for individuals with autism. This interview provides information about the individual's developmental level in four domains of everyday adaptive self help and independence skills (motor behaviours; communication; social interactions; maladaptive behaviours). This information complements direct testing (see below).

1.3.3 *Observation and individual assessments*

For children and individuals with ASD and other developmental and neurodevelopmental disorders, behaviour can vary considerably in different settings. Direct observations can be undertaken in a range of settings such as home, educational settings (including playgroup, nursery, school or college), health-based settings, other local authority and social services settings. Observations of behaviour in different settings will allow assessment of both the individual's functioning in different contexts but also how they interact with peers and adults in their usual social settings. It also provides the opportunity to assess the level of adaptability to predictable and less predictable events.

ASD-specific standardised observational assessments give complementary information that allows comparisons between individuals over time and between different clinical/research centres and samples.

Autism Diagnostic Observational Schedule (ADOS) (Lord *et al.* 2000). This assessment was first developed together with the ADI as a package of instruments for research diagnosis (Bailey *et al.* 1995; Bolton *et al.* 1994). The ADOS is a widely used semi-structured, standardised play and activities-based assessment focusing on the three behavioural domains necessary for a differential diagnosis of ASD and/or other neurodevelopmental disorders namely:

(1) communication
(2) social interaction
(3) play/imaginative use of materials and repetitive behaviours

These observations complement the information gained from other assessment procedures such as the developmental history and direct observations. It takes 30–45 minutes to administer. Training in the use of pre-determined social contexts is required and once trained regular reliability checks are necessary (de Bildt *et al.* 2004; Lord *et al.* 2001). There are four modules for use with individuals ranging from pre-school children without useful speech through to verbally able adults (Lord *et al.* 1989; 2000; 2001). The module choice controls for levels of expressive language. The ADOS publications report high levels of reliability of items across modules. The exception is coding of items such as repetitive behaviours and sensory abnormalities which may occur less frequently during a live individual assessment.

Diagnostic algorithms summarise the ratings for social behaviour and communication in relation to DSM-IV and ICD-10 diagnostic criteria with separate thresholds for autism and ASD. Until recently restricted and repetitive behaviours were not included in these diagnostic algorithms (Gotham *et al.* 2007; 2008). The ADOS is available in several languages, but further work may well be required to consider particular social and cultural factors. This assessment provides useful clinical and research information that can inform intervention planning. Although the instrument was originally developed as a diagnostic tool, it has also been used as an outcome measure (Aldred *et al.* 2004; McConachie *et al.* 2003). A new severity metric has been reported which may prove useful for evaluating the effectiveness of interventions (Gotham *et al.* 2009).

1.3.4 *Assessment of individual profile of skills and deficits*

For some individuals with ASD, co-operating with direct testing can pose particular challenges. However, since those with neurodevelopmental disorders such as ASD are likely to have unique profiles of skills and deficits (see Table 1.2), direct assessment will usually be needed. This information is important for both clinical and research purposes to inform, for example, planning of appropriate interventions for an individual, to investigate specific research hypotheses and to compare research findings across studies. Successful direct assessment inevitably requires specialist skills and experience working with people with ASD. Individual profiling of intellectual ability, neuropsychological functioning, communication, motor and sensory skills and adaptive functioning have been recommended (Johnson *et al.* 2007; Le Couteur, 2003; Ministries of Health and Education, 2008; SIGN, 2007).

1.3.5 *Neuro-cognitive assessment*

Some neuropsychological impairments may not be specific to ASD but may be more severe in individuals with ASD and the degree of impairment is likely to be influenced by several factors such as levels of communicative skills and verbal mental age. Although standardised IQ tests are considered reliable measures of functioning, direct testing of those with ASD across the age range can be challenging. For instance using the example of the assessment of verbal and non-verbal skills, this usually requires separate testing and since the age range for many tests is limited, different tests/measures are likely to be used for different age groups. This in turn means that the measures used may be different over time and indeed different centres may choose to use different measures. All these factors are likely to lead to problems with interpretation of any findings such as change in scores. This is a particular concern when evaluating the impact of an intervention for an individual and in larger scale intervention evaluation studies. Further, although many published cognitive assessment tests provide scoring protocols and norms for typically developing children, norms for different cultural groups and for individuals with ASD may not be available. Several authors have provided summaries of available tests (Howlin, 1998; The National Autism Plan for Children (Le Couteur, 2003)).

1.3.6 *Communication, speech and language assessment*

A comprehensive assessment of an individual profile of verbal and non-verbal communication skills will include a combination of targeted observations in different settings and direct assessment work. Again the choice of assessment measure(s) will depend on several factors including: the purpose of the assessment; the individual characteristics of the child/individual; other potential co-morbidities; and/or the focus of the research study (Bishop and Norbury, 2008; Botting and Conti-Ramsden, 2003; Charman *et al.* 2003; Cohen *et al.* 2003; see National Autism Plan for Children for summary of assessment tools for use with young children (Le Couteur, 2003)).

1.3.7 *Behavioural and mental health assessment*

Disturbances of behaviour, attention, activity, thought and emotion are common in individuals/children with ASD (de Bruin *et al.* 2007; Leyfer *et al.* 2006; Simonoff *et al.* 2008). Individuals with ASD can experience the same developmental, medical and mental health conditions as individuals without ASD (SIGN, 2007). Disordered sleep and food selectivity are well recognised (Bowers, 2002; Couturier *et al.* 2005; Keen, 2007; Mills and Wing, 2005; Ministries of Health and Education, 2008; Polimeni *et al.* 2005; Wigg and Stores, 2004). Problematic emotional reactions and behaviours can occur in response to a range of potentially modifiable factors such as medical conditions (for example earache) or a change in their environment. These behaviours can include self-injurious behaviour, disruptive behaviours, aggressiveness, temper tantrums, emotional lability, irritability, anxiety and a range of co-morbid mental health disorders. Co-morbidities with ASD are well recognised and have been reported to affect up to 72% of cases (de Bruin *et al.* 2007; Gillott *et al.* 2001; Green *et al.* 2000; Hutton *et al.* 2008; Leyfer *et al.* 2006; Mills and Wing, 2005; Simonoff *et al.* 2008; Witwer and Lecavalier, 2005). There is a limited evidence base for using currently available mental health diagnostic assessment tools. New instruments for individuals with ASD have been reported (Bolton and Rutter, 1994; Brereton *et al.* 2006; Hutton *et al.* 2008; Leyfer *et al.* 2006). These instruments need further testing in independent samples.

1.3.8 *Family assessment*

It has long been acknowledged that the continuity of care and attention that individuals with ASD receive has an important impact on their outcome and ability to achieve their individual potential (National Research Council, Committee on Interventions for Children with Autism Report, 2001; Schopler and Reichler, 1971; Schopler *et al.* 1982). However, the impact of caring for individuals with ASD is significant for the whole family (parents, siblings and grandparents) (Bromley *et al.* 2002; Gold, 1993; Gray, 2002; Hastings and Johnson, 2001; Margetts *et al.* 2006; Mills and Wing, 2005; National Autistic Society Report entitled 'The impact of autism on the family', 2005). Family studies have confirmed an increased genetic risk for both ASD and a broader range of qualitatively similar social, cognitive and communication traits and behaviours in relatives of individuals with autism/ASD (Bailey *et al.* 1998; Bolton *et al.* 1994; Parr *et al.* 2006; Szatmari *et al.* 1998). Studies have also reported increased rates of other psychiatric disorders (Bolton *et al.* 1998; Daniels *et al.* 2008; Murphy *et al.* 2000). Recently published clinical guidelines and practice parameter documents highlight the importance of assessing the profile of family skills and difficulties to inform both a family care plan and the individual education and therapeutic plan for the young person with ASD (Le Couteur, 2003; Ministries of Health and Education, 2008; Scottish Intercollegiate Guidelines Network, 2007; Yates and Le Couteur, 2009).

1.3.9 *Physical examination, medical investigations and other needs*

An initial general developmental assessment should be performed for all individuals when there is a concern about developmental progress. This will include a careful medical and family history and a full neurological examination. Hearing and visual impairments should be ruled out by performing appropriate assessment(s). When the differential diagnosis includes possible ASD, this medical assessment should include looking for neurocutaneous stigmata, dysmorphisms and a Wood's light examination especially in the presence of learning disability (Baird *et al.* 2003; Johnson *et al.* 2007; Scottish Intercollegiate Guidelines Network, 2007; Yates and Le Couteur, 2009). Approximately 10–15% of children with ASD have a currently recognised medical condition such as tuberous sclerosis (Barton and Volkmar, 1998; Fombonne *et al.* 1997; Kielinen *et al.* 2004; Rutter *et al.* 1994). Some disorders (for example epilepsy) are common in individuals with ASD (Billstedt *et al.* 2005; Kagan-Kushnir *et al.* 2005; Tuchman and Rapin, 2002) and at least a fifth to a third of pre-school children have a history of regression (Baird *et al.* 2008; Lord *et al.* 2004; Meilleur and Fombonne, 2009; Tuchman and Rapin 1997; Werner and Dawson, 2005). Karyotyping and DNA-specific testing for Fragile X is recommended in all individuals with other investigations guided by clinical presentation, family history and where there are specific management, treatment or genetic implications (Johnson *et al.* 2007; Ministries of Health and Education, 2008; Scottish Intercollegiate Guidelines Network, 2007; Yates and Le Couteur, 2009). Investigative yield is generally low, quoted as between 8% and 37% depending on the population studied (Challman *et al.* 2003). The yield of positive investigations is increased if there is lower IQ and dysmorphic features (Cass *et al.* 2006; Challman *et al.* 2003; Johnson *et al.* 2007).

Neuroimaging and EEGs should only be performed if there is a clinical indication, or if part of the research paradigm. Similarly evaluation of gastrointestinal tract should be guided by clinical presentation. Increasing emphasis on, and awareness of, the rates of motor, sensory and perceptual difficulties has led to specific assessments of sensory profiles and perception difficulties but this is only indicated in response to clinical and research indications (Dover and Le Couteur, 2007; Dunn 1999; Ministries of Health and Education, 2008; Scottish Intercollegiate Guidelines Network, 2007).

1.4 Best Estimate Clinical Diagnosis (BECD) and research diagnosis

Structured ASD diagnostic interviews and observational methods are often used in combination in both clinical and research practice. However, the systematic collection of information does not replace clinical judgement and further, such standardised procedures will not always resolve the problems of discrepancies between sources of information (Goodman *et al.* 1996). In most research and clinical studies all sources of information are combined to produce the 'Best Estimate' Clinical Diagnosis (BECD). This procedure is often defined as the gold standard

Table 1.3 *Example of Research Diagnosis Protocol: interview and observation*

Autism assessment
Psychometric assessment
Speech, language & communication assessment
Neurodevelopmental examination
Other assessments
Best Estimate Clinical Diagnosis (BECD)

in research and clinical guidelines (Dunn, 2000; Dover and Le Couteur, 2007; Le Couteur, 2003).

1.4.1 *ASD research diagnostic procedures*

For all research, protocols should include a detailed description of the diagnostic paradigm for ASD (see Table 1.3). This will usually comprise a developmental interview, a range of observational measures and an indication about whether or not clinical information is available to be included within a BECD procedure.

The following examples of baseline ASD assessments illustrate the use of a combination of measures (together with inclusion and exclusion criteria) to provide the details of participant characteristics required to address specific research hypotheses. The details of the specific sample recruitment, selection and study procedures are reported elsewhere.

The International Molecular Genetic Study of Autism Consortium (IMGSAC, 1998; 2001). For this multi-centre molecular genetic study, the inclusion criteria for probands with autism were very specific with the aim of minimising genetic heterogeneity. Probands had to have a clinical diagnosis of autism before the age of 12 years together with specified algorithm threshold criteria for ADI-R and ADOS; physical examination; karyotyping and specific DNA testing to exclude Fragile X; and cognitive tests. The study exclusion criteria were:

(1) Age less than 4 years at time of recruitment
(2) IQ < 35 (using specified assessments)
(3) Presence of other known medical conditions (e.g. tuberous sclerosis, Fragile X chromosomal anomaly, neurological disorders)
(4) Neonatal brain damage or incomplete obstetric information
(5) Adoptive, foster or institutional upbringing during the first 4 years (or other potential contributing circumstances, e.g. severe nutritional or psychological deprivation)
(6) Any other observational data that cast doubt on the diagnosis

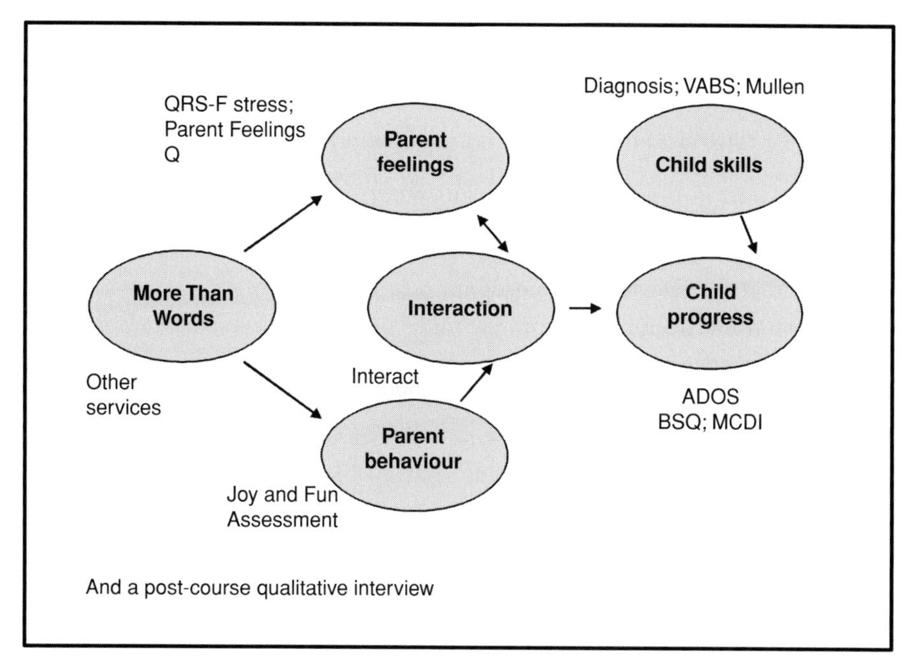

Figure 1.1 Model of Measurement for Diagnosis and the Evaluation of Outcomes of Children (used over the course of the FACTS study). BSQ – Behavior Screening Questionnaire; MCDI – MacArthur Communicative Development Inventory; QRS-F – Questionnaire on Resources and Stress-Friedrich short form. Acknowledgements to Professor Helen McConachie, Professor of Clinical Psychology and Lead Investigator for the families. For further reference please see McConachie *et al.* (2005).

Families and Communication: Training and Support (FACTS trial) (McConachie *et al.* 2003). The aim of this study was the evaluation of an early intervention group training programme for parents of pre-school children with complex social communication disorders (including suspected autism/ASD). The children did not, however, need a definite diagnosis of autism to be considered for inclusion in the parent group training programme. The main inclusion criterion was evidence of language and social or behaviour problems. The best estimate clinical diagnoses (autism, ASD and other (including those children with a speech and language disorder)) were derived from a combination of assessments (clinical accounts, ADI-R; ADOS, VABS and cognitive assessment using the Mullen Scale of Early Learning (Mullen, 1995)) (see Figure 1.1). In this study the ADOS was also used as an outcome measure.

Pre-School Children Communication Trial (PACT) (Green *et al.* 2010). This is a recently completed UK-based three-site randomised controlled trial of a parent-mediated communication-focused intervention for pre-school children with ASD added to their treatment as usual (TAU) against TAU alone. For this study all subjects have a definite clinical diagnosis of autism (using the ADI-R and ADOS algorithm thresholds) and greater than twelve months age equivalent level in non-verbal development. The exclusion criteria are severe epilepsy and twins.

Figure 1.1 illustrates the model of measurement for diagnosis and the evaluation of outcomes of the children, used over the course of the FACT study.

The Special Needs and Autism Project (SNAP) (Baird *et al.* 2006). This community-based project assessed a cohort of 1733 children in South Thames with identified special education needs and a further 255 cases known to local services, drawn from the population of just under 57 000 children born between July 1990 and December 1991. All assessed children were given a research diagnosis based on the findings from the standardised research assessment tools including ADI-R and ADOS. Each case was then reviewed by the study clinical principal investigators. Using all available information from ADI-R, ADOS, clinical vignette, IQ and language assessment and teacher reports and ICD-10 criteria, a decision was made on current presentation. This method resulted in a reported prevalence rate of 116 per 10 000. By contrast the reported prevalence rate was 143 per 10 000 using just a single diagnostic instrument such as the ADI-R: a considerable over-estimate using information derived from a single source.

These examples illustrate the significant dedicated resources needed to undertake the research procedures for assessment and diagnosis of ASD. Each study has included a combination of published standardised ASD assessments together with other measures to characterise individual functioning.

Over the last 20 years this type of combination of research instruments has been recommended for autism research although little systematic attempt has been made to evaluate how information from such instruments should be combined (Risi *et al.* 2006). In recent years more emphasis has been placed on the need to investigate the stability of ASD as well as autism (Lord *et al.* 2006; Tanguay, 2000).

Some studies have investigated the relationships both between diagnostic instruments and in combination with a BECD procedure. In 2006, Risi *et al.* proposed criteria for the combined use of ADI-R and ADOS to diagnose autism and the broader category of ASD and compared the resultant algorithms with BECD in four US and Canadian samples (Risi *et al.* 2006). Sensitivities and specificities of 75–80% and higher were obtained for autism, depending on the sample. Specificity was significantly lower using a single instrument and poor in individuals with profound intellectual disability. De Bildt *et al.* (2004) in a study of 184 children and adolescents with intellectual disability (aged 5–20 years) showed that both instruments measured autism and PDD reliably with 'fair' agreement between the instruments (63.5%). The authors had devised an ADI-R algorithm for PDD for this study. Agreement was higher for the younger children (aged 5–8 years) and most difficult for the broader diagnosis of PDD/ASD, especially in the very low-functioning individuals. The authors concluded that diagnostic instrument algorithm cut-off scores should not be used as the sole criterion and noted the additional limitation that both instruments were resource-intensive. Lord *et al.* (2006) in a follow-up study of 172 children referred for evaluation of possible autism before 36 months of age showed that both the ADI-R and PL-ADOS (pre-linguistic ADOS) had similar rates of research diagnosis of ASD but were more inclusive than clinical judgement. In this study both these instruments had been modified for use in young children under the age of 3 years. Further in a simple additive logistic regression for best estimate autism diagnosis at age 9 years, all three diagnostic measures (ADI-R, Pl-ADOS and clinical judgement) made an independent contribution to the accurate prediction of an ASD diagnosis.

Other studies from different research centres have reported fair to good concordance between the ADI-R and ADOS and made some specific recommendations for the use of the instruments in particular samples (Gray *et al.* 2008; Mazefsky and Oswald, 2006; Papanikolaou *et al.* 2009; Wiggins and Robins, 2008). The Special Needs and Autism Project (Baird *et al.* 2006) identified the limitations of using the ADI-R in isolation and the consequent impact on reported prevalence for autism if this instrument was the only source of information (Baird *et al.* 2006). Tomanik *et al.* (2007) recommended that including a measure of adaptive functioning improved classification.

Several studies using the ADI-R and ADOS in young pre-school children have noted that repetitive behaviours are reported and observed less frequently than in older age groups. These observations have implications for the validity of the existing ICD/DSM-TR diagnostic criteria for autism/ASD/PDD in this age group (Charman and Baird, 2002; Ventola *et al.* 2006; Wiggins and Robins, 2008). One recently published study (Le Couteur *et al.* 2008) has reported the utility of ADI-R and ADOS in a cohort of 101 pre-school children. In line with other studies it showed good (67%) concordance with ADI-R, ADOS and BECD for autism and less good agreement for ASD. The authors also noted that for those children where there were discrepancies between research instrument diagnoses and clinical judgement both for autism and ASD, the differences in scores were only marginal. Often the scores were just below the algorithm cut-off and yet the recorded data using the research measures were entirely consistent with the clinical evidence of difficulties across a range of settings and over time. These findings add weight to the previously reported observation that published algorithm cut-off scores should not be used in isolation. Further the authors noted that for those young children who did show evidence of repetitive behaviours during the ADOS play-based assessment, these behaviours appeared to be of diagnostic significance.

1.5 Conclusions and challenges for the early assessment and diagnosis of ASD

To progress our understanding of ASD it is essential that case definition is consistent and adequate across specialist clinical academic centres and research studies. Yet the reliable and valid diagnosis of autism/ASD has always presented a challenge both for research and clinical practice, not only in terms of the breadth of the spectrum of clinical presentation but also because of the inevitable developmental change in symptom profile for each affected individual over time. However, it is now generally agreed that the ASD spectrum extends beyond currently defined disorder(s) to a broader autism phenotype (as identified in the relatives of individuals with autism) and probably beyond even there, to qualitatively similar traits in the general population (Bailey *et al.* 1998; Bolton *et al.* 1994; Brugha, 2002; Melzer *et al.* 2002; Szatmari *et al.* 1998).

New measures have been developed such as the Social Responsiveness Scale (SRS), a parent completed postal questionnaire (Constantino *et al.* 2003), to investigate the relationship between the so-called social domain including social and communication traits and non-social domain namely rigidity, obsessive and repetitive behaviours, detail-focused behaviours and strong interests domains or characteristics of autism in different general population or at risk samples. This questionnaire has been used with a US population-based twin sample collected as part of an epidemiological study of ADHD, to assess the rates of autistic traits. The study has shown increased rates of autistic traits in children with ADHD (Reiersen *et al.* 2007). Some studies such as the Avon Longitudinal Study for Parents and Children (ALSPAC) have used existing brief ASD screening tools to record rates of autistic type behaviours; while others have devised study specific measures, for instance the 16-item parent and teacher postal/telephone questionnaire (Ronald *et al.* 2006), to investigate the genetic relationship between individual differences in the proposed social and non-social behaviours in the UK Twins Early Development Study (TEDS). Our own ASD research group in the north-east of England has focused on the repetitive behavioural domain, using the 20-item parent postal Repetitive Behaviour Questionnaire (RBQ-2) to investigate the rates of repetitive behaviours in a general population cohort of typically developing children (Leekam *et al.* 2007).

Further work is needed both to assess the validity and reliability of these various measures and to replicate the findings in independent samples. As yet we do not know whether these studies are indeed identifying components of autism in the general population. However, these findings raise important questions about the characterisation of the autism behavioural phenotype and whether or not the three domains of autistic symptomatology are more separate than the currently accepted diagnostic criteria imply. Diagnostic boundaries will inevitably be revised as our understanding of causal mechanisms for neurodevelopmental and other mental health disorders increases. In the meantime, diagnosis depends on the identification of specific behavioural characteristics in the affected individual and the skills of the professionals involved in the multidisciplinary assessment procedures.

There is an increasing awareness of autism/ASD amongst the general public, affected families and the professionals working to support them. The emphasis is for early identification, assessment and diagnosis of autism and the broader autism phenotype. Methodological constraints include the limitations of our current understanding of the underlying aetiology of these lifelong neurodevelopmental disorders and the more subtle and possibly less socially impairing manifestations of the broader autism phenotype. This awareness of the limitations of currently accepted diagnostic criteria emphasises the need for the systematic recording of clinically relevant information to contribute to the best estimate clinical diagnosis and the refinement of appropriate standardised diagnostic assessment instruments and measures to evaluate outcomes and change in presentation in the most severely affected individuals. Alongside this work with the most severely affected individuals, new epidemiological methods are needed to investigate the relevance of possible underlying component domains/factors identified in the general population that might advance knowledge of these lifelong neurodevelopmental characteristics.

1.6 References

Aldred, C., Green, J., Adams, C. (2004). A new social communication intervention for children with autism: Pilot randomised controlled treatment study suggesting effectiveness. *Journal of Child Psychology and Psychiatry*, **45**: 1420–1430.

American Psychiatric Association. (2000). *Diagnostic and Statistical Manual of Mental Disorders 4th edn. Text Revision (DSMIV TR)*. Washington DC: American Psychiatric Association.

Asperger, H. (1944). Die 'autistichen psychopathen' im kindersalter. *Archive fur psychiatrie und Nervenkrankheiten*, **117**: 76–136. (Reprinted in *Autism and Asperger Syndrome*, by U. Frith, editor, 1991, Cambridge UK: Cambridge University Press).

Atladottir, H.O., Palmer, E.T., Schendel, D., Dalsgaard, S. (2007). Time trends in reported diagnoses of childhood neuropsychiatric disorders: A Danish cohort study. *Archives of Pediatrics and Adolescent Medicine*, **16**: 193–198.

Attwood, T. (2006). *The Complete Guide to Asperger's Syndrome*. London: Jessica Kingsley Publishers.

Autism: The International Journal of Research and Practice (2008). Volume 12, No 5, September 2008: Special issue on Early Detection. Sage Publications.

Bailey, A., Parr, J. (2003). Implications of the broader phenotype for concepts of autism. In *Autism: Neural Basis and Treatment Possibilities. Novartis Foundation Symposium*, **251**. Chichester: Wiley, pp. 26–47.

Bailey, A., Le Couteur, A., Gottesman, I., *et al.* (1995). Autism as a strongly genetic disorder: Evidence from a British twin study. *Psychological Medicine*, **25**: 63–78.

Bailey, A., Palferman, S., Heavey, L., Le Couteur, A. (1998). Autism: The phenotype in relatives. *Journal of Autism and Development Disorders*, **28**: 369–392.

Baird, G., Cass, H., Slonims, V. (2003). Diagnosis of autism. *British Medical Journal*, **327**: 494–497.

Baird, G., Simonoff, E., Pickles, A., *et al.* (2006). Prevalence of disorders of the autistic spectrum in a population cohort of children in South Thames: The Special Needs and Autism Project (SNAP). *The Lancet*, **368**: 210–215.

Baird, G., Charman, T., Pickles, A., *et al.* (2008). Regression, developmental trajectory and associated problems in disorders in the autism spectrum: the SNAP study. *Journal of Autism and Developmental Disorders*, **38**: 1827–1836.

Baranek, G.T. (2004). Autism during infancy: A retrospective video analysis of sensory-motor and social behaviors at 9–12 months of age. *Journal of Autism and Developmental Disorders*, **29**: 213–224.

Barton, M., Volkmar, F. (1998). How commonly are known medical conditions associated with autism? *Journal of Autism and Developmental Disorders*, **28**: 273–278.

Billstedt, E., Gillberg, I.C., Gillberg, C. (2005). Autism after adolescence: Population-based 13–22 year follow-up study of 120 individuals with autism diagnosed in childhood. *Journal of Autism and Developmental Disorders*, **35**: 351–360.

Bishop, D.V.M., Norbury, C.F. (2008). Speech and language disorders. In *Rutter's Child and Adolescent Psychiatry*. Oxford: Blackwell, pp. 782–801.

Bolton, P.F., Rutter, M. (1994). *Schedule for Assessment of Psychiatric Problems Associated with Autism (and Other Developmental Disorders) (SAPPA): Informant Version*. Cambridge and London: University of Cambridge and Institute of Psychiatry.

Bolton, P., Macdonald, H., Pickles, A., *et al.* (1994). A case-control family history study of autism. *Journal of Child Psychology and Psychiatry*, **35**: 877–900.

Bolton, P.F., Pickles, A., Murphy, M., *et al.* (1998). Autism, affective and other psychiatric disorders: patterns of familial aggregation. *Psychological Medicine*, **28**: 385–395.

Botting, N., Conti-Ramsden, G. (2003). Autism, primary pragmatic difficulties, and specific language impairment: Can we distinguish them using psycholinguistic markers? *Developmental Medicine and Child Neurology*, **45**: 515–524.

Bowers, L. (2002). An audit of referrals of children with autism spectrum disorder to the dietetic service. *Journal of Human Nutrition and Dietetics*, **15**: 141–144.

Brereton, A.V., Tonge, B.J., Einfeld, S.L. (2006). Psychopathology in children and adolescents with autism compared to young people with intellectual disability. *Journal of Autism and Developmental Disorders*, **36**: 863–870.

Bromley, J., Hare, D., Davison, K., Emerson, E. (2002). *The Health and Social Care Needs of Families and/or Carers Supporting a Child with Autistic Spectrum Disorders*. Lancaster: Institute for Health Research. http://www.lancs.ac.uk/shm/dhr/research/learning/projects/autism.htm (accessed May 2010).

Brown, R., Hobson, R.P., Lee, A., Stevenson, J. (1997). Are there 'autistic like' features in congenitally blind children? *Journal of Child Psychology and Psychiatry*, **38**: 693–703.

Brugha, T.S. (2002). The end of the beginning: A requiem for the categorization of mental disorder? *Psychological Medicine*, **32**: 1149–1154.

Brugha, T.S., McManus, S., Meltzer, H., *et al.* (2009). *Autism Spectrum Disorders in Adults Living in Households Throughout England: Report from the Adult Psychaitric Morbidity Survey, 2007*. The NHS Information Centre for Health and Social Care (UK). Available at: http://www.ic.nhs.uk/asdpsychiatricmorbidity07.

Bryson, S.E., Rogers, S.J., Fombonne, E. (2003). Autism spectrum disorders: Early detection, intervention, education, and psychopharmacological management. *Canadian Journal of Psychiatry*, **48**: 506–516.

Bryson, S.E., Zwaigenbaum, L., Brian, J., *et al.* (2007). A prospective case series of high-risk infants who developed autism. *Journal of Autism and Developmental Disorders*, **37**: 12–24.

Buitelaar, J.K., Van Der Gaag, R., Klin, A., Volkmar, F. (1999). Exploring the boundaries of Pervasive Developmental Disorders Not Otherwise Specified: Analysis of data from the DSM-IV Autistic Disorder Field Trial. *Journal of Autism and Developmental Disorders*, **29**: 33.

Carrona, E.B., Milunsky, J.M., Tager-Flusberg, H. (2008). Autism Spectrum Disorders: clinical and research frontiers. *Archives of Disease in Childhood*, **93**: 518–523.

Carter, A.S., Volkmar, F.R., Sparrow, S.S., *et al.* (1998). The Vineland Adaptive Behavior Scales: Supplementary norms for individuals with autism. *Journal of Autism and Developmental Disorders*, **28**: 287–302.

Cass, H., Sekaran, D., Baird, G. (2006). Medical investigation of children with autistic spectrum disorders. *Child: Care, Health and Development*, **32**: 521–533.

Chakrabarti, S., Fombonne, E. (2005). Pervasive Developmental Disorders in preschool children: Confirmation of high prevalence. *American Journal of Psychiatry*, **162**: 1133–1141.

Challman, T.D., Barbaresi, W.J., Katusic, S.K., Weaver, A. (2003). The yield of the medical evaluation of children with pervasive development disorders. *Journal of Autism and Developmental Disorders*, **33**: 187–192.

Charman, T. (2003). Why is joint attention a pivotal skill in autism?. *Philosophical Transactions of The Royal Society Biological Sciences*, **358**: 315–324.

Charman, T., Baird, G. (2002). Practitioner review: Diagnosis of Autism Spectrum Disorders in 2 and 3 year old children. *Journal of Child Psychology and Psychiatry*, **43**: 289–305.

Charman, T., Swettenham, J., Baron-Cohen, S., *et al.* (1997). Infants with autism: An investigation of empathy, pretend play, joint attention and imitation. *Developmental Psychology*, **33**: 781–789.

Charman, T., Drew, A., Baird, C., Baird, G. (2003). Measuring early language development in preschool children with autism spectrum disorder using the MacArthur Communicative Development Inventory (Infant Form). *Journal of Child Language*, **30**: 213–236.

Charman, T., Taylor, E., Drew, A., *et al.* (2004). Outcome at 7 years of children diagnosed with autism at age 2: Predictive validity of assessments conducted at 2 and 3 years of age and pattern of symptom change over time. *Journal of Child Psychology and Psychiatry*, **46**: 500–513.

Chawarska, K., Klin, A., Paul, R., Volkmar, F. (2007). Autism spectrum disorder in the second year: Stability and change in syndrome expression. *Journal of Child Psychology and Psychiatry*, **48**: 128–138.

Chess, S. (1977). Follow-up report on autism in congenital rubella. *Journal of Autism and Childhood Schizophrenia*, **7**: 69–81.

Cohen, I.L., Schmidt-Lackner, S., Romanczyk, R., Sudhalter, V. (2003). The PDD behavior inventory: A rating scale for assessing response to intervention in children with pervasive developmental disorder. *Journal of Autism and Developmental Disorders*, **33**: 31–45.

Constantino, J.N., Todd, R.D. (2003). Autistic traits in the general population. *Archives of General Psychiatry*, **60**: 524–530.

Couturier, J.L., Speechley, K.N., Steele, M., *et al.* (2005). Parental perception of sleep problems in children of normal intelligence with pervasive developmental disorders: Prevalence, severity, and pattern. *Journal of the American Academy of Child and Adolescent Psychiatry*, **44**: 815–822.

Cox, A., Klein, K., Charman, T., *et al.* (1999). Autism spectrum disorders at 20 and 42 months of age: Stability of clinical and ADI-R diagnosis. *Journal of Child Psychology and Psychiatry*, **40**: 719–732.

Daniels, J., Forssen, U., Hultman, C.M., *et al.* (2008). Parental psychiatric disorders associated with autism spectrum disorders in the offspring. *Pediatrics*, **121**: 1357–1362.

Darke, J., Bushby, K., Le Couteur, A., McConachie, H. (2006). Survey of behaviour problems in children with neuromuscular diseases. *European Journal of Paediatric Neurology*, **10**: 129–134.

de Bildt, A., Systema, S., Ketelaars, C., *et al.* (2004). Inter-relationship between autism diagnostic observation schedule-generic (ADOS-G), autism diagnostic interview-revised (ADI-R) and the diagnostic and statistical manual of mental disorders (DSM-IV-TR) classification in children and adolescents with mental retardation. *Journal of Autism and Developmental Disorders*, **34**: 129–137.

de Bruin, E.I., Ferdinand, R.F., Meester, S., de Nijs, P.F.A., Verheij, F. (2007). High rates of psychiatric co-morbidity in PDD-NOS. *Journal of Autism and Developmental Disorders*, **37**: 877–886.

Dover, C., Le Couteur, A. (2007). How to diagnose autism. *Archives of Disease in Childhood*, **92**: 540–545.

Dumont-Mathieu, T., Fein, D. (2005). Screening for autism in young children: The Modified Checklist for Autism in Toddlers (M-CHAT) and other measures. *Mental Retardation and Developmental Disabilities Research Reviews*, **11**: 253–262.

Dunn, G. (2000). *Statistics in Psychiatry*. London: Arnold.

Dunn, W. (1999). *The Sensory Profile*. London: Psychological Corporation.

Filipek, P.A., Accardo, P.J., Baranek, G.T., *et al.* (1999). The screening and diagnosis of autistic spectrum disorders. *Journal of Autism and Developmental Disorders*, **29**: 439–484.

Fombonne, E. (2003). Epidemiology surveys of autism and other pervasive developmental disorders: An update. *Journal of Autism and Developmental Disorders*, **33**: 365–382.

Fombonne, E., DuMazaubrun, C., Cans, C., Grandjean, H. (1997). Autism and associated medical disorder in a French epidemiological study. *Journal of the American Academy of Child and Adolescent Psychiatry*, **36**: 1561–1569.

Frith, U. (1991). *Autism and Asperger Syndrome*. Cambridge UK: Cambridge University Press.

Frith, U. (2003). *Autism: Explaining the Enigma*, 2nd edn. Oxford: Blackwell.

Gilchrist, A., Green, J., Cox, A., Rutter, M., Le Couteur, A. (2001). Development and current functioning in adolescents with Asperger syndrome: A comparative study. *Journal of Child Psychology and Psychiatry*, **30**: 631–638.

Gillott, A., Furniss, F., Walter, A. (2001). Anxiety in high functioning children with autism. *Autism*, **5**: 277–286.

Gold, N. (1993). Depression and social adjustment in siblings of boys with autism. *Journal of Autism and Developmental Disorders*, **23**: 147–163.

Goodman, R., Yude, C., Richards, H., Taylor, E. (1996). Rating child psychiatric caseness from detailed case histories. *Journal of Child Psychology and Psychiatry*, **37**: 369–379.

Gotham, K., Risi, S., Pickles, A., Lord, C. (2007). The Autism Diagnostic Observation Schedule: Revised Algorithms for Improved Diagnostic Validity. *Journal of Autism Development Disorders*, **37**: 613–627.

Gotham, K., Risi, S., Dawson, G., *et al.* (2008). A replication of the Autism Diagnostic Observation Schedule (ADOS) Revised Algorithms. *Journal of the American Academy of Child and Adolescent Psychiatry*, **47**: 642–651.

Gotham, K., Pickles, A., Lord, C. (2009). Standardizing ADOS scores for a measure of severity in Autism Spectrum Disorders. *Journal of Autism and Developmental Disorders*, **39**: 693–705.

Gray, D.E. (2002). 'Everybody just freezes. Everybody is just embarrassed.' Felt and enacted stigma among parents of children with high functioning autism. *Sociology of Health and Illness*, **24**: 734–749.

Gray, K.M., Tonge, B.J., Sweeney, D.J. (2008). Using the Autism Diagnostic Interview-Revised and the Autism Diagnostic Observation Schedule with young children with developmental delay: Evaluating diagnostic validity. *Journal of Autism and Developmental Disorders*, **38**: 657–667.

Green, J., Gilchrist, A., Burton, D., Cox, A. (2000). Social and psychiatric functioning in adolescents with Asperger syndrome. *Journal of Autism and Developmental Disorders*, **30**: 279–293.

Green, J., Charman, T., McConachie, H., *et al.* (2010). Parent-mediated communication-focussed treatment in children with autism (PACT): a randomised control trial. *Lancet*, **375**: 2152–2160.

Hastings, R.P., Johnson, E. (2001). Stress in UK families conducting intensive home-based behavioral intervention for their young child with autism. *Journal of Autism and Developmental Disorders*, **31**: 327–336.

Honda, H., Shimizu, Y., Rutter, M. (2005). No effect of MMR withdrawal on the incidence of autism: A total population study. *The Journal of Child Psychology and Psychiatry*, **46**: 572–579.

Howlin, P. (1998). Practitioner review: Psychological and educational treatment for autism. *Journal of Child Psychology and Psychiatry*, **39**: 307–322.

Howlin, P. (2003). Outcome in high-functioning individuals with autism with and without early language delays: Implications for the differentiation between autism and Asperger syndrome. *Journal of Autism and Developmental Disorders*, **33**: 3–13.

Hutton, J., Goode, S., Murphy, M., Le Couteur, A., Rutter, M. (2008). New-onset psychiatric disorders in individuals with autism. *Autism*, **12**: 373–390.

International Molecular Genetic Study of Autism Consortium (IMGSAC). (1998). A full genome screen for autism with evidence for linkage to a region on Chromosome 7q. *Human Molecular Genetics*, **7**: 571–578.

International Molecular Genetic Study of Autism Consortium (IMGSAC). (2001). A genomewide screen for autism: Strong evidence for linkage to Chromosome 2q, 7q and 16p. *American Journal of Human Genetics*, **69**: 570–581.

Johnson, C.P., Myers, S.M., and the Council on Children with Disabilities. (2007). Identification and evaluation of children with autism spectrum disorders. *Pediatrics*, **120**: 1183–1215.

Kagan-Kushnir, T., Roberts, S.W., Snead, O.C. (2005). Screening electroencephalograms in autism spectrum disorders: Evidence-based guideline. *Journal of Child Neurology*, **20**: 197–206.

Kanner, L. (1943). Autistic disturbances of affective contact. *Nervous Child*, **2**: 217–250.

Keen, D.V. (2007). Childhood autism, feeding problems and failure to thrive in early infancy. *European Child and Adolescent Psychiatry*, **17**: 209–216.

Kerr, A. (2002). Annotation: Rett Syndrome: recent progress and implications for research and clinical practice. *Journal of Child Psychology and Psychiatry and Allied Disciplines*, **43**: 277–287.

Kielinen, M., Rantala, H., Timonen, E., Linna, S.L., Moilanen, I. (2004). Associated medical disorders and disabilities in children with autistic disorder: A population based study. *Autism*, **8**: 49–60.

Le Couteur, A. (2003). *National Autism Plan for Children (NAP-C)*. London: The National Autistic Society.

Le Couteur, A.S., Bailey, A., Goode, S., *et al.* (1996). A broader phenotype of autism: The clinical spectrum in twins. *Journal of Child Psychology and Psychiatry*, **37**: 785–801.

Le Couteur, A., Lord, C., Rutter, M. (2003). *ADI-R Autism Diagnostic Interview – Revised. Protocol*. Los Angeles: Western Psychological Services.

Le Couteur, A., Haden, G., Hammal, D., McConachie, H. (2008). Diagnosing autism spectrum disorders in pre-school children using two standardised assessment instruments: The ADI-R and the ADOS. *Journal of Autism and Developmental Disorders*, **38**: 362–372.

Lecavalier, L., Aman, M., Scahill, L., *et al.* (2006). Validity of the autism diagnostic interview-revised. *American Journal on Mental Retardation*, **111**: 199–215.

Leekam, S., Libby, S., Wing, L., Gould, J., Gillberg, C. (2000). Comparison of ICD-10 and Gillberg's criteria for Asperger syndrome. *Autism*, **4**: 11–28.

Leekam, S.R., Libby, S.J., Wing, L., Gould, J., Taylor, C. (2002). The Diagnostic Interview for Social and Communication Disorders: Algorithms for ICD-10 childhood autism and Wing and Gould autistic spectrum disorder. *Journal of Child Psychology and Psychiatry*, **43**: 327–342.

Leekam, S., Tandos, J., McConachie, H., *et al.* (2007). Repetitive behaviours in typically developing 2-year-olds. *Journal of Child Psychology and Psychiatry*, **48**: 1131–1138.

Levy, S., Mandell, D.S., Schultz, R.T. (2009). Autism. *Lancet*, **374**: 1627–1638.

Leyfer, O.T., Folstein, S.E., Bacalman, S., *et al.* (2006). Comorbid psychiatric disorders in children with autism: Interview development and rates of disorders. *Journal of Autism and Developmental Disorders*, **36**: 849–861.

Lord, C. (1995). Follow up of two year old referred for possible autism. *Journal of Child Psychology and Psychiatry*, **36**: 1365–1382.

Lord, C., Rutter, M., Goode, S., *et al.* (1989). Autism Diagnostic Observation Schedule: A standardized observation of communicative and social behaviour. *Journal of Autism and Developmental Disorders*, **19**: 185–212.

Lord, C., Rutter, M., Le Couteur, A. (1994). Autism Diagnostic Interview-Revised – A revised version of a diagnostic interview for caregivers of individuals with possible pervasive developmental disorders. *Journal of Autism and Developmental Disorders*, **24**: 659–685.

Lord, C., Risi, S., Lambrecht, L., *et al.* (2000). The Autism Diagnostic Observation Schedule – Generic: A standard measure of social and communication deficits associated with the spectrum of autism. *Journal of Autism and Developmental Disorders*, **30**: 205–224.

Lord, C., Rutter, M., DiLavore, P.D, Risi, S. (2001). *Autism Diagnostic Observation Schedule.* Los Angeles CA: Western Psychological Services.

Lord, C., Shulman, C., DiLavote, P. (2004). Regression and word loss in autistic spectrum disorders. *Journal of Child Psychology and Psychiatry*, **45**: 936–955.

Lord, C., Risi, S., DiLavore, P.S., *et al.* (2006). Autism from 2 to 9 years of age. *Archives of General Psychiatry*, **63**: 694–701.

Lotter, V. (1966). Epidemiology of autistic conditions in young children. *Social Psychiatry and Psychiatric Epidemiology*, **1**: 124–137.

Margetts, J., Le Couteur, A., Croom, S. (2006). Families in a state of flux: the experience of grandparents in autism spectrum disorder. *Child: Care, Health and Development*, **32**: 565–574.

Mazefsky, C.A., Oswald, D.P. (2006). The discriminative ability and diagnostic utility of the ADOS-G, ADI-R and GARS for children in a clinical setting. *Autism*, **10**: 533–549.

McConachie, H., Randle, V., Hammal, D., Le Couteur, A. (2003). A controlled trial of a training course for parents of children with suspected autism spectrum disorder. *The Journal of Pediatrics*, **147**: 335–340.

McConachie, H., Le Couteur, A., Honey, E. (2005). Can a diagnosis of Asperger syndrome be made in very young children with suspected Autism Spectrum Disorder? *Journal of Autism and Developmental Disorders*, **35**: 167–176.

McIntosh, K.E., Dissanayake, C. (2004). Annotation: The similarities and differences between autistic disorder and Asperger's disorder: A review of the empirical evidence. *Journal of Child Psychology and Psychiatry*, **45**: 421–434.

Meilleur, A., Fombonne, E. (2009). Regression of language and non-language skills in pervasive developmental disorders. *Journal of Intellectual Disabilities Research*, **53**: 115–124.

Melzer, D., Tom, B.D., Brugha, T.S., Fryers, T., Meltzer, H. (2002). Common mental disorder symptom counts in populations: Are there distinct case groups above epidemiological cut-offs? *Psychological Medicine*, **32**: 1195–1201.

Mills, R., Wing, L. (2005). *National Autistic Society Membership Survey*. International Conference Proceedings. London UK: National Autistic Society.

Ministries of Health and Education. (2008). *New Zealand Autism Spectrum Disorder Guideline*. Wellington: Ministry of Health.

Moore, V., Goodson, S. (2003). How well does early diagnosis of autism stand the test of time? Follow-up study of children assessed for autism at age 2 and development of an early diagnostic service. *Autism*, **7**: 47–63.

Mullen, E. (1995) *Mullen Scales of Early Learning*. Circle Pines: American Guidance Service, Inc.

Murphy, M., Bolton, P.F., Pickles, A., *et al.* (2000). Personality traits of the relatives of autistic probands. *Psychological Medicine*, **30**: 1411–1424

National Autistic Society Report. (2005). *The Impact of Autism on the Family*. Available at: http://www.autism.org.uk/en-gb/about-autism/research/information-for-pupils-and-students/families-the-impact-of-autism.aspx

National Research Council, Committee on Interventions for Children with Autism (2001). *Educating Children with Autism*. Washington DC: National Academies Press.

Newschaffer, C.J., Croen, L.A., Daniels, J., *et al.* (2007). The epidemiology of autism spectrum disorders. *Annual Review of Public Health*, **28**: 235–258.

Papanikolaou, K., Paliokosta, E., Houliaras, G., *et al.* (2009). Using the Autism Diagnostic Interview-Revised and the Autism Diagnostic Observation Schedule-Generic for the diagnosis of autism spectrum disorders in a Greek sample with a wide range of intellectual abilities. *Journal of Autism and Developmental Disorders*, **39**: 414–420.

Parr, J.R., Wallace, S., Le Couteur, A., *et al.* (2006). Characteristics of the broader phenotype in siblings and parents of affected relative pairs with autism spectrum disorder. *Archives of Disease in Childhood*, **91** (Supplement 1): A9–A10.

Pickles, A., Starr, E., Kazak, S., *et al.* (2000). Variable expression of the autism broader phenotype: Findings from extended pedigrees. *Journal of Child Psychology and Psychiatry*, **41**: 491–502.

Piven, J., Palmer, P., Jacobi, D., Childress, D., Arnott, S. (1997). Broader autism phenotype: Evidence from a family history study of multiple-incidence autism families. *American Journal of Psychiatry*, **154**: 185–190.

Polimeni, M.A., Richdale, A.L., Francis, A.J.P. (2005). A survey of sleep problems in autism, Asperger's disorder and typically developing children. *Journal of Intellectual Disability Research*, **49**: 260–268.

Reiersen, A.M., Constantino, J.N., Volk, H.E., Todd, R.D. (2007). Autistic traits in a population-based ADHD sample. *Journal of Child Psychology and Psychiatry*, **48**: 464–472.

Risi, S., Lord, C., Gotham, K., *et al.* (2006). Combining information from multiple sources in the diagnosis of autism spectrum disorders. *Journal of the American Academy of Child and Adolescent Psychiatry*, **45**: 1094–1103.

Robins, D.L., Fein, D., Barton, M.L., Green, J.A. (2001). The Modified Checklist for Autism in Toddlers: An initial study investigating the early detection of autism and pervasive developmental disorders. *Journal of Autism and Developmental Disorders*, **31**: 131–144.

Ronald, A., Happé, F., Bolton, P., *et al.* (2006). Genetic heterogeneity between the three components of the autism spectrum: A twin study. *Journal of the American Academy of Child and Adolescent Psychiatry*, **45**: 691–699

Royal College of Psychiatrists (2006). *Psychiatric Services of Adolescents and Adults with Asperger Syndrome and other Autistic Spectrum Disorders*. Council Report CR136. London: Royal College of Psychiatrists.

Rutter, M. (2005). Incidence of autism spectrum disorders: Changes over time and their meaning. *Acta Paediatrica*, **94**: 2–15.

Rutter, M. (2006). Autism: Its recognition, early diagnosis, and service implications. *Journal of Developmental and Behavioral Pediatrics*, **27** (Supplement 2): S54–S58.

Rutter, M., Bailey, A., Bolton, P., Le Couteur, A. (1994). Autism and known medical conditions: Myth and substance. *Journal of Child Psychology and Psychiatry*, **35**: 311–322.

Rutter, M., Le Couteur, A., Lord, C. (2003). *Autism Diagnostic Interview–Revised (ADI-R)*. Los Angeles CA: Western Psychological Services.

Schopler, E., Reichler, R.J. (1971). Parents as cotherapists in the treatment of psychotic children. *Journal of Autism and Childhood Schizophrenia*, **1**: 87–102.

Schopler, E., Mesibov, G.B., Baker, A. (1982). Evaluation of treatment for autistic children and their parents. *Journal of the American Academy of Child Psychiatry*, **21**: 262–267.

Scottish Intercollegiate Guidelines Network (SIGN) (2007). *Assessment, Diagnosis and Clinical Interventions for Children and Young People with Autism Spectrum Disorders*. SIGN, Edinburgh. (SIGN publication no. 98.) Available at: http://www.sign.ac.uk/pdf/sign98.pdf (accessed May 2010).

Simonoff, E., Pickles, A., Charman, T., *et al.* (2008). Psychiatric disorders in children with autism spectrum disorders: Prevalence, comorbidity and associated factors in a population derived sample. *Journal of the American Academy of Child and Adolescent Psychiatry*, **47**: 921–929.

Skuse, D., Warrington, R., Bishop, D., *et al.* (2004). The Developmental, Dimensional and Diagnostic Interview (3di): A novel computerized assessment for autism spectrum disorders. *Journal of the American Academy of Child and Adolescent Psychiatry*, **43**: 548–558.

South, M., Ozonoff, S., McMahon, W.M. (2005). Repetitive behaviour profiles in Asperger syndrome and high functioning autism. *Journal of Autism and Developmental Disorders*, **35**: 145–158.

Sparrow, S.S., Balla, D.A., Cicchetti, D.V., Doll, E.A. (1984). *Vineland Adaptive Behavior Scales: Interview Edition, Survey Form Manual*. Circle Pines, Minnesota: American Guidance Service.

Stone, W.L., Lee, E.B., Ashford, L., *et al.* (1999). Can autism be diagnosed accurately in children under 3 years? *Journal of Child Psychology and Psychiatry and Allied Disciplines*, **40**: 219–226.

Swinkels, S.H.N., Dietz, C., van Daalen, E., *et al.* (2006). Screening for autistic spectrum in children aged 14–15 months. I: The development of the Early Screening of Autistic Traits Questionnaire (ESAT). *Journal of Autism and Developmental Disorders*, **36**: 723–732.

Szatmari, P., Jones, M.B., Zwaigenbaum, L., MacLean, J.E. (1998). Genetics of autism: Overview and new directions. *Journal of Autism and Developmental Disorders*, **28**: 351–368.

Szatmari, P., Bryson, S.E., Boyle, M.H., Streiner, D.L., Duku, E. (2003). Predictors of outcome among high functioning children with autism and Asperger Syndrome. *Journal of Child Psychology and Psychiatry*, **44**: 520–528.

Tanguay, P.E. (2000). Pervasive developmental disorders: A 10-year review. *Journal of the American Academy of Child and Adolescent Psychiatry*, **39**: 1079–1095.

Tomanik, S.S., Pearson, D.A., Loveland, K.A., Lane, D.M., Shaw, J.B. (2007). Improving the reliability of autism diagnoses: Examining the utility of adaptive behavior. *Journal of Autism and Developmental Disorders*, **37**: 921–918.

Tuchman, R.F., Rapin, I. (1997). Regression in pervasive developmental disorders: Seizures and epileptiform electroencephalogram correlates. *Pediatrics*, **99**: 560–566.

Tuchman, R.F., Rapin, I. (2002). Epilepsy in autism. *Lancet Neurology*, **1**: 352–358.

Turner, L.M., Stone, W.L., Pozdol, S.L., Coonrod, E.E. (2006). Follow-up of children with autism spectrum disorders from age two to age nine. *Autism*, **10**: 243–265.

Ventola, P., Kleinman, J., Pandei, J., *et al.* (2006). Agreement among four diagnostic instruments for autism spectrum disorders in toddlers. *Journal of Autism and Developmental Disorders*, **36**: 839–847.

Volkmar, F.R. (1998). Categorical approaches to the diagnosis of autism. *Autism*, **2**: 45–59.

Volkmar, F.R., Lord, C., Bailey, A., Schultz, R.T., Klin, A. (2004). Autism and Pervasive Developmental Disorders. *Journal of Child Psychology and Psychiatry*, **45**: 135–170.

Werner, E., Dawson, G. (2005). Validation of the phenomenon of autistic regression using home videotapes. *Archives of General Psychiatry*, **62**: 889–895.

Wigg, L., Stores, G. (2004). Sleep patterns and sleep disorders in children with autistic spectrum disorders: Insights using parent report and actigraphy. *Developmental Medicine and Child Neurology*, **46**: 372–380.

Wiggins, L.D., **Robins, D.L.** (2008). Brief report: Excluding the ADI-R behavioral domain improves diagnostic agreement in toddlers. *Journal of Autism and Developmental Disorders*, **38**: 972–976.

Wing, L. (1978). Social, behavioral, and cognitive characteristics: An epidemiological approach. In *Autism: A Reappraisal of Concepts and Treatment*. New York: Plenum Press, pp. 27–46.

Wing, L. (1981). Asperger's syndrome: A clinical account. *Psychological Medicine*, **11**: 115–129.

Wing, L., **Gould, J.** (1978). Systematic recording of behaviors and skills of retarded and psychotic children. *Journal of Autism and Developmental Disorders*, **8**: 79–97.

Wing, L., **Gould, J.** (1979). Severe impairments of social interaction and associated abnormalities in children: Epidemiology and classification. *Journal of Autism and Developmental Disorders*, **9**: 11–29.

Wing, L., **Leekam, S.**, **Libby, S.J.**, **Gould, J.**, **Larcombe, J.** (2002). The Diagnostic Interview for Social and Communication Disorders: Background, inter-rater reliability and clinical use. *Journal of Child Psychology and Psychiatry and Allied Disciplines*, **43**: 307–326.

Witwer, A., **Lecavalier, L.** (2005). Treatment incidence and patterns in children and adolescents with autism spectrum disorders. *Journal of Child and Adolescent Psychopharmacology*, **15**: 671–681.

World Health Organisation (1993). *The ICD-10 Classification of Mental and Behavioural Disorders: Diagnostic Criteria for Research*. Geneva: World Health Organization.

Yates, K., **Le Couteur, A.** (2009). Diagnosing Autism. *Paediatrics and Child Health*, **19**: 55–59.

PART II GENETICS, NEUROLOGY AND BIOCHEMISTRY

2

Unravelling the genetics of autism spectrum disorders

INÊS DE SOUSA, RICHARD HOLT, ALISTAIR PAGNAMENTA AND ANTHONY MONACO

Since autism was first described in 1943, it has become evident that the condition is one of the most heritable of all the childhood onset neurodevelopmental disorders. In this chapter we chart the progress of researchers' attempts to understand the genetic components of autism spectrum disorders and how these studies have tracked the advances in technology and knowledge in the field of genetics in general. We start by describing the evidence that autism spectrum disorders have such a strong genetic component. We then consider approaches to identify susceptibility genes such as linkage, candidate gene studies and association analysis. Various epigenetic mechanisms of potential relevance to autism as well as the expanding area of copy number variations are also highlighted. Some of the theoretical background to each of these approaches is given and findings from each approach are summarized and discussed. In addition, several specific examples are given for each method to demonstrate in detail the way in which they have been employed to yield key successes within the field of autism genetics. Finally, we look towards the future and suggest possible further avenues of investigation, as well as newly arising challenges, in this difficult, yet exciting field of study.

2.1 Evidence for genetic liability and the multifactorial model for autism

In 1943, Leo Kanner, an Austrian psychiatrist, was the first to describe a condition observed in a group of eleven children with developmental abnormalities, a disorder that today is known as autism (Kanner, 1943). Autism (OMIM 209850) is a severe complex neurodevelopmental disorder, characterised by impairments in (1) reciprocal social interaction and (2) communication, and (3)

Researching the Autism Spectrum: Contemporary Perspectives, ed. I. Roth and P. Rezaie. Published by Cambridge University Press.

restricted and stereotyped patterns of interests and behaviours (Lord *et al.* 2000). It is an extremely heterogeneous condition, predominantly affecting males (with a sex ratio of about 4:1), and the severity of symptoms and intellectual ability varies greatly in a continuum along these three main areas (Fombonne, 2005; Santangelo and Tsatsanis, 2005). Family and twin studies have demonstrated over the years that genetic factors are the major cause of idiopathic autism, broadening our understanding of the disorder, although the major causative variants/genes and their mode of transmission remain elusive even today.

Family studies are commonly used to assess familial clustering and thus the genetic component of a certain trait. The latter can be quantified by comparing the disease frequency in family members of one proband (the first person in the family to be brought to medical attention) in relation to the observed frequency in the general population. The prevalence of autism and other pervasive developmental disorders (PDDs) in siblings of autistic individuals was estimated to be approximately 2.2% and 3.6% respectively (Bailey *et al.* 1998; Maestrini *et al.* 1998; Szatmari *et al.* 1998). However, this prevalence could be an underestimate since some parents may decide not to have any more children after their first autistic child is born (the stoppage effect) (Szatmari *et al.* 1998; 1999). To overcome this constraint and avoid its effects, the siblings recurrence risk (λ_S, also called the Dahlberg's later-sib method) can be calculated (Maestrini *et al.* 1998). The recurrence risk estimates the likelihood that each sibling born after an autistic child will develop autism and is far higher among siblings of individuals with autism (2–8%) than the general population prevalence (0.5% for autism spectrum disorders (ASD) (Rutter, 2005)); however, it is much lower than for monogenic diseases (Fombonne, 2005; Muhle *et al.* 2004; Rutter, 2005). Nevertheless, for complex diseases, such as autism, having an elevated λ_S in a certain population does not necessarily mean that the identification of genetic factors is a straightforward task, since this value can be the result of several genetic factors of weak effect, rather than a single gene of major effect.

A marked reduction has been observed in autism prevalence in second and third degree family members compared to first degree relatives. The risk for autism in these family members decreases by nearly half as degrees of genetic relatedness become more distant, pointing to the involvement of multiple interacting genes in autism aetiology (Maestrini *et al.* 1998; Szatmari *et al.* 1998). Autistic related traits, such as obsessive-compulsive disorder, communication disorders and social phobias, are more frequently found in non-autistic parents and family members of the patients than in the general population (Bailey *et al.* 1996; 1998; Folstein and Rosen-Sheidley, 2001). These individuals show milder behaviour/personality characteristics from the traditional triad of autistic symptoms (social interaction, communication and/or stereotyped and repetitive behaviours), showing a broader phenotypic spectrum even when a common genetic background is present (Bailey *et al.* 1998).

The high degree of familial aggregation in autism can reflect common environmental factors, but especially suggests the involvement of genetic factors (Maestrini *et al.* 1998). One powerful tool to estimate the relative contribution of genetic and environmental factors is to compare the concordance rate of autism in monozygotic twins (MZ, that are genetically identical) with dizygotic twins (DZ, that share approximately half of the genome identical by descent), measuring the percentage of cases where both twins present with autism. Several studies in idiopathic cases of ASD have shown that the concordance rate for MZ twins is much higher than for DZ pairs (Bailey *et al.* 1995; Folstein and Rutter, 1977; Rutter, 2005; Steffenburg *et al.* 1989). The first study for autism carried out in the UK reported a 36% concordance in MZ twins compared to 0% in DZ twins, providing further evidence for a key role of genetic factors (Folstein *et al.* 1977). A following study conducted in the UK showed a concordance rate of 60% and 0% for MZ and DZ twins, respectively (Bailey *et al.* 1995). However, when concordance is examined for a broader phenotype that includes not only autism but also milder ASD impairments, 82–92% of MZ twins compared to 10% of DZ pairs are concordant (Bailey *et al.* 1995; Folstein and Rosen-Sheidley, 2001). This higher concordance rate indicates that genetic factors have a prominent role in increasing the susceptibility to autism and ASD when compared to environmental factors, since both MZ and DZ twins tend to share common environments (MacGregor *et al.* 2000). These studies also show, based on the different concordance rates, that the heritability estimates are especially high (approximately 90%), showing autism is one of the most heritable of all neuropsychiatric disorders (Bailey *et al.* 1995; Rutter, 2000). Heritability is strongly related with familial correlations and corresponds in the broad sense to the proportion of the total phenotypic variance that can be explained by genetic factors (Folstein and Rosen-Sheidley, 2001; Yashin and Iachine, 1995).

The transmission mode of autism seems to be non-Mendelian since the concordance between MZ twins is below 100% if full penetrance (which is the the conditional probability that an individual with a given genotype expresses a specific phenotype) is assumed, even accounting for twin pairs affected with other PDDs. Also, both the lower concordance rates of DZ compared to MZ twins and the recurrence risk estimates being lower than expected for single gene diseases are not consistent with an autosomal dominant or recessive mode of transmission. Therefore, autism is classified as a complex disorder, because it is a genetic condition whose mode of inheritance does not follow any of the simple Mendelian laws. Furthermore, studies report a higher recurrence risk for siblings of female probands than for siblings of male probands (Ritvo *et al.* 1989) and, as mentioned earlier, autism is more frequent in males than females (Fombonne, 2005). This suggests different genetic or epigenetic factors in male and female patients, with a higher penetrance or genetic susceptibility in males. One possible explanation would be the involvement of genes on the sex chromosomes, as males only have one copy of the X chromosome. The contribution of weak effect X-linked mutations and rare variants are possible. However, a mode of inheritance linked to the X chromosome has been ruled out by the analysis of extended pedigrees and evidence of male-to-male transmission in a number of family studies (Hallmayer *et al.* 1996a; 1996b). This gender bias could also be explained by epigenetic factors (which modify expression of the genome and gene function, without changing the DNA sequence; see Section 2.5) (Knickmeyer and Baron-Cohen, 2006).

Several alternatives have been suggested over the years as possible models for the genetic aetiology of autism. Among others, reduced penetrance, variable expression (different outcomes for the same genotype), locus and allele heterogeneity (variations in different genes, or different variations within the same gene, respectively producing the same characteristic) or the combined action of several genes have been suggested (Cook *et al.* 1997a; O'Roak and State, 2008). These genes could act epistatically (epistasis generally being defined as the interaction between different genes), and even maternal effects and gestation complications could interact with some of these genes affecting their expression (Cook *et al.* 1997a; Szatmari *et al.* 1998). In an analysis of twin (Bailey *et al.* 1995) and family data (Bolton *et al.* 1994), Pickles *et al.* (1995) suggested a multilocus model involving two to ten epistatic loci. Other results are explained by different models that include more than twenty different loci, each with a minor effect (Maestrini *et al.* 1998; Risch, 1990; Stoltenberg and Burmeister, 2000). Thus, depending on the set of variants/genes present and their variable expression, each individual could develop either the full autistic phenotype or just part of the spectrum of impairments. It is currently believed that multiple interacting genes of weak effect are likely involved, in which alterations in one gene may not be necessary or sufficient to cause disease (Maestrini *et al.* 1998; Szatmari *et al.* 1998). There is still little agreement regarding several questions about the aetiology of this disorder, such as the number of genes involved or whether we are looking for relevant common (common disease – common variant hypothesis) or rare (rare variant – common disease hypothesis) risk variants/genes. It is likely that both hypotheses will be relevant and that gene contributions may alter in different families. Genetic susceptibility may result from the combined action of several common genetic variants, or it may arise from rare mutations in single genes, such as the recently identified mutations in *neuroligins* (*NLGN3* and *NLGN4*), *neurexin 1* (*NRXN1*) and *SHANK3* (Durand *et al.* 2007; Feng *et al.* 2006; Jamain *et al.* 2003).

It has also recently been suggested that we are addressing genetically different classes with distinct underlying aetiologies. The first hypothesis is that autism in singleton families is more likely to be due to *de novo* spontaneous mutations, and multiplex families have a higher chance of containing common inherited genetic predisposing factors (O'Roak and State, 2008; Risch, 2001; Sebat *et al.* 2007). Zhao *et al.* (2007) propose another model for multiplex families, in which high risk families (where male offspring have an approximate risk of nearly 50% for developing autism) originate from offspring that carry and transmit a new causative mutation in a dominant way. In contrast, sporadic autism in low-risk families would mainly be caused by spontaneous mutations with high penetrance in males and relatively poor penetrance in females (Zhao *et al.* 2007). Both models account for the importance of common and rare factors contributing in different manners to disease susceptibility, confirming once more that autism is an extremely genetically heterogeneous disorder.

2.2 Linkage studies

Linkage was first observed in the early 1900s by Bateson and Punnet (Darden, 2005). It can be described as the tendency of genes or other DNA segments at a specific *locus* to be inherited together on the same chromosome, as a consequence of their physical proximity. The further apart two loci are, the higher the probability of recombination events (crossing-over, a process by which pre-existing genetic variation is reshuffled) occurring during meiosis. Therefore, the closer two loci are, the smaller the frequency of recombination will be, and the larger the probability of co-segregation compared to independent assortment. Thus, linked loci are inherited together as a 'block'. Linkage studies are designed to test for co-segregation between a well characterised polymorphic genetic marker and an unknown locus influencing the disease susceptibility, using affected sibling pairs (ASPs) or extended families (Lewis, 2007; Maestrini *et al.* 2000; Strachan and Read, 1996).

Genetic linkage methods can be model-based (parametric) or model-free (non-parametric), the former of which requires knowledge of the mode of inheritance of the trait and relevant initial parameters (such as number of alleles at each locus, allele frequencies and genotype penetrances, among others). While the traditional model-based tests are very powerful tools for monogenic disorders, model-free tests, based on allele-sharing methods, are more useful for complex traits in which the mode of inheritance is not known (O'Roak and State, 2008). Model-free linkage methods aim at the identification of genomic regions that are shared more often by affected siblings or affected relative pairs, or less often in discordant family members, than expected by chance, that is, where alleles at different loci are inherited together. In contrast to parametric methods, this approach does not require such large numbers of extended families with multiple affected members across several generations; however, a greater number of affected relative pairs is required. Furthermore, for both methods identification of the locus of interest is not precise; it could be a broad region in the order of megabases. Therefore, the identified area has to be subsequently refined by fine-mapping approaches for the identification of the gene(s) of interest (Elston and Thompson, 2000; Maestrini *et al.* 2000).

Genome-wide linkage screens were frequently the first choice adopted by most studies to locate unknown susceptibility genes in ASD. Typically, this approach would involve hundreds of evenly spaced polymorphic satellite markers screened across the genome in multiple families (Klauck, 2006). This information is used to calculate a logarithm (base 10) of the odds score (LOD score) for each marker and to estimate the multipoint maximum LOD score (MLS), constructing a profile across all chromosomes. The profile peaks correspond to regions of increased sharing between ASPs and subsequently can identify possible locations for susceptibility variants or genes (Maestrini *et al.* 2000).

The LOD score, introduced by Morton in 1955, is then a useful measure of linkage that represents the ratio between the likelihood of linkage for a certain recombination fraction and the expected likelihood of no linkage, in the families under study. Conventionally, a LOD score of 3.3 or greater can be interpreted as significant evidence for linkage, meaning that the observed data are 1000 times more likely to have occurred if the variants/genes are in physical proximity, than by chance (Lander and Kruglyak, 1995). In contrast, if it is less than −2 the hypothesis of linkage can be rejected. LOD scores between −2 and 3 are generally inconclusive (Strachan and Read, 1996). Linkage studies are powerful and specific for the discovery of genes of main effect on the phenotype, although genes of weak effect may not be detected. So, when studying complex diseases, where several genes are probably involved, a modest maximum LOD score is expected and should not be disregarded (Elston and Thompson, 2000; Lewis, 2007; Maestrini *et al.* 1998; Strachan and Read, 1996).

In the case of ASD the mode of inheritance is uncertain. Therefore parametric linkage studies are rarely reported in the literature, compared to non-parametric studies (O'Roak and State, 2008). Since the first published genome-wide linkage screen in 1998 (carried out by the IMGSAC [International Molecular Genetic Study of Autism Consortium]) several independent studies for autism and many follow-ups have been conducted. However, suggestive evidence for linkage has been found on almost all chromosomes, with little concordance between studies (Figure 2.1). This supports the hypothesis that autism aetiology contains extensive genetic heterogeneity, possibly with the involvement of a few genes of major effect and/or the interaction of multiple genes of weak effect. The interpretation of the results obtained can become more difficult due to lack of consistency of the data, which in turn can be the result of a combination of factors such as sample size, inclusion–exclusion criteria, the statistical approach taken and markers genotyped by each group (Bacchelli and Maestrini, 2006).

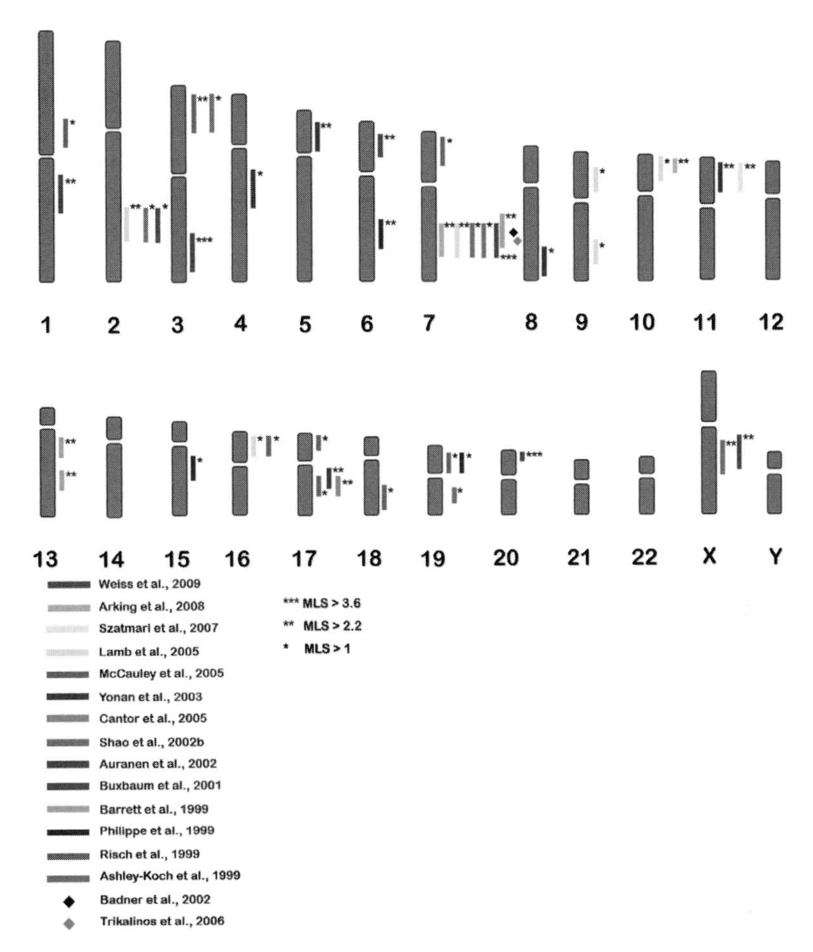

Figure 2.1 Ideogram representing linkage findings in eleven genome-wide screens for autism. Each scan is represented by differently coloured bars in the respective chromosomal regions and the two meta-analyses by diamond shaped symbols. The results indicated are followed by *** if MLS > 3.6, by ** if MLS > 2.2, and by * if MLS > 1. See plate section for colour version.

The most consistently replicated loci, with greatest evidence of linkage, are on chromosomes 2q, 7q and 17q (see Figure 2.1). These overlapping regions likely contain autism susceptibility variants or genes.

The Autism Susceptibility Locus 1 (AUTS1), identified by the IMGSAC on chromosome 7q with an MLS of 2.53 in 99 families from the UK (IMGSAC, 1998), was further established in two following studies conducted by the IMGSAC using additional families and markers (IMGSAC, 2001; Lamb *et al.* 2005). It has also shown more consistent positive results, with evidence of increased haplotype sharing seen in several studies (Alarcón *et al.* 2002; Arking *et al.* 2008; Ashley-Koch *et al.* 1999;

Auranen *et al.* 2002; Barrett *et al.* 1999; Molloy *et al.* 2005; Philippe *et al.* 1999; Risch *et al.* 1999; Shao *et al.* 2002a). However, the linkage significance and location of the peak varies between studies. Thus the peak of linkage in this area remains broad, spanning more than 40 Mb and containing over two hundred mapped genes.

Another region that shows frequent overlap is located on chromosome 2q (Buxbaum *et al.* 2001; IMGSAC, 2001; Lamb *et al.* 2005; Philippe *et al.* 1999; Shao *et al.* 2002a).

It is a similar story for the chromosome 17q region, where a linkage peak at 17q11–17q21 with an MLS of 2.04 was found in 345 AGRE (Autism Genetic Resource Exchange) consortium families (Yonan *et al.* 2003), and afterwards reported in other studies (Cantor *et al.* 2005; Lamb *et al.* 2005; McCauley *et al.* 2005; Stone *et al.* 2004).

Another approach taken in parallel to resolve discrepancies between studies is to conduct a statistical analysis that integrates the available results of several independent analyses, called a meta-analysis. To date, there have been two meta-analyses performed for autism. The first, a regional meta-analysis, combined the reported results from the first four autism genome scans (from the IMGSAC, Stanford group, PARIS [Paris Autism Research International Sibpair Study] group and CLSA [Collaborative Linkage Study of Autism]), the 7q locus being the most significant finding and replicating the individual evidence reported previously for the region (Badner and Gershon, 2002). The second meta-analysis used data from six independent genome-wide screens and confirmed evidence for linkage at 7q22–q32 (containing the AUTS1 locus). Moreover, suggestive linkage was also met for the regions 17p11.2–q12 and 10p12–q11.1 in weighted analyses (Trikalinos *et al.* 2006).

Decreasing sample heterogeneity, for instance by studying specific trait components or phenotypic subsets associated with disease that tend to be shared by family members, increases the probability of gene identification. These traits (endophenotypes) are then commonly used to refine specific linkage regions. However, with this type of analysis, statistical power is reduced because of the smaller sample size in each subgroup, so this must be taken into account when designing this sort of study (Bacchelli and Maestrini, 2006; Veenstra-VanderWeele and Cook, 2004). Genome screens that restricted the analysis to autistic families with phrase-speech delay (onset of phrase speech later than 3 years of age) or other language problems found increased evidence for linkage to 7q (Alarcon *et al.* 2002; Bradford *et al.* 2001), 2q (Buxbaum *et al.* 2001; Shao *et al.* 2002b), 3q and two regions on chromosome 17 (17p13–q21 and 17q23–q25) (Alarcon *et al.* 2005). Other reports employed repetitive and stereotyped behaviours as a covariate to partition their sample sets (Hauser *et al.* 2004). Thus families sharing high scores of 'insistence on sameness' were used and resulted in increased evidence for linkage to autism at 15q11–q13 (Shao *et al.* 2003) (a region of common cytogenetic abnormalities). Evidence for linkage to regions 7q and 21q was found for autism using a subset of autistic families presenting a history of developmental regression (loss of pre-existing communication skills) (Molloy *et al.* 2005). Moreover, support for linkage on chromosome 1q (Buxbaum *et al.* 2004) was found using affected relative pairs with more severe obsessive-compulsive behaviours as a criterion for linkage analysis. This suggests that restricting the original sample may create more genetically homogeneous population sets and lead to the identification of genes that are closely related to these specific traits.

Sex-specific linkage analysis, separating the sample according to the sex of the affected individuals (male only versus female containing groups) was another criterion used to reduce genetic heterogeneity. Since autism is more frequent in males, some genetic susceptibility factors could possibly be different between males and females. A male-specific effect has been identified for the locus on 17q11, where linkage was greatly increased compared to the original signal identified in the whole AGRE cohort (Stone *et al.* 2004; Yonan *et al.* 2003). Likewise, in the IMGSAC sample, male ASPs largely contribute to the linkage evidence found on chromosomes 7q and 16p, whereas the linkage on 15q derived from the female-containing ASPs (Lamb *et al.* 2005). The latter study also looked at parent-of-origin effects and discovered what seem to be two different peaks at the 7q region, with paternal and maternal contributions, respectively. This could possibly implicate an imprinted gene(s) underlying the susceptibility in these locations (Lamb *et al.* 2005).

The 2007 linkage scan by the Autism Genome Project Consortium (AGP, www.autismgenome.org) found significant linkage to a novel region on chromosome 11p12 (LOD score of 3.57), using 1181 multiplex families and 10 000 markers (Szatmari *et al.* 2007). Despite the high power of this study, attained by collaboration between over fifty different research groups, there was an absence of a major locus for autism, confirming the heterogeneity within the disorder.

2.3 Association studies

An alternative method to identify ASD susceptibility genes is genetic association studies. These attempt to identify alleles of polymorphisms that are present in affected individuals more often than would be expected by chance based on the frequency of the polymorphism in the general population. Such polymorphisms are said to be associated with the disorder. Currently the most commonly used polymorphisms for such studies are single nucleotide polymorphisms (SNPs) that consist of a single base change in the DNA. One of the main advantages of association studies over linkage studies is that they allow finer mapping of disease genes (Hirschhorn and Daly, 2005).

Association studies are typically performed by genotyping SNPs in groups of affected (case) and typical (control) individuals, although other classes of polymorphism, such as insertion/deletions, may also be used. Such case–control association study designs are able to detect more subtle effects than family-based cohorts of similar size. However, if the controls used are not well matched to the cases for variables such as sex, age, geographical location and ethnicity, the study can suffer from population substructure (differences between the genotypes of the case and control populations for reasons other than affection status). This can then lead to an increased incidence of false-positive results. However, statistical methods are now available to address this possible source of error (Hirschhorn and Daly, 2005; Ober and Hoffjan, 2006). Alternatively, family-based study designs can be used, based on the frequency of transmission of alleles to affected children. Under the null hypothesis (i.e. if the alleles under study are not associated with disease), then they will have an equal probability of transmission (50%). Significantly elevated transmission rates may suggest the allele in question is indexing a susceptibility gene. One of the most widely used family-based tests is the transmission disequilibrium test (TDT), as implemented by Spielman (Spielman *et al.* 1993). These types of association tests offer the advantage of immunity to population substructure, controlling for environmental effects and allowing the identification of parent-of-origin effects (Hirschhorn and Daly, 2005).

Typically, polymorphisms are chosen for association studies by one of four methods. The first is by the identification of polymorphisms within the region of interest, such as by the sequencing of the locus in several affected individuals. This has the advantage of identifying polymorphisms that may be of direct relevance to the disorder in the population being studied. However, sequencing can be costly and time consuming. Alternatively, polymorphisms may be obtained by interrogation of databases, such as the freely available dbSNP on the NCBI website (http://www.ncbi.nlm.nih.gov/) (Hirschhorn and Daly, 2005). This is cheaper and quicker, but care is required to choose verified polymorphisms. Third, the phenomenon of linkage disequilibrium (LD) may be used. LD is when the alleles of two or more polymorphisms occur together more frequently than expected by chance due to their physical proximity in the genome (Hirschhorn and Daly, 2005). If the level of LD between two polymorphisms is high, then by genotyping one polymorphism, the genotype of the other can be predicted with a high degree of certainty (The International HapMap Project, 2003). Therefore, by knowing the pattern of LD across the region it is possible to capture the variation by genotyping fewer polymorphisms (Hirschhorn and Daly, 2005; The International HapMap Project, 2003), with consequent savings in time, cost, and quantity of DNA required per sample. The human HapMap project (http://www.hapmap.org/) (2003) has identified such blocks of SNPs in regions of high LD, thus allowing researchers to tactically choose SNPs for genotyping that capture all or most of the variation in their target region. These so called 'tagging' approaches again reduce costs and time, but may fail to capture the whole variation in the region if the LD is not strong enough (The International HapMap Project, 2003). Finally, companies such as Illumina®

and Affymetrix® currently produce standard panels of SNPs for use with high throughput genotyping technologies. While providing good cost efficiency, such panels of SNPs are most appropriate for genome-wide investigations rather than targeted association studies of candidate genes.

If a polymorphism is associated with the disorder, it can be for one of three reasons. First, the result may be a false positive. Therefore, care must be taken in designing the experiment to ensure it is as statistically powerful as possible, and to correct results for the effect of seeking association with multiple polymorphisms or multiple subphenotypes (Hirschhorn and Daly, 2005; Risch and Merikangas, 1996). Second, the polymorphism may be associated because it is a direct cause of susceptibility to the disorder. However, the third possibility is that the polymorphism is not itself causing susceptibility, but rather is in LD with the true susceptibility variant. Therefore, it is important to know both the extent of LD within a region showing association, so as to localise the area in which to search for a true susceptibility allele, and to perform extensive functional experiments to verify that such an allele is truly responsible for increasing susceptibility to the disorder (Hirschhorn and Daly, 2005).

Association studies have typically been performed on candidate genes, due to technological and financial limitations on the number of polymorphisms which could be genotyped (Risch and Merikangas, 1996). However, with the rise of cost-effective high throughput genotyping methods, genome-wide association studies have become a reality (Seng and Seng, 2008). Such projects are currently being employed for ASD.

A large amount of effort has been spent carrying out association studies for candidate genes for ASD susceptibility. Such genes are chosen due to an implied role in ASD, either on account of their putative function or location in a region previously implicated in ASD susceptibility. A literature search between 1995 and late 2009 revealed that more than 200 genes have been investigated for association with ASD, with approximately 100 reported as showing a positive result (Table 2.1). However, there is a large amount of variability in terms of the power of the studies, strength of association and the amount of positive replication that has been observed. It is beyond the scope of this chapter to cover in detail each of these genes, but instead three of the ASD candidate genes most highly studied using association, *RELN*, *SLC6A4* and *GABRB3*, will be described, together with a gene more recently identified as a strong candidate, *CNTNAP2*.

2.3.1 *RELN*

The first study to show association between *RELN* and autism was performed by Persico *et al.* (2001). *RELN* was chosen as a candidate due to three lines of evidence indicating its possible involvement in autism susceptibility.

Table 2.1 *Candidate genes reported as having positive association to autism (1995–2009)*

Chromosome	Genes*	References
1	***DISC1*** (disrupted in schizophrenia 1)	Kilpinen *et al.* 2008
	GSTM1 (glutathione S-transferase M1)	Buyske *et al.* 2006
	MARK1 (MAP/microtubule affinity-regulating kinase 1)	Maussion *et al.* 2008
	MTF1 (metal-regulatory transcription factor 1)	Serajee *et al.* 2004
	PTGS2 (prostaglandin-endoperoxide synthase 1)	Yoo *et al.* 2008
2	***DLX1*** (distal-less homeobox 1)	Liu *et al.* 2009
	DLX2 (distal-less homeobox 2)	Liu *et al.* 2009
	INPP1 (inositol polyphosphate-1-phosphatase)	Serajee *et al.* 2003b
	ITGA4 (integrin, alpha 4)	Conroy *et al.* 2009; Correia *et al.* 2009; Ramoz *et al.* 2008
	NPAS2 (neuronal PAS domain protein 2)	Nicholas *et al.* 2007
	NRP2 (neuropilin 2)	Wu *et al.* 2007
	NRXN1 (neurexin 1)	Feng *et al.* 2006; Szatmari *et al.* 2007
	SLC25A12 (solute carrier family 25 (mitochondrial carrier, Aralar), member 12)	Segurado *et al.* 2005; Ramoz *et al.* 2008; Turunen *et al.* 2008
	STK39 (serine threonine kinase 39)	Ramoz *et al.* 2008
3	***DRD3*** (dopamine receptor D3)	de Krom *et al.* 2009
	HTR3C (5-hydroxytryptamine (serotonin) receptor 3, family member C)	Rehnström *et al.* 2009
	GPX1 (glutathione peroxidise 1)	Ming *et al.* 2010
	NLGN1 (neuroligin 1)	Ylisaukko-oja *et al.* 2005
	OXTR (oxytocin receptor)	Jacob *et al.* 2007; Lerer *et al.* 2008; Wu *et al.* 2005b; Yrigollen *et al.* 2008
4	***EGF*** (epidermal growth factor (beta-urogastrone))	Toyoda *et al.* 2007
	GABRA2 (gamma-aminobutyric acid (GABA) A receptor, alpha 2)	Ma *et al.* 2005
	GABRA4 (gamma-aminobutyric acid (GABA) A receptor, alpha 4)	Collins *et al.* 2006; Ma *et al.* 2005
	GABRB1 (gamma-aminobutyric acid (GABA) A receptor, beta 1)	Collins *et al.* 2006; Ma *et al.* 2005
	GABRG1 (gamma-aminobutyric acid (GABA) A receptor, gamma 1)	Ma *et al.* 2005
	TDO2 (tryptophan 2,3-dioxygenase)	Nabi *et al.* 2004
5	***ADRB2*** (adrenergic, beta-2-, receptor, surface)	Connors *et al.* 2005
	APC (adenomatous polyposis coli)	Zhou *et al.* 2007
	DHFR (dihydrofolate reductase)	Adams *et al.* 2007

Table 2.1 *(cont.)*

Chromosome	Genes*	References
	DRD1 (dopamine receptor D1)	Hettinger *et al.* 2008a
	PITX1 (paired-like homeodomain 1)	Philippi *et al.* 2007
	PRLR (prolactin receptor)	Yrigollen *et al.* 2008
6	***AHI1*** (Abelson helper integration site 1)	Alvarez Retuerto *et al.* 2008
	C4B (complement component 4B (Childo blood group))	Odell *et al.* 2005
	GLO1 (glyoxalase I)	Junaid *et al.* 2004
	GRIK2 (glutamate receptor, ionotropic, kainate 2)	Jamain *et al.* 2002; Kim *et al.* 2007; Shuang *et al.* 2004
	HLA-A (major histocompatibility complex, class I, A)	Torres *et al.* 2006
	HLA-DRB1 (major histocompatibility complex, class II, DR beta 1)	Johnson *et al.* 2009
	HTR1B (5-hydroxytryptamine (serotonin) receptor 1B)	Orabona *et al.* 2009
	MHC (major histocompatibility complex) genes	Warren *et al.* 1996
	PRL (prolactin)	Yrigollen *et al.* 2008
7	***DOCK4*** (dedicator of cytokinesis 4)	Maestrini *et al.* 2009
	EN2 (engrailed homeobox 2)	Benayed *et al.* 2005, 2009; Wang *et al.* 2008
	FOXP2 (forkhead box P2)	Li *et al.* 2005
	GRM8 (glutamate receptor, metabotropic 8)	Serajee *et al.* 2003a
	HOXA1 (homeobox A1)	Conciatori *et al.* 2004; Ingram *et al.* 2000; Tischfield *et al.* 2005
	HTR5A (5-hydroxytryptamine (serotonin) receptor 5A)	Coutinho *et al.* 2007
	LAMB1 (laminin, beta 1)	Bonora *et al.* 2005; Hutcheson *et al.* 2004
	MET (proto-oncogene hepatocyte growth factor receptor)	Campbell *et al.* 2006, 2009; Jackson *et al.* 2009; Sousa *et al.* 2009
	NRCAM (neuronal cell adhesion molecule)	Bonora *et al.* 2005; Marui *et al.* 2009b
	PIK3CG (phosphoinositide-3-kinase, catalytic, gamma polypeptide)	Serajee *et al.* 2003a
	PON1 (paraoxonase 1)	D'Amelio *et al.* 2005
	RELN (reelin)	Dutta *et al.* 2007; Persico *et al.* 2001; Skaar *et al.* 2005; Serajee *et al.* 2006; Zhang *et al.* 2002

(cont.)

Table 2.1 *(cont.)*

Chromosome	Genes*	References
	SERPINE1 (serpin peptidase inhibitor, clade E, member 1)	Campbell *et al.* 2008
	STX1A (syntaxin 1A (brain))	Nakamura *et al.* 2008
	UBE2H (ubiquitin-conjugating enzyme E2H (UBC8 homologue, yeast))	Vourc'h *et al.* 2003
	WNT2 (wingless-type MMTV integration site family member 2)	Marui *et al.* 2009a; Wassink *et al.* 2001
	CNTNAP2 (contactin associated protein-like 2)	Alarcon *et al.* 2008; Arking *et al.* 2008
9	***DBH*** (dopamine beta-hydroxylase, plasma)	Robinson *et al.* 2001
10	***PTEN*** (phosphatase and tensin homologue (mutated in multiple advanced cancers 1))	Butler *et al.* 2005
11	***BDNF*** (brain-derived neurotrophic factor)	Cheng *et al.* 2009; Nishimura *et al.* 2007
	HRAS (v-Ha-ras Harvey rat sarcoma viral oncogene homologue)	Herault *et al.* 1995
	HTR3A (5-hydroxytryptamine (serotonin) receptor 3A)	Anderson *et al.* 2009
	ROBO3 (roundabout, axon guidance receptor, homologue 3)	Anitha *et al.* 2008
	ROBO4 (roundabout homologue 4, magic roundabout)	Anitha *et al.* 2008
12	***AVPR1A*** (arginine vasopressin receptor 1A)	Kim *et al.* 2002; Wassink *et al.* 2004; Yirmiya *et al.* 2006
	DAO (D-amino-acid oxidase)	Chung *et al.* 2007
	NOS-I (nitric oxide synthase 1 (neuronal))	Kim *et al.* 2009
	TPH2 (tryptophan hydroxylase 2)	Coon *et al.* 2005
13	***HTR2A*** (5-hydroxytryptamine (serotonin) receptor 2A)	Cho *et al.* 2007
15	***ATP10A***** (ATPase, class V, type 10A)	Nurmi *et al.* 2003
	ATP10C (ATPase, class V, type 10C)	Kato *et al.* 2008
	GABRA5 (gamma-aminobutyric acid (GABA) A receptor, alpha 5)	Kim *et al.* 2008a; McCauley *et al.* 2004b
	GABRB3 (gamma-aminobutyric acid (GABA) A receptor, beta 3)	Buxbaum *et al.* 2002; Cook *et al.* 1998; Curran *et al.* 2006; Kim *et al.* 2008a; McCauley *et al.* 2004b; Yoo *et al.* 2009b
	GABRG3 (gamma-aminobutyric acid (GABA) A receptor, gamma 3)	Kim *et al.* 2008a; Menold *et al.* 2001
	SNRPN (small nuclear ribonucleoprotein polypeptide N)	Kato *et al.* 2008

Table 2.1 *(cont.)*

Chromosome	Genes*	References
16	***A2BP1*** (ataxin 2-binding protein 1)	Martin *et al.* 2007
	CACNA1H (calcium channel, voltage-dependent, T type, alpha 1H subunit)	Splawski *et al.* 2006
	GRIN2A (glutamate receptor, ionotropic, *N*-methyl D-aspartate 2A)	Barnby *et al.* 2005
	PRKCB1 (protein kinase C, beta 1)	Lintas *et al.* 2009; Philippi *et al.* 2005
	TSC2 (tuberous sclerosis 2)	Serajee *et al.* 2003b
17	***ACCN1*** (amiloride-sensitive cation channel 1, neuronal (degenerin))	Stone *et al.* 2007
	CACNA1G (calcium channel, voltage-dependent, T type, alpha 1G subunit)	Strom *et al.* 2009
	DHRS7B (dehydrogenase/reductase (SDR family) member 7B)	Stone *et al.* 2007
	DKF204340047	Stone *et al.* 2007
	ITGB3 (integrin, beta 3 (platelet glycoprotein IIIa, antigen CD61))	Coutinho *et al.* 2007; Ma *et al.* 2009
	LASP1 (LIM and SH3 protein 1)	Stone *et al.* 2007
	LOC440421	Stone *et al.* 2007
	LOC440422	Stone *et al.* 2007
	LOC636202	Stone *et al.* 2007
	LOC645435	Stone *et al.* 2007
	LOC646157	Stone *et al.* 2007
	MGC33894	Stone *et al.* 2007
	MYO1D (myosin ID)	Stone *et al.* 2007
	NA (protein kinase, lysine-deficient 4)	Stone *et al.* 2007
	NF1 (neurofibromatosis, Type 1)	Marui *et al.* 2004
	NOS-II (nitric oxide synthase 2, inducible)	Kim *et al.* 2009
	PER1 (period homologue 1 (*Drosophila*))	Nicholas *et al.* 2007
	PIPOX (pipecolic acid oxidase)	Stone *et al.* 2007
	PSMD11 (proteasome (prosome, macropain) 26S subunit, non-ATPase, 11)	Stone *et al.* 2007
	SLC6A4 (solute carrier family 6 (neurotransmitter transporter, serotonin), member 4)	Cho *et al.* 2007; Coutinho *et al.* 2004; 2007; Guhathakurta *et al.* 2006; 2008; Ma *et al.* 2010; Mulder *et al.* 2005
	TMEM98 (transmembrane protein 98)	Stone *et al.* 2007

(cont.)

Table 2.1 *(cont.)*

Chromosome	Genes*	References
19	***APOE2*** (apolipoprotein E like-2)	Persico *et al.* 2004
	FOSB (FBJ murine osteosarcoma viral oncogene homologue B)	Yrigollen *et al.* 2008
	PLAUR (plasminogen activator, urokinase receptor)	Campbell *et al.* 2008
20	***ADA*** (adenosine deaminase)	Hettinger *et al.* 2008b
	OXT (oxytocin, prepro – (neurophysin I))	Yrigollen *et al.* 2008
22	***ADORA2A*** (adenosine A2a receptor)	Freitag *et al.* 2010
	MIF (macrophage migration inhibitory factor)	Grigorenko *et al.* 2008
X	***AR*** (androgen receptor)	Henningsson *et al.* 2009
	FMR1 (fragile X mental retardation 1)	Vincent *et al.* 1996
	HTR2C (5-hydroxytryptamine (serotonin) receptor 2C)	Orabona *et al.* 2009
	MAOA (monoamine oxidase A)	Yoo *et al.* 2009a
	MECP2 (methyl CpG binding protein 2 (Rett syndrome))	Loat *et al.* 2008; Shibayama *et al.* 2004
	NLGN3 (neuroligin 3)	Ylisaukko-oja *et al.* 2005
	NLGN4 (neuroligin 4, X-linked)	Ylisaukko-oja *et al.* 2005

* Names were checked using the HUGO Gene Nomenclature Committee Database (http://www.genenames.org/index.html).

** ***ATP10A*** – previously called ***ATP10C***.

First, the Reelin protein is involved in neuronal migration, functionally implying a possible role in autism (Persico *et al.* 2001). Second, regions of brain alteration in autistic individuals overlap those of male reeler mutant mice, who lack expression of the *reln* gene. Finally, *RELN* is located either close to or within the region of chromosome 7 that has repeatedly shown linkage to autism. These three lines of evidence made *RELN* an attractive candidate gene to investigate using association studies. In their study, Persico *et al.* identified polymorphisms within *RELN*, including a triplet repeat (GGC) in the 5' untranslated region (UTR) of the gene. The identified polymorphisms were genotyped in 95 autistic participants and 186 matched non-autistic individuals for a case–control analysis. The results indicated that the frequency of long alleles ($\geq$11 repeats) of the triplet repeat in individuals with autism was more than double that of controls ($P < 0.001$). To confirm the result, genotyping was performed in a further 172 complete and 12 incomplete trios in a family-based test. This confirmed the preferential transmission of long alleles to autistic individuals ($P < 0.05$). It was concluded that the GGC repeat polymorphism probably directly conferred susceptibility to autism, although the authors were unable to rule out the possibility that it was in LD with an alternative susceptibility polymorphism (Persico *et al.* 2001).

Since the original study, a further ten association studies for *RELN* with ASD have been performed (Ashley-Koch *et al.* 2007; Bonora *et al.* 2003; Devlin *et al.* 2004; Dutta *et al.* 2007; 2008; Krebs *et al.* 2002; Li *et al.* 2004; Serajee *et al.* 2006; Skaar *et al.* 2005; Zhang *et al.* 2002). The success of these studies in replicating the initial finding has been mixed. Five of the studies failed to find association (Bonora *et al.* 2003; Devlin *et al.* 2004; Dutta *et al.* 2008; Krebs *et al.* 2002; Li *et al.* 2004). However, the remaining five did find evidence for the role of *RELN* in ASD susceptibility (Ashley-Koch *et al.* 2007; Dutta *et al.* 2007; Skaar *et al.* 2005; Serajee *et al.* 2006; Zhang *et al.* 2002). Therefore, *RELN* remains an intriguing candidate gene for ASD.

2.3.2 *SLC6A4*

The serotonin transporter gene *SLC6A4* (also known as *5-HTT*), located on chromosome 17, was initially chosen as a candidate gene solely based upon its function. It was known that mean whole blood serotonin levels are increased in autistic cohorts compared to the general population and serotonin transporter inhibitors had been shown to effectively reduce routines that are part of autistic behaviour (Anderson *et al.* 1987; Cook *et al.* 1997b). Some studies show that higher levels of serotonin are more significant in multiplex families (Piven *et al.* 1991), while other studies show a unimodal increase. Therefore, *SLC6A4* was considered a very good functional candidate gene for autism. The first association study performed between the gene and autism was by Cook *et al.* (1997b). Two polymorphisms, a VNTR (variable number tandem repeat) in the second intron and an insertion/deletion polymorphism in the promoter region, were genotyped in 86 trios. A significant preferential transmission of the promoter deletion variant to autistic children was observed ($P = 0.03$), although the VNTR was non-significant. When both polymorphisms were analysed as a two-marker haplotype, a significant result was again obtained ($P = 0.018$). It was concluded that the research showed preliminary evidence for a role of *SLC6A4* in autism, but that further study was required to replicate the finding and to determine whether the polymorphisms genotyped were themselves causal or acting as markers in LD with causal variants.

Later that year, a second association study was published by Klauck *et al.* (1997). The polymorphisms genotyped were again the promoter insertion/deletion and intron 2 VNTR, in an initial group of 52 trios and an extended set of 65 trios. A significant over-transmission of the long allele of the promoter variant was observed in the extended population ($P = 0.032$), opposite to the previous result of Cook *et al.* (1997b). Haplotype analysis also gave a weakly significant result in the extended population ($P = 0.049$). Therefore, although a significant result was obtained, it is difficult to view these findings as a replication of those of Cook *et al.*, due to the opposite alleles of the same polymorphism being found to be significantly associated. Klauck *et al.* considered reasons such as small sample size, differences in geographical and ethnic background and differences in ascertainment of the patients as possibly explaining the discrepancy in results (Klauck *et al.* 1997).

Since these initial two studies, a further 21 have been performed on *SLC6A4* for autism or ASD, of which twelve have found evidence for association (Cho *et al.* 2007; Conroy *et al.* 2004; Coutinho *et al.* 2004; 2007; Devlin *et al.* 2005; Guhathakurta *et al.* 2008; Ma *et al.* 2010; McCauley *et al.* 2004a; Mulder *et al.* 2005; Sutcliffe *et al.* 2005; Tordjman *et al.* 2001; Yirmiya *et al.* 2001) while nine have not (Betancur *et al.* 2002; Guhathakurta *et al.* 2006; Koishi *et al.* 2006; Longo *et al.* 2009; Maestrini *et al.* 1999; Persico *et al.* 2002; Ramoz *et al.* 2006; Zhong *et al.* 1999; Wu *et al.* 2005a). This makes *SLC6A4* the most studied ASD candidate gene to date.

2.3.3 GABRB3

The first study reporting association between autism and *GABRB3* was performed by Cook *et al.* Due to the repeated identification of 15q11–13 duplications in autistic individuals, they used markers in this region to create a LD map for autism in 138 families. This resulted in the marker 155CA-2 in *GABRB3* showing significant association ($P = 0.0014$), with no evidence of parent-of-origin effects (Cook *et al.* 1998).

As with the previously discussed genes, subsequent attempts to replicate the association between *GABRB3* and ASD have been mixed. The first four studies that attempted to confirm Cook *et al.*'s result failed to do so (Maestrini *et al.* 1999; Martin *et al.* 2000; Nurmi *et al.* 2001; Salmon *et al.* 1999). Since then, six studies have presented data offering support for an association between *GABRB3* and ASD (Buxbaum *et al.* 2002; Curran *et al.* 2006; Kim *et al.* 2006; Kim *et al.* 2008a; McCauley *et al.* 2004b; Yoo *et al.* 2009b), but an additional three negative results have also been published (Ashley-Koch *et al.* 2006; Ma *et al.* 2005; Tochigi *et al.* 2007). In addition to differences between populations used and the estimated powers of the studies, it has been suggested that a possible reason for the difficulty to replicate the positive result is the difference in statistical methods used (Buxbaum *et al.* 2002).

Despite this, *GABRB3* remains a good ASD candidate gene for several reasons. First, it is located in the 15q11–13 region, maternal duplications of which can lead to ASD (Shao *et al.* 2003). Second, there is evidence that the GABA neurotransmitter system is involved in ASD. This includes findings of reduced $GABA_A$ ligand binding in the brains of individuals with autism, together with reduced $GABA_A$ receptors and increased levels of circulating GABA and its precursor molecule in these individuals (McCauley *et al.* 2004b). $GABA_A$ receptor agonists have also been useful for treating seizures and anxiety disorders found in a significant proportion of individuals with autism (McCauley *et al.* 2004b). Finally, linkage to autism has also been shown in this region (Shao *et al.* 2003).

2.3.4 *CNTNAP2*

A recent gene to be implicated in ASD susceptibility is *CNTNAP2*, a neuronal cell adhesion molecule known to interact with *Contactin 2* (Bakkaloglu *et al.* 2008), and a member of the neurexin gene family (Alarcón *et al.* 2008). Two studies (Alarcón *et al.* 2008; Arking *et al.* 2008) were published concurrently, both utilising, at least in part, association study designs to identify *CNTNAP2* as an ASD susceptibility gene.

Alarcón *et al.* (2008) performed a two-stage association study in a 15 Mb region of 7q35, including a 10 Mb region thought to be a language related autism quantitative trait locus (QTL), and approximately 200 known genes. In the first stage of the study 172 trios were genotyped for 2758 SNPs across the region and association to age at first word sought. This identified four genes worthy of further study, *KIAA1549*, *PRKAG2*, *FLJ42291* and *CNTNAP2*. In stage two, six tagging and two non-tagging SNPs across the four genes were genotyped in 304 independent trios, again seeking association to age at first word. The only significant result observed was with a tagging SNP in *CNTNAP2*, rs2710102, the association being driven by trios containing male probands. The authors concluded that *CNTNAP2* was a good candidate for autism susceptibility and that common variants were important in language acquisition in autistic individuals. The authors further supported the role of *CNTNAP2* functionally by demonstrating that its transcripts are restricted to regions of the brain thought to be important for verbal communication and language development (Alarcón *et al.* 2008).

Concurrently, Arking *et al.* (2008) published a two-stage study, also implicating *CNTNAP2* in autism. The first stage of the study consisted of a joint genome-wide linkage and association screen genotyping 500 000 SNPs in 72 autism multiplex families. The affected individuals were required to be positive for autism using both the ADI-R and ADOS instruments, an inclusion criterion stricter than any previously reported study on the genetics of autism. This was designed to reduce phenotypic heterogeneity within the cohort. No genome-wide significant result was identified by the association analysis, but two regions of linkage were found, on 7q35 and 10p13–14. The SNP under the 7q35 linkage peak, rs7794745, showed association to autism, including after the result was corrected for the number of SNPs contained within the linkage peak, and lay within *CNTNAP2*. This SNP was then genotyped in a further 1295 more broadly defined autism trios, yielding a significant association, with parent-of-origin and gender effects. An additional ten SNPs flanking rs7794745 and tagging the LD block in which it lies were genotyped in all trios from stage one and two, but no increase in significance was obtained (Arking *et al.* 2008).

An issue raised by Arking *et al.* concerning the two studies was the occurrence of overlap of the samples used (70 of the 72 trios from stage one and one third of trios from stage two had been used by Alarcón *et al.*). Arking *et al.* do not think that this invalidates the results of either study due to the use of alternative phenotypes, different polymorphisms being implicated and the SNPs being located > 1 Mb apart with no evidence of LD between them. In addition, rs7794745 remained significant in the study by Arking *et al.* even with the removal of overlapping samples in stage two (Arking *et al.* 2008).

CNTNAP2 is a good candidate gene for autism and ASD due to the region of the genome in which it resides showing linkage to autism and also because of functional work which has been performed. *CNTNAP2* is a neurexin, members of which have been implicated in autism (Feng *et al.* 2006; Kim *et al.* 2008b; Szatmari *et al.* 2007), and are known to interact with genes shown to be mutated in some instances of ASD. Mutations in *CNTNAP2* have been identified in an Amish family with seizures, language regression and PDD (Alarcón *et al.* 2008). The gene also segregates with a seizure disorder that is itself associated with autism and language delay (Alarcón *et al.* 2008). Finally, *CNTNAP2* has been shown to be expressed in regions of the brain believed to be relevant in autism (Bakkaloglu *et al.* 2008).

2.3.5 *Genome-wide association studies*

As molecular genetic genotyping technologies have advanced, they have increased throughput while simultaneously decreasing the cost per genotype and the quantity of DNA per sample needed for experiments. This has made genome-wide association studies for complex diseases a possibility, enabling the identification of common polymorphisms with small to moderate effects on disease susceptibility, such as for asthma (Moffatt *et al.* 2007). The resolution of genome-wide association studies is sufficient to enable fine-mapping of single genes, in contrast to linkage studies which are rarely capable of doing so.

To date, five genome-wide association studies examining ASD have been published. The first can be considered a bridge between earlier genome-wide linkage studies and the later SNP-based genome-wide association studies described below. It examined association across the genome in a case–control study using individuals from the Faroe islands genotyped for a total of 601 microsatellite markers. Evidence of association at six loci (2q, 3p, 6q, 15q, 16p, 18q) was found, with the strongest result being on 3p25.3. Therefore, the results provided support for loci identified by earlier linkage studies. However, the study suffered from limited sample size (12 cases, three with an uncertain diagnosis of ASD, and 44 controls) and marker density (Lauritsen *et al.* 2006).

Arking *et al.* genotyped approximately 500 000 SNPs, but in a small number of families, 72 in total (Arking *et al.* 2008). Despite the affected children having a strict diagnosis of autism, this was a very low number of families for such a study. Therefore, it was not surprising that no significant association results were identified, although other findings of interest were observed with the data using different analyses (Section 2.3.4).

Since then, studies involving larger numbers of individuals have been reported. Wang *et al.* (2009) identified a region of association on chromosome 5p14.1. Initially, 780 families were genotyped for 550 000 SNPs and a family-based association analysis performed. However, no significant results were obtained after taking into account the number of tests performed. Subsequently, a further 1453 cases and 7070 controls were genotyped for the same SNPs and a case–control analysis performed, but still no genome-wide significant results were identified. However, when the two data sets were combined a single SNP on chromosome 5p14.1 reached genome-wide significance, with another five SNPs at the locus reaching nominal significance. Two further cohorts were examined for association in order to replicate this result. The first consisted of 447 families genotyped for 1 million SNPs, while the second was 108 cases and 540 controls genotyped for 300 000 SNPs. Taking nominal significance as replication, the authors took the findings from their combined analysis to be confirmed. The associated region on 5p14.1 lies between two genes, *CDH9* and *CDH10*, in a region containing conserved elements, hinting at a possible regulatory role for the region. In addition to this major finding, several other interesting results were obtained, including multiple cell adhesion genes, already of interest in ASD genetics, being implicated (Wang *et al.* 2009). Concurrently, a genome-wide association paper was published by Ma *et al.* They also reported the presence of a risk locus on 5p14.1, but due to the considerable overlap of data with the study of Wang *et al.*, this cannot be considered an independent replication of this risk locus (Ma *et al.* 2009).

The most recent genome-wide association study for ASD was published by Weiss *et al.* (2009). The initial analysis was comprised of a TDT analysis of association on 1031 families genotyped for ~500 000 SNPs, but no genome-wide significant results were found. However, an excess of nominally significant results compared to that expected by chance was observed, indicating a lack of power to identify the associated variants. A case–control analysis using 90 additional cases and 1476 controls was performed for all the SNPs of interest from the original analysis and these data combined with that of the TDT. This resulted in the identification of seven regions of interest, one SNP at each of 4q13 between *CENPC1* and *EPHA5*, 5p15 between *SEMA5A* and *TAS2R1*, 6p23 in *JARID2*, 9p24 between *PTPRD* and *JMJD2C*, 9q21 between *ZCCHC6* and *GAS1*, and 10q21 in *CTNNA3*, and 2 SNPs on 11p14 in *GAS2*. By including data from the Autism Genome Consortium (AGC, 318 trios),

Autism Genome Project (AGP), Finland and Iran (1755 trios in total), they found an increased signal at the chromosome 5 locus. The associated region is ~80 kb upstream of *SEMA5A*, a strong candidate for ASD as it is involved in axon guidance, is downregulated in autistic lymphoblastoid cell lines, has lower expression in the brains of individuals with autism than in controls and is in a pathway involving *MET*, a gene shown to have association with ASD in multiple studies (Campbell *et al.* 2006; Sousa *et al.* 2009; Weiss *et al.* 2009).

These studies demonstrate both the difficulties encountered in trying to identify common variants of moderate effect in ASD, the need for data from large cohorts, the importance of replication in independent samples and the benefit of pursuing results that do not necessarily meet strict criteria for genome-wide significance. They are also examples of co-operation between researchers in the field of ASD genetics, as the latter three studies used data generated by multiple consortia.

2.4 Rare single gene mutations in autism

In addition to common variants being associated with autism and ASD, there is a body of evidence indicating that in some cases the disorder can be due to rare mutations of large effect in single genes. These include the genes *Neurexin 1* (*NRXN1*), *SH3 and Multiple Repeat Domains 3* (*SHANK3*, also known as *ProSAP2*), *Neuroligin 3* (*NLGN3*) and *Neuroligin 4* (*NLGN4*).

Jamain *et al.* (2003) were the first to identify single mutations in neuroligin genes likely to be causal in individuals with ASD. They noted that two regions of the X chromosome likely to be associated with autism, Xp22.3 and Xq13, contained the neuroligin genes *NLGN4* and *NLGN3*, respectively. They therefore decided to screen *NLGN3*, *NLGN4X* and *NLGN4Y* for mutations in 36 sibling pairs and 122 trios with autism or Asperger syndrome. In one Swedish family a mutation in *NLGN4* resulting in a premature stop codon (a mutation that leads to a truncated protein) was observed in two brothers, one with autism and the second with Asperger syndrome. The mutation was shown to have occurred *de novo* in the mother and was not present in an unaffected brother or 350 control individuals. In a second family, a C/T transition in *NLGN3* was identified in two brothers, again one autistic and one with Asperger syndrome. This mutation was inherited from the mother, but was absent in 200 controls and predicted to affect a highly conserved amino acid which could result in altered binding to neurexins. Therefore, it was concluded that in these two families the alterations in the neuroligin genes were leading to the development of ASD (Jamain *et al.* 2003).

In a large French pedigree Laumonnier *et al.* identified a 2 bp deletion in exon 5 of *NLGN4*, resulting in a premature stop codon. This mutation was present in all male members of the pedigree affected by autism, intellectual disability or PDD, but absent in the healthy males of the family and 200 healthy male controls.

The authors stated that the deletion was therefore likely to be a rare causative mutation for cognitive disorders (Laumonnier *et al.* 2004). Other possible evidence for the role of missense mutations in *NLGN4* (Yan *et al.* 2005) and alternative splice isoforms of *NLGN3* and *NLGN4* (Talebizadeh *et al.* 2006) as causative in individual cases of autism has been gathered. In addition, copy number variants (CNVs) (Section 2.6.1) affecting *NLGN3* have been found in individuals with ASD (Glessner *et al.* 2009; Marshall *et al.* 2008). However, several studies have been unable to identify mutations within the neuroligin genes likely to play a causal role in autism development (Blasi *et al.* 2006; Gauthier *et al.* 2005; Talebizadeh *et al.* 2006; Vincent *et al.* 2004; Wermter *et al.* 2008; Ylisaukko-oja *et al.* 2005), or association between these genes and autism or ASD (Wermter *et al.* 2008; Ylisaukko-oja *et al.* 2005), reinforcing the view that these genes only rarely play a role in ASD development, estimated as 0.4% of cases (Ylisaukko-oja *et al.* 2005).

The neuroligin genes encode post-synaptic membrane cell-adhesion molecules which bind β-neurexins, which are themselves encoded by three neurexin genes *NRXN1*, *NRXN2* and *NRXN3*. Each neurexin gene also encodes a longer α variant (Feng *et al.* 2006). Due to the interaction between *NRXN1* and the neuroligins (Figure 2.2A), Feng *et al.* scanned the exons and splice junctions of the three neurexin genes for mutations in 72 Caucasian autistic individuals. No structural variants were identified in *NRXN2* or *NRXN3*. However, two putative missense mutations in exon 1 of *NRXN1* were observed which were not present in 535 non-autistic Caucasian controls ($P = 0.0056$). Further sequencing in both the Caucasian and an additional 194 African-American controls identified no further changes in exon 1. Feng *et al.* suggested that the variants may affect signalling function, thereby resulting in autism susceptibility, but that there might be incomplete penetrance based on family data (Feng *et al.* 2006). In a paper published by the AGP, a CNV which removed the paternal coding exons of *NRXN1* was identified in two autistic children from one family. The CNV was not present in the parents, was likely inherited due to paternal gonadal mosaicism and might be a causative variant (Szatmari *et al.* 2007). In addition, Glessner *et al.* (2009) found deletions in 10 of 2195 ASD cases, but in none of 2519 controls, a statistically significant result of $P = 4.7 \times 10^{-4}$ ($P = 0.002$ after correcting for multiple testing). This striking result was also observed by Bucan *et al.* while analysing the same data, although they also noted the lack of perfect segregation of the CNVs with affected status. This indicates the lack of total penetrance of the deletions of this gene and the importance of other factors in ASD susceptibility (Bucan *et al.* 2009). Marshall *et al.* have also published a report implicating CNVs involving *NRXN1* in ASD (Marshall *et al.* 2008). Recently, Kim *et al.* have identified two independent individuals with ASD and chromosomal aberration breakpoints at 2p16.3. In the first proband there is an 8.9 Mb non-reciprocal translocation involving chromosomes 2 and 16, with one breakpoint occurring in intron 5 of *NRXN1*. This mutation affects the transcription

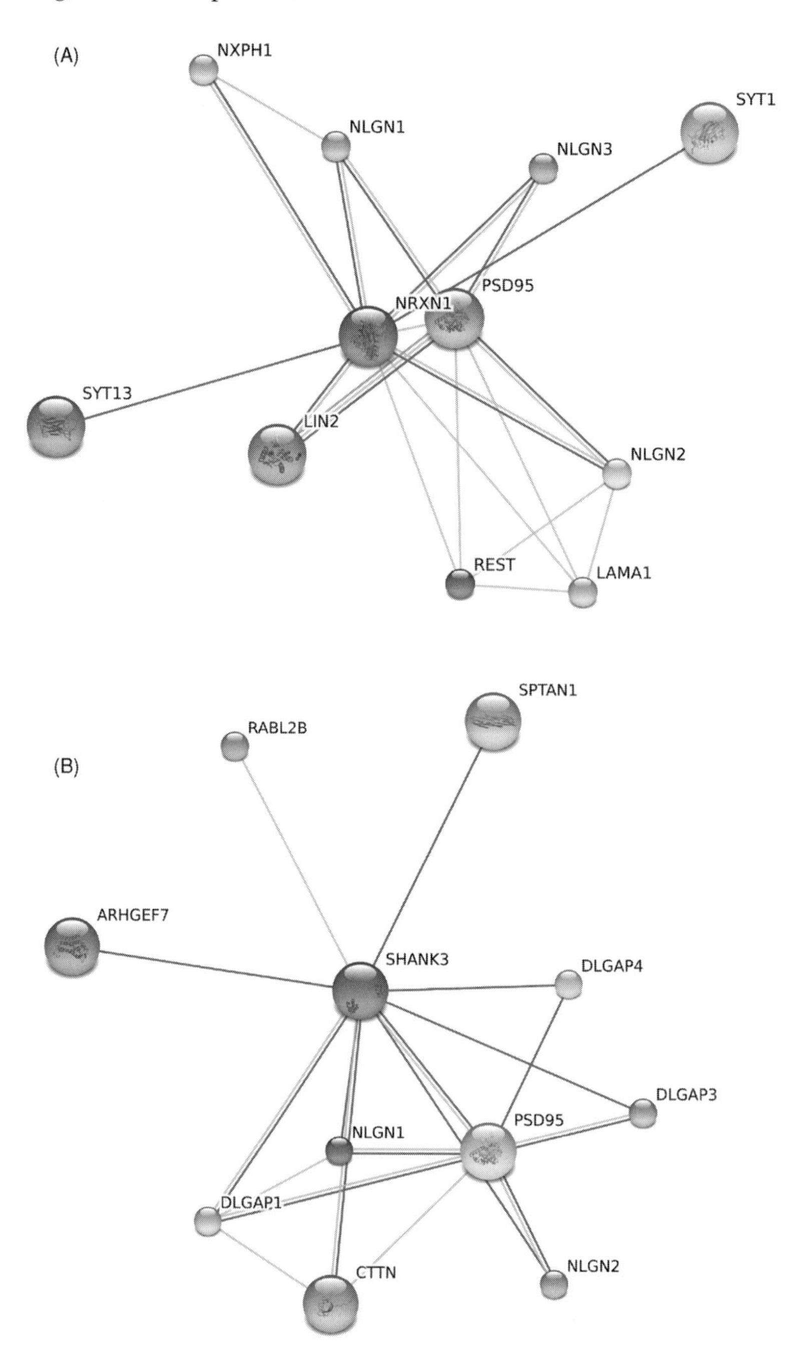

Figure 2.2 Data from Search Tool for the Retrieval of Interacting Genes/Proteins (http://string.embl.de/). Spheres represent specific genes/proteins. Lines represent evidence for associations from experimental data (pink), text mining (green) or homology studies (blue). (**A**) Network of proteins that interact with *NRXN1*. (**B**) Network of proteins interacting with *SHANK3* (von Mering *et al.* 2007). See plate section for colour version.

of *α-NRXN1*, while *β-NRXN1* is unaffected. The father also carries the polymorphism, but is unaffected, so that if the mutation is causal it is not fully penetrant. In the second proband a *de novo* balanced translocation was identified with a breakpoint approximately 750 kb 5' of exon 1 of *α-NRXN1* in a region containing no other known genes, but predicted to have strong regulatory potential. The translocation therefore has the potential to affect *NRXN1* expression. Due to the identification of two independent subjects with the same phenotype and chromosomal aberrations potentially affecting the same gene, Kim *et al.* concluded that *NRXN1* is a causal gene in autism susceptibility in some individuals (Kim *et al.* 2008b).

Finally, rare mutations in a third gene involved in the function of the synapse have been implicated in ASD susceptibility. One of the common chromosomal alterations found in autism involves 22q. Microdeletion of chromosome 22q12.3 leads to cognitive deficits with the minimal deleted region containing three genes, *ACR*, *RABL2B* and *SHANK3*. The latter is the strongest candidate to be involved in autism due to its encoding a scaffolding protein found in the synapse which can also bind to the neuroligin proteins (Figure 2.2B) (Durand *et al.* 2007). Therefore, Durand *et al.* used a combination of FISH (fluorescent *in situ* hybridisation) and direct sequencing to search for alterations of *SHANK3* in families containing children with ASD. This led to three *SHANK3* alterations being observed. One family contained an autistic proband with absent language and moderate intellectual disability who had a *de novo* 22q13 deletion containing *SHANK3*. A second family contained two autistic brothers, both of whom were heterozygous for a single base pair insertion in exon 21 of *SHANK3* inherited on the mother's haplotype. The insertion caused a frameshift leading to a truncated version of the protein. Both brothers had severely impaired speech and intellectual disability. No unaffected members of the family carried the mutation, including the mother, indicating that it was inherited due to maternal gonadal mosaicism. The third family contained a girl with autism and severe language delay who had a 22q deletion. Her brother suffered from Asperger syndrome, although with precocious language and fluent speech, and had a 22qter trisomy. Both aberrations were paternally inherited and affected *SHANK3*. Durand *et al.* concluded that these three families demonstrated the importance of alterations in *SHANK3* causing susceptibility to ASD (Durand *et al.* 2007). A second study by Moessner *et al.* (2007) looked at the frequency of CNVs in *SHANK3* in 400 ASD subjects. They found a single *de novo* non-synonymous mutation and two chromosomal deletions within their cohort. The non-synonymous mutation occurred in exon 8 of *SHANK3* and was not observed in either the parents and unaffected siblings of the proband, or in controls. Of the chromosomal deletions, one resulted in the loss of approximately 277 kb of DNA, including *SHANK3*. The deletion was present in the proband, but not in the unaffected siblings or parents. The second deletion was of 3.2 Mb of 22q13.31–33 in a proband with autism from a second family (Moessner *et al.* 2007). In addition Moessner *et al.* characterised a deletion including *SHANK3* in a family previously characterised by Szatmari *et al.* (2007). Within the family, a 4.4 Mb deletion of the maternal chromosome was present in an affected brother and sister, but not in either parent, indicating that it had been inherited due to gonadal mosaicism (Moessner *et al.* 2007). Moessner *et al.* failed to identify any CNVs in controls, indicating that those observed were autism specific. By combining the frequency of causal *SHANK3* alterations observed by both themselves and Durand *et al.*, Moessner *et al.* concluded that mutations in the gene accounted for approximately 1% of autism cases (Moessner *et al.* 2007). A further study identified a missense and splice site mutation in *SHANK3* not present in controls. However, seven other missense mutations were also identified which either occurred in cases and controls, or controls alone (Gauthier *et al.* 2009). Additional CNV studies have also been mixed, with one implicating CNVs in ASD (Marshall *et al.* 2008), whereas work by Sykes *et al.* failed to identify any in their cohort (Sykes *et al.* 2009). Therefore, as with other genes discussed, it appears that mutations involving *SHANK3* may not be fully penetrant or sufficient to cause ASD in isolation.

In conclusion, it seems that in some rare cases, ASD is due to single gene changes of major effect. Also of interest is that the genes in the work presented are all involved in the function of the synapse, suggesting that this pathway is of importance in the development of ASD.

2.5 Epigenetics

Epigenetics are heritable changes in gene expression that are not due to alterations in the sequence of the genome. Epigenetic changes have been implicated in a variety of complex diseases, including ASD. They can be caused by methylation of CpG dinucleotides, post-translational modification of histone proteins or by non-coding RNA (ncRNA) based gene silencing. These multiple types of epigenetics can interact and stabilise each other (van Vliet *et al.* 2007).

2.5.1 DNA methylation

In mammalian genomes, approximately 80% of CpG dinucleotides are methylated (van Vliet *et al.* 2007). Such alterations of the genome are associated with increased chromatin stability and gene silencing (van Vliet *et al.* 2007). Methylation may result in gene silencing by recruiting proteins such as MeCP2 to the region, which in turn interact with co-repressors and histone deacetylases resulting in repression of transcription (Persico and Bourgeron, 2006; Samaco *et al.* 2004; Schanen, 2006; van Vliet *et al.* 2007). *MeCP2* has been implicated in ASD susceptibility. Decreased expression of its protein has been observed in the brains of autistic individuals (Samaco *et al.* 2004). *MeCP2* is also mutated in Rett syndrome, an ASD (Persico and Bourgeron, 2006; Schanen, 2006; van Vliet *et al.* 2007), and variants have been implicated as a rare cause of idiopathic autism (Lam *et al.* 2000). The resulting decrease in activity of MeCP2 causes derepression of specific promoters, including some for genes involved in brain development and plasticity, such as *BDNF*, *DLX5*, *UBE3A* and *GABRB3* (Persico and Bourgeron, 2006), the latter of which has itself been well studied as an ASD candidate gene (Section 2.3.3). In addition, *MeCP2* null mice lack normal expression patterns for imprinted genes, including *UBE3A* (Samaco *et al.* 2005).

Regions of the human genome that have shown linkage to autism overlap with, or are close to, areas that are also imprinted, i.e. regions where either the maternal or paternal allele is silenced by epigenetic mechanisms. These include chromosome 15q and two areas of chromosome 7q (Persico and Bourgeron, 2006; Schanen, 2006). The linkage region of chromosome 15 includes the gene *UBE3A*, which, in addition to its relationship with *MeCP2*, has itself been shown to have abnormal methylation in post-mortem brain tissue from individuals with autism (Jiang *et al.* 2004; van Vliet *et al.* 2007). Also, *UBE3A* shows decreased expression in autism, Asperger syndrome and Rett syndrome (Jiang *et al.* 2004; Samaco *et al.* 2005). Therefore, *UBE3A* misexpression may be of importance in ASD.

Other lines of evidence also indicate that epigenetic modification of the chromosome 7q and 15q loci may also be of importance in ASD. Maternally derived duplications of chromosome 15q11–13 are associated with increased ASD risk and regulation of the region is controlled by methylation and non-coding RNAs (nc-RNAs) (Schanen, 2006). Approximately 5% of cases of ASD have these duplications, which include the gene *UBE3A* (van Vliet *et al.* 2007). The region also contains paternally expressed genes which may be good candidates for autism, including *NDN* and *MAGEL2*. *NDN* is involved in controlling the expression of *DLX5*, a maternally expressed gene on chromosome 7 which is itself a possible autism susceptibility gene (Schanen, 2006). Specifically on chromosome 7, Lamb *et al.* have shown an excess of paternal allele sharing in individuals with autism near an imprinted gene cluster (Lamb *et al.* 2005; Schanen, 2006). This cluster includes the paternally expressed genes *SGCE* and *PEG10*, both of which are targets of MeCP2.

2.5.2 *Histone modification*

DNA is packaged by winding around nucleosomes, which consist of histone proteins. These histone proteins have a globular region and a tail, the latter of which can be modified in a variety of ways, including acetylation, methylation, phosphorylation, ubiquitination, sumoylation, ADP ribosylation and glycosylation. The combination of modifications of the histone tail forms a code which is recognised by proteins that modify the chromatin structure, such as HP1, and so

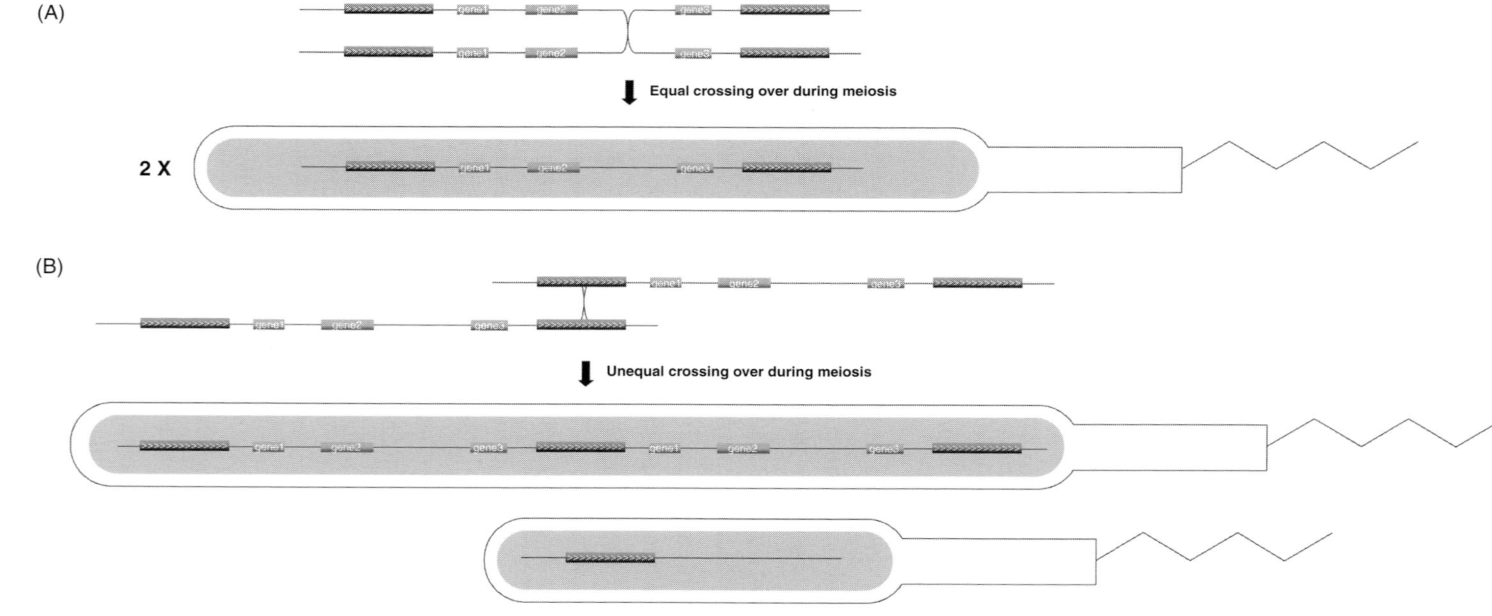

Figure 2.3 CNVs often arise by unequal crossing over during meiosis. Schematic diagram showing 3 genes in green, flanked by segmental duplications in orange. (A) Equal crossing over leads to gametes with a single copy of the three genes. (B) Unequal crossing over results in gametes with 0 or 2 copies of these genes. See plate section for colour version.

modify gene expression (van Vliet *et al.* 2007). Evidence has been presented showing that increased prenatal exposure to *HDAC* (a histone deacetylase) can increase susceptibility to autism, indicating a possible role for this type of epigenetic change in autism (van Vliet *et al.* 2007).

2.6 Copy number variation (CNV) associated with ASD

2.6.1 *What are CNVs?*

With the exception of genes localised on the sex chromosomes and multicopy genes such as the ribosomal RNAs, the vast majority of human genes are represented twice; once on each chromosome of a homologous pair. However, due to sporadic deletion or duplication events, two copies can become zero, one, three, four, or greater. These genetic regions are collectively termed CNVs. The size of the genetic fragment that is deleted or amplified typically ranges from a few thousand to many million base pairs.

CNVs can be inherited in a Mendelian fashion, arise during gametogenesis or as somatic mutations. The genetic regions that flank CNVs often contain segmental repeats, suggesting that the principal underlying mechanism is unequal crossing-over during meiosis (also known as non-allelic homologous recombination, Figure 2.3). The duplication architecture of the human genome can even be used to predict CNV hotspots and this method has been successfully employed to identify novel CNVs associated with intellectual disability (Sharp *et al.* 2006).

For many recessive genes, a single functional copy is enough to protect against a particular trait or disease. However, other genes can affect phenotype in a dosage-dependent manner. Therefore, the effect of any particular CNV depends on which dosage-sensitive genes are contained therein. Large CNVs are likely to contain more dosage-sensitive genes than smaller ones and thus tend to have a greater effect on phenotype. For example, trisomy 21 (Down's syndrome) can be thought of as a CNV comprising the whole of chromosome 21 and causes a severe, multifaceted disorder. In contrast, a 64 kb segmental duplication CNV encompassing *CCL3L1* and *CCL4L1* has a smaller direct phenotypic effect relating solely to immune function (Burns *et al.* 2005; Mamtani *et al.* 2007; McKinney *et al.* 2008), such as influencing susceptibility to AIDS (Gonzalez *et al.* 2005).

2.6.2 *Methods used to detect CNVs*

Due to the role of chromosomal rearrangements in oncogenesis, plus the increasingly acknowledged impact of CNVs on human disease and normal phenotypic diversity, there has been a proliferation of methods developed for studying genomic imbalances.

The resolution of standard karyotyping is approximately 5 Mb (reviewed along with recent developments by de Ravel *et al.* (2007)), so this approach will pick up only the largest of CNVs. However, it does have an advantage over array-based approaches of being able to identify balanced translocations.

Another traditional approach used to detect CNVs is comparative genomic hybridisation (CGH). This involves differential labelling of test and reference DNA samples, for example with cyanine dyes Cy3/Cy5 or with FITC/Texas Red, and hybridising this DNA onto a normal human metaphase spread. Alternatively, for increased resolution, in array-based CGH (aCGH), the fluorescently labelled DNA is hybridised onto a microarray containing thousands of single-stranded DNA probes. Differences in the fluorescence ratio found between test and reference samples indicate regions of the genomes differing in copy number and can be confirmed by simple dye-swap experiments.

Commercial SNP arrays are now available which can target over a million polymorphic and potentially polymorphic sites in the human genome. As well as determining SNP genotypes for use in whole genome association studies (Section 2.3.5), regions of uniparental disomy and homozygosity-by-descent can be detected. In addition, by combining the B-allele frequency and log R ratio (Figure 2.4), data can be used to identify CNVs (Collela *et al.* 2007; Peiffer *et al.* 2006; Szatmari *et al.* 2007).

Representational oligonucleotide microarray analysis (ROMA) is another commonly used method for detecting copy number aberrations. This method is a form of CGH involving restriction digestion of sample and reference DNA. Adaptors are then ligated to the resulting sticky-ended fragments. PCR is then used to amplify a selection of these fragments using primers complementary to the adaptor sequence. Because only fragments of a certain size will amplify efficiently, this reduces the complexity of the resulting DNA and subsequently aids hybridisation to the custom microarray. PCR fragments from the two genomes are labelled with different fluorophores and, as with aCGH, differences in the fluorescence ratio at a specific feature on the microarray indicate copy number changes relative to the reference sample. Copy number changes can be verified using a different genomic representation, by using an alternative restriction enzyme for the procedure.

For verification of novel CNVs, or for large-scale screening of a particular gene for CNVs, other methods such as multiplex ligation-dependent probe amplification (MLPA) have been developed (Slater *et al.* 2003). In MLPA, a pair of oligonucleotide probes are designed that can bind immediately adjacent to each other on the same genomic template strand. Pairs of oligonucleotides can be multiplexed for analysis of 40 or more target sites (for example each exon in a large gene). Once annealed, the ends of these two oligonucleotides are close enough to be ligated. The amount of ligation is dependent on the number of oligonucleotide pairs to have annealed and hence on the amount of genomic template present for that

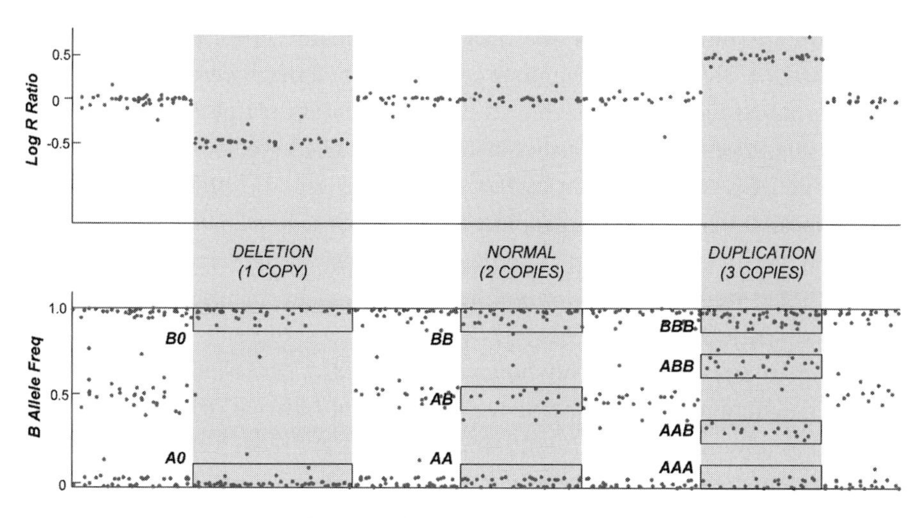

Figure 2.4 Hypothetical data along an autosome demonstrating how results from SNP arrays can be used to detect CNVs. A drop in the log R ratio, combined with a lack of heterozygous SNP calls is suggestive of a deletion. In contrast, segments which demonstrate increased log R ratios and B allele frequencies clustering around 1/3 and 2/3 suggest a duplication. Real experimental data are usually noisier than this schematic diagram, and moving window average analysis of log R ratio is often carried out to detect changes. 'Log R Ratio' is a measure of the combined fluorescent intensity signals from both sets of probes/alleles at each SNP, whereas 'B Allele Frequency' is the relative ratio of fluorescent signals between the two probes/alleles. See plate section for colour version.

target sequence. The oligonucleotides have a universal primer sequence tail and a 'stuffer' fragment that allows size-based identification of fluorescently labelled PCR fragments. Following capillary electrophoresis, peak detection and normalisation of samples, CNV changes are identified by relative changes in peak heights.

Finally, fluorescence *in situ* hybridisation (FISH), where a specific fluorescently labelled DNA probe (usually a bacterial artificial chromosome [BAC], P1-derived artificial chromosome [PAC] or fosmid) is hybridised to interphase or metaphase chromosome spreads, is also another commonly used method to confirm CNVs.

2.6.3 *Presence of CNVs in the general population*

Sebat and colleagues used ROMA analysis of 20 unrelated individuals from a variety of geographical backgrounds to determine the extent of CNVs found in the normal population (Sebat *et al.* 2004). Using a *Bgl*II representation with 35 kb resolution arrays, 71 unique CNVs were detected. Over 90% of these CNVs could be verified using another technique. In addition, many of these changes were confirmed by running two of the DNA samples again with a *Hin*dIII genomic representation. Five additional unique copy number changes were detected using this alternative restriction enzyme. This non-redundant set of 76 CNVs had an average length of 465 kb and only 5 had been described previously. The average number of CNVs found between any two individuals was 11. Although CNVs were widely distributed through the genome, some hotspot regions, such as on chromosome 15q (near the Prader-Willi and Angelman locus), were overrepresented. The importance of these findings was highlighted by the fact that there are 70 genes contained within this set of CNVs.

A more comprehensive CNV study of the HapMap DNA samples from four human populations using both SNP arrays and clone-based aCGH suggested that as much as 12% of the genome (360 Mb) contains CNVs (Redon *et al.* 2006). Even though recent data suggest this figure is possibly an overestimate (Perry *et al.* 2008), these regions are still likely to comprise more nucleotide content per genome than do SNPs – for instance there were a total of 3.1 million SNPs in the 2007 release of HapMap (Frazer *et al.* 2007) – thus highlighting the importance of CNVs in genetic diversity and human evolution. The average combined length of CNV regions per genome was more than 20 million base pairs. Two-thirds of the 1447 CNV regions detected have been replicated, either on both CNV detection platforms, using a locus-specific platform, or by virtue of being present in more than one sample or in a previous study. Approximately 8% were estimated to be false positives. In more than half overlap genes, however, deletions were less likely to encompass genes than were duplications. CNVs were spread throughout the genome, with the proportion of any given chromosome being susceptible to CNV ranging from 6% to 19%. However, gaps in the human genome reference sequence (build 35) had an increased likelihood of being associated with CNVs. In addition, the paucity of HapMap phase I SNPs in regions surrounding CNVs meant that few could be efficiently tagged for potential analysis in genome-wide association studies.

CNVs from the two studies described above are available as Structural Variation tracks on the UCSC genome browser (http://genome.ucsc.edu/), along with copy number data from seven other studies (Conrad *et al.* 2006; Hinds *et al.* 2006; Iafrate *et al.* 2004; Locke *et al.* 2006; McCarroll *et al.* 2006; Sharp *et al.* 2005; Tuzun *et al.* 2005). CNVs found in controls are also listed in the Database of Genomic Variants (DGV) (http://projects.tcag.ca/variation/).

2.6.4 *Whole genome CNV screens in ASD*

Despite the unexpectedly high CNV rate found in controls, there has been much effort directed towards identifying autism-associated copy number changes that might confer susceptibility to this disorder. Seven notable whole genome CNV studies in autism cohorts are summarised below and in Table 2.2.

Table 2.2 *Summary of seven notable whole genome CNV screens in autism*

Sample cohort	Method	Autism specific / *de novo* / clinically relevant CNVs detected	Total CNVs detected in probands	Reference
29 syndromic ASD cases	aCGH with 1M resolution BAC and PACs	7/29 *de novo* 1/29 inherited with skewed X inactivation in mother	33 200 kb to 16 Mb	Jacquemont *et al.* 2006
1168 multiplex ASD	Affymetrix 10K array	10 *de novo* 126 recurrent or overlapping 18 overlapped rearrangements found in the ACRD*	254 in 173 families, average size 3.4 Mb**	Szatmari *et al.* 2007
118 simplex ASD, 49 multiplex ASD and 99 controls	ROMA, 35 kb resolution	17 *de novo* CNVs in 16 individuals in 12/118 sporadic cases in 2/77 multiplex families in 2/196 controls	NA	Sebat *et al.* 2007
751 multiplex AGRE families, 2814 bipolar/control samples	Affymetrix 5.0 arrays for patients, 500K arrays for controls	32 loci found in 3 or more patients but variant in <1% of parents, 8 of these regions had at least one *de novo* event**	NA	Weiss *et al.* 2008
237 simplex ASD, 189 multiplex ASD 500 controls	Affymetrix 500K array and karyotyping	277 autism-specific CNVs, 27 cases with *de novo* CNV, 13 recurrent loci	1315, average size 603 kb**	Marshall *et al.* 2008
397 ASD cases from AGRE and 372 controls	aCGH with 19K BACs, 200 kb resolution	51 autism specific CNVs in 46 patients 9 *de novo*	NA	Christian *et al.* 2008
859/1336 ASD cases and 1409/1110 controls	Illumina 550K SNP array	CNVs enriched in ubiquitin pathway (*UBE3A*, *PARK2*, *RFWD2* and *FBXO40*) and neuron development genes (*NRXN1*, *CNTN4*, *ASTN2* and *NLGN1*)	78 490	Glessner *et al.* 2009

*ACRD – The Autism Chromosome Rearrangement Database: http://projects.tcag.ca/autism/

**Highest confidence data; NA – not available.

A French study of 29 cases of syndromic ASD used aCGH with a resolution of 1 Mb and identified clinically relevant CNVs in eight patients (Jacquemont *et al.* 2006). These rearrangements comprised six deletions and two duplications and ranged from 1.4 to 16 Mb in size. Seven of these CNVs were *de novo* and the eighth was a duplication of Xq25, inherited from a mother who exhibited skewed X-inactivation. Although none of these CNVs was recurrent in this small sample group, the 1 in 4 detection rate underscores the value of copy number analysis, especially in cases of syndromic autism.

The AGP study used Affymetrix 10K SNP arrays to analyse copy number changes in over a thousand multiplex families with idiopathic ASD (Szatmari *et al.* 2007). Using the most stringent cut-off values, 254 CNVs with an average size of 3.4 Mb were detected in 196 probands from 173 families. Two-thirds of copy number changes found were increases. Of these CNVs, 126 were recurrent or overlapping while another 18 overlapped with previously mapped chromosome rearrangements annotated in the Autism Chromosome Rearrangement Database (http://projects.tcag.ca/autism/). Apparent *de novo* rearrangements were seen in ten families, in three of which both affected sibs harboured the CNV, suggesting parental gonadal mosaicism. One of these CNVs on chromosome 2p16, found in two affected sisters, encompasses the *neurexin 1* (*NRXN1*) gene. Based on its interaction with *SHANK3* and the neuroligins (Feng *et al.* 2006), plus its role in synaptogenesis, this gene is a good functional candidate for autism. Another of these CNVs was a 1.1 Mb gain on the long arm of chromosome 1. This variant was detected in three families and overlaps a region implicated in intellectual disability (Sharp *et al.* 2006).

Another study has compared the association of CNVs with ASD in simplex and multiplex families (Sebat *et al.* 2007). High resolution ROMA was performed on 118 simplex, 47 multiplex and 99 control families with an array consisting of 85 000 probes. Seventeen *de novo* CNVs, found in 16 individuals (14 patients and two controls), were validated by other techniques. Only four of 17 CNVs had been reported previously and these were all > 4 Mb. The overall rates of spontaneous mutation were 10% (12/118) in sporadic cases of autism, 3% (2/77) in multiplex families and only 1% (2/196) in controls/unaffected siblings. Both *de novo* CNVs found in controls were duplications, whereas most CNVs in autism cases were deletions. The male to female ratio in patients with *de novo* CNVs was 1.8:1 compared to 5:1 for the study group as a whole. These data led the authors to propose that these spontaneous mutations detected in sporadic cases have a relatively high penetrance and so contribute more equally to disease between males and females. In contrast, unless germline mosaicism is present in one of the parents, multiplex families are unlikely to be explained by *de novo* CNV events. These families are more likely to harbour numerous heritable risk factors, each with a smaller effect on susceptibility.

In the first component of a CNV and genetic association scan using Affymetrix 5.0 arrays, Weiss *et al.* (2008) analysed copy number in probands from 751 multiplex families. By searching for CNV loci shared by three or more patients and variant in $< 1\%$ of parents, they identified 32 high confidence CNV regions, of which eight contained at least one *de novo* event. The one region that particularly stood out was a single recurrent deletion on chromosome 16, detected in five cases from four independent families and is discussed in more detail in Section 2.6.6.

Marshall and colleagues have used the Affymetrix 500K platform together with karyotyping to study 427 unrelated ASD cases (Marshall *et al.* 2008). Using their most stringent CNV calling algorithm, they identified a set of 1315 CNVs, with an average of three per genome and mean size of 603 kb, a similar number being observed in the set of 500 controls. Of these, 277 were found to be autism-specific. *De novo* CNVs were detected in 7.1% and 2.0% of simplex and multiplex families, respectively, consistent with the findings of Sebat *et al.* that association of *de novo* CNVs is increased for sporadic cases. Some of the loci described have previously been detected in cohorts of patients with intellectual disability. In addition, the karyotype analysis of idiopathic cases detected 3.5% with balanced translocations (not detected in the primary CNV analysis) and 2.2% unbalanced translocations (all detectable as CNVs).

An aCGH study of 397 ASD probands and 372 controls using ~19 000 BAC DNA probes identified autism-specific CNVs in approximately 12% of cases (Christian *et al.* 2008). Nine CNVs were *de novo*, whilst 42 were inherited. This set of autism-specific CNVs overlaps with about 270 genes, many of which may now be considered candidate genes. CNVs ranged in size from 189 kb to 6.1 Mb. This set of CNVs included three cases of the well-characterised maternally-derived 15q11–13 duplication (Section 2.6.5) and four cases of the 16p11.2 deletion, a finding which was investigated further (Section 2.6.6) (Kumar *et al.* 2007). In the multiplex families with an inherited CNV, the concordance rate was 21/33 for the presence of the autism-specific CNV in affected sibs. These CNVs were enriched in female cases; changes were detected in 25 females and 21 males in a study group comprising 165 females and 232 males. In this study, only around 30% of CNVs detected in control samples were found in the DGV. This low rate highlights the importance of using an identical method of CNV detection together with a suitable number of control subjects for comparison.

Finally, a recent genome-wide CNV study using the Illumina 550K SNP array analysed 859 ASD cases and 1409 non-autistic controls for discovery (Glessner *et al.* 2009). A further 1336 AGRE cases and 1110 controls were then used for replication. On average, 15.5 CNVs were detected in each individual, for both case and control cohorts. However, it was notable that four genes that were significantly enriched for CNVs in ASD cases (*UBE3A, PARK2, RFWD2* and *FBXO40*) are all involved in the ubiquitin pathway. Although this pathway has not previously been associated with autism susceptibility, the *UBE3A* gene lies within the previously identified 15q11–13 region (Section 2.6.5). Novel ASD candidate genes involved in neuronal cell-adhesion, such as *NLGN1* and *ASTN2*, were also identified.

2.6.5 *The 15q11–13 duplication*

Proximal 15q11–13 duplications have long been associated with autism (Baker *et al.* 1994; Christian *et al.* 2008; Gillberg *et al.* 1991). In probands, they can be inherited or sporadic, but in either case the duplication is usually derived from the maternal chromosome. In contrast, inheritance from the paternal chromosome leads to a normal phenotype (Cook *et al.* 1997b). The duplication is variable in size and so is sometimes missed by karyotype analysis. For example, the AGP study detected chromosome 15q gains in seven samples from three families, at least two of which were missed in earlier karyotype analysis (Szatmari *et al.* 2007). In the other whole genome screens described (Section 2.6.4), *de novo* duplications of this locus were detected in 1/29 cases of syndromic ASD (Jacquemont *et al.* 2006), 1/264 ASD families assayed with ROMA (Sebat *et al.* 2007) and in 2/427 ASD cases assayed with Affymetrix SNP arrays (Marshall *et al.* 2008). Duplications at 15q11–13 ranging from 1.4 Mb to 7.6 Mb were also detected in 5/751 multiplex AGRE families (Weiss *et al.* 2008). The smallest of these contained only two genes, so may help prioritise candidate gene selection in this region.

2.6.6 *ASD-specific CNVs at the 16p11.2 locus*

One of the spontaneous CNVs detected by Sebat *et al.* was an ~500 kb loss at 16p11.2 found in a female Asperger syndrome patient (Sebat *et al.* 2007). Although not detected by the 10K AGP scan (Szatmari *et al.* 2007), the importance of this locus has rapidly been verified in three subsequent studies (Section 2.6.4).

The 16p11.2 deletion was found in two of the first 180 samples to be run in the 19K BAC aCGH study (Christian *et al.* 2008). The significance of this deletion was further assessed by quantitative PCR screening of a further 532 probands and 465 controls. The deletion was detected in two additional individuals with autism, but was not present in controls (Kumar *et al.* 2007). These deletions were verified with FISH and microsatellite analysis and a custom designed oligonucleotide array was used to map the breakpoints to the edges of 147 kb segmental duplications with 99.5% sequence identity. This deletion contains 25 genes and is similar to a deletion reported in identical twins presenting with mild intellectual disability, heart defects and seizures (Ghebranious *et al.* 2007). It also overlaps with a previously described microdeletion syndrome involved with developmental disabilities (Ballif *et al.* 2007). Detailed phenotype analysis of autistic individuals with this 16p11.2 deletion could not detect any striking features that suggest this group of individuals are a distinct autism subtype. The reciprocal duplication product was identified in one subject with autism, but unlike the deletions was found to be inherited. The duplication was also detected in two controls, so its significance to autism susceptibility is uncertain. The deletion segregated with autism in one family; the proband's affected brother carried the deletion and unaffected sister did not. However, affected sibs in the three other families did not harbour the deletion, demonstrating how there can be different autism susceptibility factors involved even within the same family.

Weiss *et al.* found *de novo* 16p11.2 deletions (see Figure 2.5) in five cases from 751 multiplex AGRE families (Weiss *et al.* 2008). Deletions were confirmed by MLPA in all cases. This deletion was only detected in 3/2814 controls. The association of this deletion with autism was subsequently confirmed in two other participant cohorts; being identified in 5/512 cases referred for developmental delay, intellectual disability or ASD, and in 3/299 cases of autism from an isolated Icelandic population. In two families from the replication cohorts for which the deletion was inherited, parents carrying the 16p11.2 abnormality exhibited mild intellectual disability or attention deficit hyperactivity disorder. The rate of the deletion was also elevated among Icelandic patients with a psychiatric or language disorder, although to a lesser extent than for autism. These findings are typical of microdeletion syndromes which often show a wide range of phenotypic variability. The reciprocal duplication (see Figure 2.5) was also elevated in two of the three ASD cohorts, but these were predominantly inherited. In this study, 16p11.2 events were mostly associated with early-onset cases.

In the study by Marshall *et al.*, the 16p11.2 CNVs were detected in four ASD families (two gains and two losses) out of 427 (Marshall *et al.* 2008). Both deletions were *de novo*, whereas one of the duplications was maternally inherited. One of the deletions was found in a multiplex family where an affected brother did not harbour the CNV, again demonstrating the presence of multiple autism susceptibility factors even within the same family.

Finally, the study by Glessner *et al.* (2009) also detected 16p11.2 CNVs in probands which did not co-segregate with ASD in the rest of the family. In contrast to earlier studies, the similar frequencies seen in cases and controls did not provide additional support for this locus being involved in ASD susceptibility.

In contrast to the autism-associated 15q11–13 duplication, which is predominantly maternal in origin, cases of the 16p11.2 deletion both paternal and maternal in origin have been documented (Christian *et al.* 2008; Weiss *et al.* 2008), making any parent-of-origin effects unlikely.

Some of these autism sample cohorts overlap (for example the AGRE cohort was used in four of the studies described above: Christian *et al.* 2008; Glessner

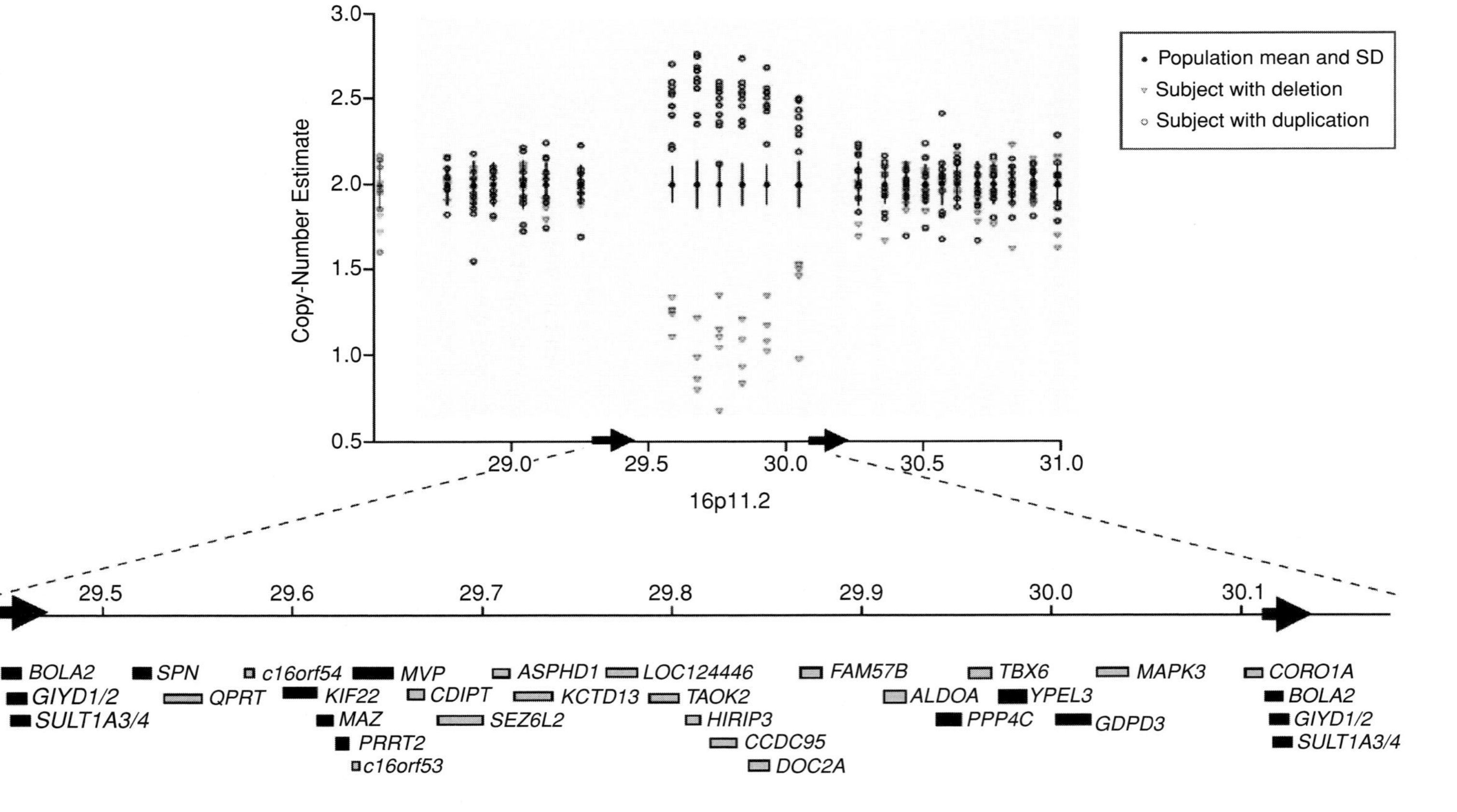

Figure 2.5 Regions of microdeletion and microduplication on chromosome 16p11.2 (Weiss *et al.* 2008). Normalised intensity data from Affymetrix SNP arrays averaged every 11 to 12 probes across a 2 Mb region on chromosome 16. Means (closed circles) and standard deviations (vertical bars) for subjects with normal copy numbers are depicted in blue; subjects with duplications are denoted with red open circles, and those with deletions are denoted with green triangles. Annotated genes in the region of interest are shown (not to scale), with grey denoting brain expression and black denoting unknown or little brain expression. Arrows represent the segmental duplications mediating the rearrangements, with three genes located within the segmental duplication. Reproduced with kind permission. See plate section for colour version.

et al. 2009; Sebat *et al.* 2007; Weiss *et al.* 2008), thus giving the false impression of independent replication. This problem is not unique to autism genetics (Chinnery, 2007) and can be resolved by further independent replication. Nevertheless, these studies indicate that this locus on chromosome 16 is implicated in 0.3–1% of cases of ASD. As there are ~25 genes in this region, it remains to be determined which gene, or combinations of genes, are implicated. Detection of smaller CNVs, or balanced translocations overlapping this region, and searching for rare ASD-specific sequence variants in this set of genes may shed light on the matter.

2.6.7 *CNVs in schizophrenia and overlap with autism*

CNVs have also been implicated in the aetiology of other psychiatric disorders such as schizophrenia. Using ROMA 85K and Affymetrix 500K SNP arrays, Walsh *et al.* screened two independent cohorts for structural variants not present in the DGV and over 100 kb in size (Walsh *et al.* 2008). In both cohorts they detected a significant increase in the number of these CNVs that alter genes, when comparing individuals with schizophrenia to control subjects. In the primary cohort, almost all rare variants detected were different. However, in the replication cohort, they detected two cases of 16p11.2 duplication, at the same locus that has recently been associated with autism (Section 2.6.6). In addition, a 115 kb deletion was detected on chromosome 2 which disrupts *NRXN1*, further demonstrating the genetic overlap between autism and schizophrenia.

A more recent meta-analysis has since confirmed the 16p11.2 duplication as a schizophrenia susceptibility factor, with an odds ratio of 8.4 (McCarthy *et al.* 2009). These new data also show that 16p11.2 dosage is inversely correlated with head circumference, suggesting that early brain growth rate may be a possible mechanism to explain the role of this CNV in neurodevelopmental disorders.

A larger study looking specifically for *de novo* variants associated with schizophrenia identified three loci: 1p21.1, 15q11.2 and 15q13.3 (Stefansson *et al.* 2008). The last of these CNVs is situated at the distal end of the Prader-Willi/Angelman locus, between breakpoints 4 (BP4) and 5 (BP5) and also has been detected in ASD cohorts (Miller *et al.* 2008) and was demonstrated to segregate in a multiplex autism family (Pagnamenta *et al.* 2008). A further study describing smaller (680 kb) recurrent deletions within the BP4-BP5 region, suggests that haploinsufficiency of *CHRNA7* is most likely to underlie the neurodevelopmental phenotypes seen in the 15q13.3 microdeletion syndrome (Shinawi *et al.* 2009).

2.7 Final remarks

As molecular genetic technologies and knowledge of the genetics of ASD advance, so will the strategies used to further investigate the aetiology of these disorders. Genotyping technology has rapidly progressed, providing increased throughput and decreased cost per genotype and quantity of DNA per sample needed for experiments. This has made genome-wide association studies for ASD and other complex diseases a reality, enabling the identification of common polymorphisms with small to moderate effects on disease susceptibility. However, the need for increased cohort size for such studies is still a pressing issue.

New sequencing technologies, such as the 454 and Genome Analyser systems of Roche and Illumina respectively, allow sequencing at a scale not previously possible. Therefore, research is now progressing towards the resequencing of megabase quantities of DNA, including whole exomes (the total coding sequence in the genome) in many individuals. As costs inevitably continue to decrease, this will eventually lead to the sequencing of the entire genomes of individuals with ASD, allowing the identification of all variation within their DNA. Such studies will aid the identification of rare mutations of strong effect, as well as providing data for association and linkage analyses. Such studies are in the foreseeable future, and will usher in an exciting new age of ASD genetics research.

The direction of research into ASD is also likely to increasingly change. Already, a change in focus to CNV variation has been possible due to advances in microarray technology and the methods of SNP genotyping currently being employed. Although unexpectedly high levels of CNVs in controls make interpretation of results difficult, the seven genome-wide studies described paint a picture that highlights the importance of CNVs in relation to ASD. Clinical diagnosis may soon become possible for the most abundant and penetrant of these CNVs. CNVs will also aid identification of genes involved in the molecular mechanisms underlying ASD. In addition, high resolution CNV screening of ASD cohorts prior to further genetic analyses will give future linkage and association studies more power by leading to cohorts which are less heterogeneous.

Although many genes have been implicated as possible candidates for ASD susceptibility, verification has been achieved for only a small number of these. As described previously, a combination of genomic deletions plus other deleterious sequence variants has led to *SHANK3* being considered a *bone fide* ASD susceptibility factor (Durand *et al.* 2007; Moessner *et al.* 2007). *NRXN1* has also been validated as an ASD susceptibility locus. As well as being present in single-gene ASD-associated CNVs (Szatmari *et al.* 2007), it has been interrupted in balanced translocations, and rare sequence variants have also been identified (Kim *et al.* 2008b). More effort is also likely to be spent on understanding the epigenetics of those genes proving to be strong candidates for ASD, as it is becoming increasingly clear that the regulation of genes is a highly complex process.

Another pressing need is for an increase in the number of available samples for these genetic experiments. In order to have sufficient power to detect genes of weak effect (or very rare variants with moderate to strong effects), it has been estimated that 10 to 20 times more samples are needed than are presently available for use in ASD studies (around 20–40 000 samples in total) (O'Roak and State, 2008). While collection of samples is ongoing, the time and effort needed to carry out the diagnostics is not trivial.

Within the framework of a genetically complex heterogeneous disorder such as ASD, common genetic predisposing factors are likely to be enriched in multiplex families, whereas sporadic cases are more likely to be caused by rare *de novo* chromosomal rearrangements or environmental factors (Risch, 2001). These two classes are assumed to be genetically distinct with different underlying aetiologies (two different genetic mechanisms contributing to risk: spontaneous mutation and inheritance, with the latter being more frequent in families that have multiple affected children) (Sebat *et al.* 2007). Therefore, such differences should be accounted for in future studies. In addition, syndromic autism (where other syndromes such as Fragile X, tuberous sclerosis, amongst others, are the cause of autism) and non-syndromic autism should also be addressed differently, since they have different aetiologies.

The need to use different strategies reflects the complex aetiology of ASD with multiple interacting genes and pathways possibly involved. Several approaches such as association studies, whole genome screens, candidate gene studies taking different endophenotypes into account, and large scale sequencing efforts will be essential to discover the causal variants involved in ASD. In the near future, it is hoped that new experiments, especially those as part of large collaborative efforts such as the AGP, will achieve these goals.

2.8 References

Adams, M., Lucock, M., Stuart, J., *et al.* (2007). Preliminary evidence for involvement of the folate gene polymorphism 19bp deletion-DHFR in occurrence of autism. *Neuroscience Letters*, **422**: 24–29.

Alarcón, M., Cantor, R.M., Liu, J., Gilliam, T.C., Geschwind, D.H. and the Autism Genetic Research Exchange Consortium. (2002). Evidence for a language quantitative trait locus on chromosome 7q in multiplex autism families. *American Journal of Human Genetics*, **70**: 60–71.

Alarcón, M., Yonan, A.L., Gilliam, T.C., Cantor, R.M., Geschwind, D.H. (2005). Quantitative genome scan and Ordered-Subsets Analysis of autism endophenotypes support language QTLs. *Molecular Psychiatry*, **10**: 747–757.

Alarcón, M., Abrahams, B.S., Stone, J.L., *et al.* (2008). Linkage, association, and gene-expression analyses identify CNTNAP2 as an autism-susceptibility gene. *American Journal of Human Genetics*, **82**: 150–159.

Alvarez Retuerto, A.I., Cantor, R.M., Gleeson, J.G., *et al.* (2008). Association of common variants in the Joubert syndrome gene (AHI1) with autism. *Human Molecular Genetics*, **17**: 3887–3896.

Anderson, B.M., Schnetz-Boutaud, N.C., Bartlett, J., *et al.* (2009). Examination of association of genes in the serotonin system to autism. *Neurogenetics*, **10**: 209–216.

Anderson, G.M., Freedman, D.X., Cohen, D.J., *et al.* (1987). Whole blood serotonin in autistic and normal subjects. *Journal of Child Psychology and Psychiatry*, **28**: 885–900.

Anitha, A., Nakamura, K., Yamada, K., *et al.* (2008). Genetic analyses of roundabout (ROBO) axon guidance receptors in autism. *American Journal of Medical Genetics Part B: Neuropsychiatric Genetics*, **147B**: 1019–1027.

Arking, D.E., Cutler, D.J., Brune, C.W., *et al.* (2008). A common genetic variant in the neurexin superfamily member CNTNAP2 increases familial risk of autism. *American Journal of Human Genetics*, **82**: 160–164.

Ashley-Koch, A., Wolpert, C.M., Menold, M.M., *et al.* (1999). Genetic studies of autistic disorder and chromosome 7. *Genomics*, **61**: 227–236.

Ashley-Koch, A.E., Mei, H., Jaworski, J., *et al.* (2006). An analysis paradigm for investigating multi-locus effects in complex disease: examination of three GABA receptor subunit genes on 15q11-q13 as risk factors for autistic disorder. *Annals of Human Genetics*, **70**: 281–292.

Ashley-Koch, A.E., Jaworski, J., Ma de, Q., *et al.* (2007). Investigation of potential gene-gene interactions between APOE and RELN contributing to autism risk. *Psychiatric Genetics*, **17**: 221–226.

Auranen, M., Vanhala, R., Varilo, T., *et al.* (2002). A genomewide screen for autism-spectrum disorders: evidence for a major susceptibility locus on chromosome 3q25–27. *American Journal of Human Genetics*, **71**: 777–790.

Bacchelli, E., Maestrini, E. (2006). Autism spectrum disorders: molecular genetic advances. *American Journal of Medical Genetics Part C: Seminars in Medical Genetics*, **142**: 13–23.

Badner, J.A., Gershon, E.S. (2002). Regional meta-analysis of published data supports linkage of autism with markers on chromosome 7. *Molecular Psychiatry*, **7**: 56–66.

Baker, P., Piven, J., Schwartz, S., Patil, S. (1994). Brief report: duplication of chromosome 15q11–13 in two individuals with autistic disorder. *Journal of Autism and Developmental Disorders*, **24**: 529–535.

Bailey, A., Le Couteur, A., Gottesman, I., *et al.* (1995). Autism as a strongly genetic disorder: evidence from a British twin study. *Psychological Medicine*, **25**: 63–77.

Bailey, A., Phillips, W., Rutter, M. (1996). Autism: towards an integration of clinical, genetic, neuropsychological and neurobiological perspectives. *Journal of Child Psychology and Psychiatry*, **37**: 89–126.

Bailey, A., Palferman, S., Heavey, L., Le Couteur, A. (1998). Autism: the phenotype in relatives. *Journal of Autism and Developmental Disorders*, **28**: 369–392.

Bakkaloglu, B., O'Roak, B.J., Louvi, A., *et al.* (2008). Cytogenetic analysis and resequencing of Contactin Associated Protein-Like 2 in Autism Spectrum Disorders. *American Journal of Human Genetics*, **82**: 165–173.

Ballif, B.C., Hornor, S.A., Jenkins, E., *et al.* (2007). Discovery of a previously unrecognized microdeletion syndrome of 16p11.2–p12.2. *Nature Genetics*, **39**: 1071–1073.

Barnby, G., Abbott, A., Sykes, N., *et al.* (2005). Candidate-gene screening and association analysis at the autism-susceptibility locus on chromosome 16p: evidence of association at GRIN2A and ABAT. *American Journal of Human Genetics*, **76**: 950–966.

Barrett, S., Beck, J.C., Bernier, R., *et al.* (1999). An autosomal genomic screen for autism. Collaborative linkage study of autism. *American Journal of Medical Genetics*, **88**: 609–615.

Benayed, R., Gharani, N., Rossman, I., *et al.* (2005). Support for the homeobox transcription factor gene ENGRAILED 2 as an autism spectrum disorder susceptibility locus. *American Journal of Human Genetics*, **77**: 851–868.

Benayed, R., Choi, J., Matteson, P.G., *et al.* (2009). Autism-associated haplotype affects the regulation of the homeobox gene, ENGRAILED 2. *Biological Psychiatry*, **66**: 911–917.

Betancur, C., Corbex, M., Spielewoy, C., *et al.* (2002). Serotonin transporter gene polymorphisms and hyperserotonemia in autistic disorder. *Molecular Psychiatry*, **7**: 67–71.

Blasi, F., Bacchelli, E., Pesaresi, G., *et al.* (2006). Absence of coding mutations in the X-linked genes neuroligin 3 and neuroligin 4 in individuals with autism from the IMGSAC collection. *American Journal of Medical Genetics Part B: Neuropsychiatric Genetics*, **141**: 220–221.

Bolton, P., Macdonald, H., Pickles, A., *et al.* (1994). A case-control family history study of autism. *Journal of Child Psychology and Psychiatry*, **35**: 877–900.

Bonora, E., Bayer, K.S., Lamb, J.A., *et al.* (2003). Analysis of reelin as a candidate gene for autism. *Molecular Psychiatry*, **8**: 885–892.

Bonora, E., Lamb, J.A., Barnby, G., *et al.* (2005). Mutation screening and association analysis of six candidate genes for autism on chromosome 7q. *European Journal of Human Genetics*, **13**: 198–207.

Bradford, Y., Haines, J., Hutcheson, H., *et al.* (2001). Incorporating language phenotypes strengthens evidence of linkage to autism. *American Journal of Medical Genetics*, **105**: 539–547.

Bucan, M., Abrahams, B.S., Wang, K., *et al.* (2009). Genome-wide analyses of exonic copy number variants in a family-based study point to novel autism susceptibility genes. *PLoS Genetics*, **5**: e1000536.

Burns, J.C., Shimizu, C., Gonzalez, E., *et al.* (2005). Genetic variations in the receptor-ligand pair CCR5 and CCL3L1 are important determinants of susceptibility to Kawasaki disease. *Journal of Infectious Diseases*, **192**: 344–349.

Butler, M.G., Dasouki, M.J., Zhou, X.P., *et al.* (2005). Subset of individuals with autism spectrum disorders and extreme macrocephaly associated with germline PTEN tumour suppressor gene mutations. *Journal of Medical Genetics*, **42**: 318–321.

Buxbaum, J.D., Silverman, J.M., Smith, C.J., *et al.* (2001). Evidence for a susceptibility gene for autism on chromosome 2 and for genetic heterogeneity. *American Journal of Human Genetics*, **68**: 1514–1520.

Buxbaum, J.D., Silverman, J.M., Smith, C.J., *et al.* (2002). Association between a GABRB3 polymorphism and autism. *Molecular Psychiatry*, **7**: 311–316.

Buxbaum, J.D., Silverman, J., Keddache, M., *et al.* (2004). Linkage analysis for autism in a subset of families with obsessive-compulsive behaviors: evidence for an autism susceptibility gene on chromosome 1 and further support for susceptibility genes on chromosomes 6 and 19. *Molecular Psychiatry*, **9**: 144–150.

Buyske, S., Williams, T.A., Mars, A.E., *et al.* (2006). Analysis of case-parent trios at a locus with a deletion allele: association of GSTM1 with autism. *BMC Genetics*, **7**: 8.

Campbell, D.B., Sutcliffe, J.S., Ebert, P.J. *et al.* (2006). A genetic variant that disrupts MET transcription is associated with autism. *Proceedings of the National Academy of Sciences USA*, **103**: 16834–16839.

Campbell, D.B., Li, C., Sutcliffe, J.S., Persico, A.M., Levitt, P. (2008). Genetic evidence implicating multiple genes in the MET receptor tyrosine kinase pathway in autism spectrum disorder. *Autism Research*, **1**: 159–168.

Campbell, D.B., Buie, T.M., Winter, H., *et al.* (2009). Distinct genetic risk based on association of MET in families with co-occurring autism and gastrointestinal conditions. *Pediatrics*, **123**: 1018–1024.

Cantor, R.M., Kono, N., Duvall, J.A., *et al.* (2005). Replication of autism linkage: fine-mapping peak at 17q21. *American Journal of Human Genetics*, **76**: 1050–1056.

Cheng, L., Ge, Q., Xiao, P., *et al.* (2009). Association study between BDNF gene polymorphisms and autism by three-dimensional gel-based microarray. *International Journal of Molecular Science*, **10**: 2487–2500.

Chinnery, P.F. (2007). Mutations in SUCLA2: a tandem ride back to the Krebs cycle. *Brain*, **130**: 606–609.

Cho, I.H., Yoo, H.J., Park, M., Lee, Y.S., Kim, S.A. (2007). Family-based association study of 5-HTTLPR and the 5-HT2A receptor gene polymorphisms with autism spectrum disorder in Korean trios. *Brain Research*, **1139**: 34–41.

Christian, S.L., Brune, C.W., Sudi, J., *et al.* (2008). Novel submicroscopic chromosomal abnormalities detected in autism spectrum disorder. *Biological Psychiatry*, **63**: 1111–1117.

Chung, S., Hong, J.P., Yoo, H.K. (2007). Association of the DAO and DAOA gene polymorphisms with autism spectrum disorders in boys in Korea: a preliminary study. *Psychiatry Research*, **153**: 179–182.

Colella, S., Yau, C., Taylor, J.M., *et al.* (2007). QuantiSNP: an Objective Bayes Hidden-Markov Model to detect and accurately map copy number variation using SNP genotyping data. *Nucleic Acids Research*, **35**: 2013–2025.

Collins, A.L., Ma, D., Whitehead, P.L., *et al.* (2006). Investigation of autism and GABA receptor subunit genes in multiple ethnic groups. *Neurogenetics*, **7**: 167–174.

Conciatori, M., Stodgell, C.J., Hyman, S.L., *et al.* (2004). Association between the HOXA1 A218G polymorphism and increased head circumference in patients with autism. *Biological Psychiatry*, **55**: 413–419.

Connors, S.L., Crowell, D.E., Eberhart, C.G., *et al.* (2005). Beta2-adrenergic receptor activation and genetic polymorphisms in autism: data from dizygotic twins. *Journal of Child Neurology*, **20**: 876–884.

Conrad, D.F., Andrews, T.D., Carter, N.P., Hurles, M.E., Pritchard, J.K. (2006). A high-resolution survey of deletion polymorphism in the human genome. *Nature Genetics*, **38**: 75–81.

Conroy, J., Meally, E., Kearney, G., *et al.* (2004). Serotonin transporter gene and autism: a haplotype analysis in an Irish autistic population. *Molecular Psychiatry*, **9**: 587–593.

Conroy, J., Cochrane, L., Anney, R.J., *et al.* (2009). Fine mapping and association studies in a candidate region for autism on chromosome 2q31–q32. *American Journal of Medical Genetics Part B: Neuropsychiatric Genetics*, **150B**: 535–544.

Cook, E.H. Jr., Lindgren, V., Leventhal, B.L., *et al.* (1997a). Autism or atypical autism in maternally but not paternally derived proximal 15q duplication. *American Journal of Human Genetics*, **60**: 928–934.

Cook, E.H. Jr., Courchesne, R., Lord, C., *et al.* (1997b). Evidence of linkage between the serotonin transporter and autistic disorder. *Molecular Psychiatry*, **2**: 247–250.

Cook, E.H. Jr., Courchesne, R.Y., Cox, N.J., *et al.* (1998). Linkage-disequilibrium mapping of autistic disorder, with 15q11–13 markers. *American Journal of Human Genetics*, **62**: 1077–1083.

Coon, H., Dunn, D., Lainhart, J., *et al.* (2005). Possible association between autism and variants in the brain-expressed tryptophan hydroxylase gene (TPH2). *American Journal of Medical Genetics Part B: Neuropsychiatric Genetics*, **135**: 42–46.

Correia, C., Coutinho, A.M., Almeida, J., *et al.* (2009). Association of the alpha4 integrin subunit gene (ITGA4) with autism. *American Journal of Medical Genetics Part B: Neuropsychiatric Genetics*, **150B**: 1147–1151.

Coutinho, A.M., Oliveira, G., Morgadinho, T., *et al.* (2004). Variants of the serotonin transporter gene (SLC6A4) significantly contribute to hyperserotonemia in autism. *Molecular Psychiatry*, **9**: 264–271.

Coutinho, A.M., Sousa, I., Martins, M., *et al.* (2007). Evidence for epistasis between SLC6A4 and ITGB3 in autism etiology and in the determination of platelet serotonin levels. *Human Genetics*, **121**: 243–256.

Curran, S., Powell, J., Neale, B.M., *et al.* (2006). An association analysis of candidate genes on chromosome 15 q11–13 and autism spectrum disorder. *Molecular Psychiatry*, **11**: 709–713.

D'Amelio, M., Ricci, I., Sacco, R., *et al.* (2005). Paraoxonase gene variants are associated with autism in North America, but not in Italy: possible regional specificity in gene-environment interactions. *Molecular Psychiatry*, **10**: 1006–1016.

Darden, L. (2005). Relations among fields: Mendelian, cytological and molecular mechanisms. *Studies in History and Philosophy of Biological and Biomedical Sciences*, **36**: 349–371.

de Krom, M., Staal, W.G., Ophoff, R.A., *et al.* (2009). A common variant in DRD3 receptor is associated with autism spectrum disorder. *Biological Psychiatry*, **65**: 625–630.

de Ravel, T.J., Devriendt, K., Fryns, J.P., Vermeesch, J.R. (2007). What's new in karyotyping? The move towards array comparative genomic hybridisation (CGH). *European Journal of Pediatrics*, **166**: 637–643.

Devlin, B., Bennett, P., Dawson, G., *et al.* (2004). Alleles of a reelin CGG repeat do not convey liability to autism in a sample from the CPEA network. *American Journal of Medical Genetics Part B: Neuropsychiatric Genetics*, **126**: 46–40.

Devlin, B., Cook, E.H. Jr., Coon, H., *et al.* (2005). Autism and the serotonin transporter: the long and short of it. *Molecular Psychiatry*, **10**: 1110–1116.

Durand, C.M., Betancur, C., Boeckers, T.M., *et al.* (2007). Mutations in the gene encoding the synaptic scaffolding protein SHANK3 are associated with autism spectrum disorders. *Nature Genetics*, **39**: 25–27.

Dutta, S., Guhathakurta, S., Sinha, S., *et al.* (2007). Reelin gene polymorphisms in the Indian population: a possible paternal 5'UTR-CGG-repeat-allele effect on autism. *American Journal of Medical Genetics Part B: Neuropsychiatric Genetics*, **144**: 106–112.

Dutta, S., Sinha, S., Ghosh, S., *et al.* (2008). Genetic analysis of reelin gene (RELN) SNPs: no association with autism spectrum disorder in the Indian population. *Neuroscience Letters*, **441**: 56–60.

Elston, R.C., Thompson, E.A. (2000). A century of biometrical genetics. *Biometrics*, **56**: 659–666.

Feng, J. *et al.* (2006). High frequency of neurexin-1beta signal peptide structural variants in patients with autism. *Neuroscience Letters*, **409**: 10–13.

Folstein, S.E., Rosen-Sheidley, B. (2001). Genetics of autism: complex aetiology for a heterogeneous disorder. *Nature Reviews Genetics*, **21**: 943–955.

Folstein, S., Rutter, M. (1977). Infantile autism: a genetic study of 21 twin pairs. *Journal of Child Psychology and Psychiatry*, **18**: 297–321.

Fombonne, E. (2005). Epidemiology of autistic disorder and other pervasive developmental disorders. *Journal of Clinical Psychiatry*, **66** (Suppl. 10): 3–8.

Frazer, K.A., Ballinger D.G., Cox, D.R. and the International HapMap Consortium. (2007). A second generation human haplotype map of over 3.1 million SNPs. *Nature*, **449**: 851–861.

Freitag, C.M., Agelopoulos, K., Huy, E., *et al.* (2010). Adenosine A(2A) receptor gene (ADORA2A) variants may increase autistic symptoms and anxiety in autism spectrum disorder. *European Child and Adolescent Psychiatry*, **19**: 67–74.

Gauthier, J., Bonnel, A., St-Onge, J., *et al.* (2005). NLGN3/NLGN4 gene mutations are not responsible for autism in the Quebec population. *American Journal of Medical Genetics Part B: Neuropsychiatric Genetics*, **132**: 74–75.

Gauthier, J., Spiegelman, D., Piton, A., *et al.* (2009). Novel de novo SHANK3 mutation in autistic patients. *American Journal of Medical Genetics Part B: Neuropsychiatric Genetics*, **150B**: 421–424.

Ghebranious, N., Giampietro, P.F., Wesbrook, F.P., Reazkalla, S.H. (2007). A novel microdeletion at 16p11.2 harbors candidate genes for aortic valve development, seizure disorder, and mild mental retardation. *American Journal of Medical Genetics*, **143**: 1462–1471.

Gillberg, C., Steffenburg, S., Wahlstrom, J., *et al.* (1991). Autism associated with marker chromosome. *Journal of the American Academy of Child and Adolescent Psychiatry*, **30**: 489–494.

Glessner, J., Wang, K., Cai, G., *et al.* (2009). Autism genome-wide copy number variation reveals ubiquitin and neuronal genes. *Nature*, **459**: 569–573.

Gonzalez, E., Kulkarni, H., Bolivar, H., *et al.* (2005). The influence of CCL3L1 gene-containing segmental duplications on HIV-1/AIDS susceptibility. *Science*, **307**: 1434–1440.

Grigorenko, E.L., Han, S.S., Yrigollen, C.M., *et al.* (2008): Macrophage migration inhibitory factor and autism spectrum disorders. *Pediatrics*, **122**: e438–445.

Guhathakurta, S., Ghosh, S., Sinha, S., *et al.* (2006). Serotonin transporter promoter variants: Analysis in Indian autistic and control population. *Brain Research*, **1092**: 28–35.

Guhathakurta, S., Sinha, S., Ghosh, S., *et al.* (2008). Population-based association study and contrasting linkage disequilibrium pattern reveal genetic association of SLC6A4 with autism in the Indian population from West Bengal. *Brain Research*, **1240**: 12–21.

Hallmayer, J., Herbert, J.M., Spiker, D., *et al.* (1996a). Autism and the X chromosome. Multipoint sib-pair analysis. *Archives of General Psychiatry*, **53**: 985–989.

Hallmayer, J., Spiker, D., Lotspeich, L., *et al.* (1996b). Male-to-male transmission in extended pedigrees with multiple cases of autism. *American Journal of Medical Genetics*, **67**: 13–18.

Hauser, E.R., Watanabe, R.M., Duren, W.L., *et al.* (2004). Ordered subset analysis in genetic linkage mapping of complex traits. *Genetic Epidemiology*, **27**: 53–63.

Henningsson, S., Jonsson, L., Ljunggren, E., *et al.* (2009). Possible association between the androgen receptor gene and autism spectrum disorder. *Psychoneuroendocrinology*, **34**: 752–761.

Herault, J., Petit, E., Martineau, J., *et al.* (1995). Autism and genetics: clinical approach and association study with two markers of HRAS gene. *American Journal of Medical Genetics*, **60**: 276–281.

Hettinger, J.A., Liu, X., Schwartz, C.E., Michaelis, R.C., Holden, J.J. (2008a). A DRD1 haplotype is associated with risk for autism spectrum disorders in male-only affected sib-pair families. *American Journal of Medical Genetics Part B: Neuropsychiatric Genetics*, **147B**: 628–636.

Hettinger, J.A., Liu, X., Holden, J.J. (2008b). The G22A polymorphism of the ADA gene and susceptibility to autism spectrum disorders. *Journal of Autism and Developmental Disorders*, **38**: 14–19.

Hinds, D.A., Kloek, A.P., Jen, M., Chen, X., Frazer, K.A. (2006). Common deletions and SNPs are in linkage disequilibrium in the human genome. *Nature Genetics*, **38**: 82–85.

Hirschhorn, J.N., Daly, M.J. (2005). Genome-wide association studies for common diseases and complex traits. *Nature Reviews Genetics*, **6**: 95–108.

Hutcheson, H.B., Olson, L.M., Bradford, Y., *et al.* (2004). Examination of NRCAM, LRRN3, KIAA0716, and LAMB1 as autism candidate genes. *BMC Medical Genetics*, **5**: 12.

Iafrate, A.J., Feuk, L., Rivera, M.N., *et al.* (2004). Detection of large-scale variation in the human genome. *Nature Genetics*, **36**: 949–951.

IMGSAC – International Molecular Genetic Study of Autism Consortium. (1998). A full genome screen for autism with evidence for linkage to a region on chromosome 7q. *Human Molecular Genetics*, **7**: 571–578.

IMGSAC – International Molecular Genetic Study of Autism Consortium. (2001). A genomewide screen for autism: Strong evidence for linkage to chromosomes 2q, 7q, and 16p. *American Journal of Human Genetics*, **69**: 570–581.

Ingram, J.L., Stodgell, C.J., Hyman, S.L., *et al.* (2000). Discovery of allelic variants of HOXA1 and HOXB1: genetic susceptibility to autism spectrum disorders. *Teratology*, **62**: 393–405.

Jackson, P.B., Boccuto, L., Skinner, C., *et al.* (2009). Further evidence that the rs1858830 C variant in the promoter region of the MET gene is associated with autistic disorder. *Autism Research*, **2**: 232–236.

Jacob, S., Brune, C.W., Carter, C.S., *et al.* (2007). Association of the oxytocin receptor gene (OXTR) in Caucasian children and adolescents with autism. *Neuroscience Letters*, **417**: 6–9.

Jacquemont, M.L., Sanlaville, D., Redon, R., *et al.* (2006). Array-based comparative genomic hybridisation identifies high frequency of cryptic chromosomal rearrangements in patients with syndromic autism spectrum disorders. *Journal of Medical Genetics*, **43**: 843–849.

Jamain, S., Betancur, C., Quach, H., *et al.* (2002). Linkage and association of the glutamate receptor 6 gene with autism. *Molecular Psychiatry*, **7**: 302–310.

Jamain, S., Quach, H., Betancur, C., *et al.* (2003). Mutations of the X-linked genes encoding neuroligins NLGN3 and NLGN4 are associated with autism. *Nature Genetics*, **34**: 27–29.

Jiang, Y.H., Sahoo, T., Michaelis, R.C., *et al.* (2004). A mixed epigenetic/genetic model for oligogenic inheritance of autism with a limited role for UBE3A. *American Journal of Medical Genetics*, **131**: 1–10.

Johnson, W.G., Buyske, S., Mars, A.E., *et al.* (2009). HLA-DR4 as a risk allele for autism acting in mothers of probands possibly during pregnancy. *Archives of Pediatrics and Adolescent Medicine*, **163**: 542–546.

Junaid, M.A., Kowal, D., Barua, M., *et al.* (2004). Proteomic studies identified a single nucleotide polymorphism in glyoxalase I as autism susceptibility factor. *American Journal of Medical Genetics*, **131**: 11–17.

Kanner, L. (1943). Autistic disturbances of affective contact. *Nervous Child*, **2**: 217–250.

Kato, C., Tochigi, M., Ohashi, J., *et al.* (2008). Association study of the 15q11–q13 maternal expression domain in Japanese autistic patients. *American Journal of Medical Genetics Part B: Neuropsychiatric Genetics*, **147B**: 1008–1012.

Kilpinen, H., Ylisaukko-oja, T., Hennah, W., *et al.* (2008). Association of DISC1 with autism and Asperger syndrome. *Molecular Psychiatry*, **13**: 187–196.

Kim, H.G., Kishikawa, S., Higgins, A.W., *et al.* (2008b). Disruption of neurexin 1 associated with autism spectrum disorder. *American Journal of Human Genetics*, **82**: 199–207.

Kim, H.W., Cho, S.C., Kim, J.W., *et al.* (2009). Family-based association study between NOS-I and -IIA polymorphisms and autism spectrum disorders in Korean trios. *American Journal of Medical Genetics Part B: Neuropsychiatric Genetics*, **150B**: 300–306.

Kim, S.A., Kim, J.H., Park, M., Cho, I.H., Yoo, H.J. (2006). Association of GABRB3 polymorphisms with autism spectrum disorders in Korean trios. *Neuropsychobiology*, **54**: 160–165.

Kim, S.A., Kim, J.H., Park, M., Cho, I.H., Yoo, H.J. (2007). Family-based association study between GRIK2 polymorphisms and autism spectrum disorders in the Korean trios. *Neuroscience Research*, **58**: 332–335.

Kim, S.J., Young, L.J., Gonen, D., *et al.* (2002). Transmission disequilibrium testing of arginine vasopressin receptor 1A (AVPR1A) polymorphisms in autism. *Molecular Psychiatry*, **7**: 503–507.

Kim, S.J., Brune, C.W., Kistner, E.O., *et al.* (2008a). Transmission disequilibrium testing of the chromosome 15q11–q13 region in autism. *American Journal of Medical Genetics Part B:Neuropsychiatric Genetics*, **147B**: 1116–1125.

Klauck, S.M. (2006). Genetics of autism spectrum disorder. *European Journal of Human Genetics*, **14**: 714–720.

Klauck, S.M., Poustka, F., Benner, A., Lesch, K.P., Poustka, A. (1997). Serotonin transporter (5-HTT) gene variants associated with autism? *Human Molecular Genetics*, **6**: 2233–2238.

Knickmeyer, R.C., Baron-Cohen, S. (2006). Fetal testosterone and sex differences in typical social development and in autism. *Journal of Child Neurology*, **21**: 825–845.

Koishi, S., Yamamoto, K., Matsumoto, H., *et al.* (2006). Serotonin transporter gene promoter polymorphism and autism: a family-based genetic association study in Japanese population. *Brain and Development*, **28**: 257–260.

Krebs, M.O., Betancur, C., Leroy, S., *et al.* (2002). Absence of association between a polymorphic GGC repeat in the 5' untranslated region of the reelin gene and autism. *Molecular Psychiatry*, **7**: 801–804.

Kumar, R.A., KaraMohamed, S., Sudi, J., *et al.* (2007). Recurrent 16p11.2 microdeletions in autism. *Human Molecular Genetics*, **17**: 628–638.

Lam, C.W., Yeung, W.L., Ko, C.H., *et al.* (2000). Spectrum of mutations in the MECP2 gene in patients with infantile autism and Rett syndrome. *Journal of Medical Genetics*, **37**: e41.

Lamb, J.A., Barnby G., Bonora, E., *et al.* (2005). Analysis of IMGSAC autism susceptibility loci: evidence for sex limited and parent of origin specific effects. *Journal of Medical Genetics*, **42**: 132–137.

Lander, E., Kruglyak, L. (1995). Genetic dissection of complex traits: guidelines for interpreting and reporting linkage results. *Nature Genetics*, **11**: 241–247.

Laumonnier, F., Bonnet-Brilhault, F., Gomot, M., *et al.* (2004). X-linked mental retardation and autism are associated with a mutation in the NLGN4 gene, a member of the neuroligin family. *American Journal of Human Genetics*, **74**: 552–557.

Lauritsen, M.B., Als, T.D., Dahl, H.A., *et al.* (2006). A genome-wide search for alleles and haplotypes associated with autism and related pervasive developmental disorders on the Faroe Islands. *Molecular Psychiatry*, **11**: 37–46.

Lerer, E., Levi, S., Salomon, S., *et al.* (2008). Association between the oxytocin receptor (OXTR) gene and autism: relationship to Vineland Adaptive Behavior Scales and cognition. *Molecular Psychiatry*, **13**: 980–988.

Lewis, R. (2007). *Human Genetics – Concepts and Applications*, 7th edn. New York: McGraw-Hill.

Li, H., Yamagata, T., Mori, M., Momoi, M.Y. (2005). Absence of causative mutations and presence of autism-related allele in FOXP2 in Japanese autistic patients. *Brain and Development*, **27**: 207–210.

Li, J., Nguyen, L., Gleason, C., *et al.* (2004). Lack of evidence for an association between WNT2 and RELN polymorphisms and autism. *American Journal of Medical Genetics Part B: Neuropsychiatric Genetics*, **126**: 51–57.

Lintas, C., Sacco, R., Garbett, K., *et al.* (2009). Involvement of the PRKCB1 gene in autistic disorder: significant genetic association and reduced neocortical gene expression. *Molecular Psychiatry*, **14**: 705–718.

Liu, X., Novosedlik, N., Wang, A., *et al.* (2009). The DLX1 and DLX2 genes and susceptibility to autism spectrum disorders. *European Journal of Human Genetics*, **17**: 228–235.

Loat, C.S., Curran, S., Lewis, C.M., *et al.* (2008). Methyl-CpG-binding protein 2 polymorphisms and vulnerability to autism. *Genes Brain and Behavior*, **7**: 754–760.

Locke, D.P., Sharp, A.J., McCarroll, S.A., *et al.* (2006). Linkage disequilibrium and heritability of copy-number polymorphisms within duplicated regions of the human genome. *American Journal of Human Genetics*, **79**: 275–290.

Longo, D., Schuler-Faccini, L., Brandalize, A.P., dos Santos Riesgo, R., Bau, C.H. (2009). Influence of the 5-HTTLPR polymorphism and environmental risk factors in a Brazilian sample of patients with autism spectrum disorders. *Brain Research*, **1267**: 9–17.

Lord, C., Cook, E.H., Leventhal, B.L., Amaral, D.G. (2000). Autism spectrum disorders. *Neuron*, **28**: 355–363.

Ma, D.Q., Whitehead, P.L., Menold, M.M., *et al.* (2005). Identification of significant association and gene-gene interaction of GABA receptor subunit genes in autism. *American Journal of Human Genetics*, **77**: 377–388.

Ma, D., Salyakina, D., Jaworski, J.M., *et al.* (2009). A genome-wide association study of autism reveals a common novel risk locus at 5p14.*1*. *Annals of Human Genetics*, **73**: 263–273.

Ma, D.Q., Rabionet, R., Konidari, I., *et al.* (2010). Association and gene-gene interaction of SLC6A4 and ITGB3 in autism. *American Journal of Medical Genetics Part B: Neuropsychiatric Genetics*, **153B**: 477–483.

MacGregor, A.J., Snieder, H., Schork, N.J., Spector, T.D. (2000). Twins. Novel uses to study complex traits and genetic diseases. *Trends in Genetics*, **16**: 131–134.

Maestrini, E., Marlow, A.J., Weeks, D.E., Monaco, A.P. (1998). Molecular genetic investigations of autism. *Journal of Autism and Developmental Disorders*, **28**: 427–437.

Maestrini, E., Lai, C., Marlow, A., *et al.* (1999). Serotonin transporter (5-HTT) and gamma-aminobutyric acid receptor subunit beta3 (GABRB3) gene polymorphisms are not associated with autism in the IMGSA families. The International Molecular Genetic Study of Autism Consortium. *American Journal of Medical Genetics*, **88**: 492–496.

Maestrini, E., Paul, A., Monaco, A.P., Bailey, A. (2000). Identifying autism susceptibility genes. *Neuron*, **28**: 19–24.

Maestrini, E., Pagnamenta, A.T., Lamb, J.A., *et al.* (2009). High-density SNP association study and copy number variation analysis of the AUTS1 and AUTS5 loci implicate the IMMP2L-DOCK4 gene region in autism susceptibility. *Molecular Psychiatry*, Epub ahead of print doi: **10**.1038/mp.2009.34

Mamtani, M., Rovin, B., Brey. R., *et al.* (2007). CCL3L1 gene-containing segmental duplications and polymorphisms in CCR5 affect risk of systemic lupus erythematosus. *Annals of the Rheumatic Diseases*, **67**: 1076–1083.

Marshall, C.R., Noor, A., Vincent, J.B., *et al.* (2008). Structural variation of chromosomes in autism spectrum disorder. *American Journal of Human Genetics*, **82**: 477–488.

Martin, C.L., Duvall, J.A., Ilkin, Y., *et al.* (2007). Cytogenetic and molecular characterization of A2BP1/FOX1 as a candidate gene for autism. *American Journal of Medical Genetics Part B: Neuropsychiatric Genetics*, **144**: 869–876.

Martin, E.R., Menold, M.M., Wolpert, C.M., *et al.* (2000). Analysis of linkage disequilibrium in gamma-aminobutyric acid receptor subunit genes in autistic disorder. *American Journal of Medical Genetics*, **96**: 43–48.

Marui, T., Hashimoto, O., Nanba, E., *et al.* (2004). Association between the neurofibromatosis-1 (NF1) locus and autism in the Japanese population. *American Journal of Medical Genetics Part B: Neuropsychiatric Genetics*, **131**: 43–47.

Marui, T., Funatogawa, I., Koishi, S., *et al.* (2009a). Association between autism and variants in the wingless-type MMTV integration site family member 2 (WNT2) gene. *International Journal of Neuropsychopharmacology*, Epub ahead of print doi: **10**.1017/S1461145709990903.

Marui, T., Funatogawa, I., Koishi, S., *et al.* (2009b). Association of the neuronal cell adhesion molecule (NRCAM) gene variants with autism. *International Journal of Neuropsychopharmacology*, **12**: 1–10.

Maussion, G., Carayol, J., Lepagnol-Bestel, A.M., *et al.* (2008). Convergent evidence identifying MAP/microtubule affinity-regulating kinase 1 (MARK1) as a susceptibility gene for autism. *Human Molecular Genetics*, **17**: 2541–2551.

McCarroll, S.A., Hadnott, T.N., Perry, G.H., *et al.* (2006). Common deletion polymorphisms in the human genome. *Nature Genetics*, **38**: 86–92.

McCarthy, S.E., Makarov, V., Kirov, G., *et al.* (2009). Microduplications of 16p11.2 are associated with schizophrenia. *Nature Genetics*, **41**: 1223–1227.

McCauley, J.L., Olson, L.M., Dowd, M., *et al.* (2004a). Linkage and association analysis at the serotonin transporter (SLC6A4) locus in a rigid-compulsive subset of autism. *American Journal of Medical Genetics Part B: Neuropsychiatric Genetics*, **127**: 104–112.

McCauley, J.L., Olson, L.M., Delahanty, R., *et al.* (2004b). A linkage disequilibrium map of the 1-Mb 15q12 GABA(A) receptor subunit cluster and association to autism. *American Journal of Medical Genetics Part B: Neuropsychiatric Genetics*, **131**: 51–59.

McCauley, J.L., Li, C., Jiang, L., *et al.* (2005). Genome-wide and Ordered-Subset linkage analyses provide support for autism loci on 17q and 19p with evidence of phenotypic and interlocus genetic correlates. *BMC Medical Genetics*, **6**: 1.

McKinney, C., Merriman, M.E., Chapman, P.T., *et al.* (2008). Evidence for an influence of chemokine ligand 3-like 1 (CCL3L1) gene copy number on susceptibility to rheumatoid arthritis. *Annals of the Rheumatic Diseases*, **67**: 409–413.

Menold, M.M., Shao, Y., Wolpert, C.M., *et al.* (2001). Association analysis of chromosome 15 $GABA_A$ receptor subunit genes in autistic disorder. *Journal of Neurogenetics*, **15**: 245–259.

Miller, D.T., Shen, Y., Weiss, L.A., *et al.* (2008). Microdeletion/duplication at 15q13.2q13.3 among individuals with features of autism and other neuropsychiatric disorders. *Journal of Medical Genetics*, **46**: 242–248.

Ming, X., Johnson, W.G., Stenroos, E.S., *et al.* (2010). Genetic variant of glutathione peroxidase 1 in autism. *Brain and Development*, **32**: 105–109.

Moessner, R., Marshall, C.R., Sutcliffe, J.S., *et al.* (2007). Contribution of SHANK3 mutations to autism spectrum disorder. *American Journal of Human Genetics*, **81**: 1289–1297.

Moffatt, M.F., Kabesch, M., Liang, L., *et al.* (2007). Genetic variants regulating ORMDL3 expression contribute to the risk of childhood asthma. *Nature*, **448**: 470–473.

Molloy, C.A., Keddache, M., Martin, L.J. (2005). Evidence for linkage on 21q and 7q in a subset of autism characterized by developmental regression. *Molecular Psychiatry*, **10**: 741–746.

Muhle, R., Trentacoste, S.V., Rapin, I. (2004). The genetics of autism. *Pediatrics*, **113**: 472–486.

Mulder, E.J., Anderson, G.M., Kema, I.P., *et al.* (2005). Serotonin transporter intron 2 polymorphism associated with rigid-compulsive behaviors in Dutch individuals with pervasive developmental disorder. *American Journal of Medical Genetics Part B: Neuropsychiatric Genetics*, **133**: 93–96.

Nabi, R., Serajee, F.J., Chugani, D.C., Zhong, H., Huq, A.H. (2004). Association of tryptophan 2,3 dioxygenase gene polymorphism with autism. *American Journal of Medical Genetics Part B: Neuropsychiatric Genetics*, **125**: 63–68.

Nakamura, K., Anitha, A., Yamada, K., *et al.* (2008). Genetic and expression analyses reveal elevated expression of syntaxin 1A (STX1A) in high functioning autism. *International Journal of Neuropsychopharmacology*, **11**: 1073–1084.

Nicholas, B., Rudrasingham, V., Nash, S., *et al.* (2007). Association of Per1 and Npas2 with autistic disorder: support for the clock genes/social timing hypothesis. *Molecular Psychiatry*, **12**: 581–592.

Nishimura, K., Nakamura, K., Anitha, A., *et al.* (2007). Genetic analyses of the brain-derived neurotrophic factor (BDNF) gene in autism. *Biochemical and Biophysical Research Communications*, **356**: 200–206.

Nurmi, E.L., Bradford, Y., Chen, Y., *et al.* (2001). Linkage disequilibrium at the Angelman syndrome gene UBE3A in autism families. *Genomics*, **77**: 105–113.

Nurmi, E.L., Amin, T., Olson, L.M., *et al.* (2003). Dense linkage disequilibrium mapping in the 15q11–q13 maternal expression domain yields evidence for association in autism. *Molecular Psychiatry*, **8**: 624–634.

Ober, C., Hoffjan, S. (2006). Asthma genetics 2006: the long and winding road to gene discovery. *Genes and Immunity*, **7**: 95–100.

Odell, D., Maciulis, A., Cutler, A., *et al.* (2005). Confirmation of the association of the C4B null allele in autism. *Human Immunology*, **66**: 140–145.

Orabona, G.M., Griesi-Oliveira, K., Vadasz, E., *et al.* (2009). HTR1B and HTR2C in autism spectrum disorders in Brazilian families. *Brain Research*, **1250**: 14–19.

O'Roak, BJ, State, M.W. (2008). Autism genetics: strategies, challenges and opportunities. *Autism Research*, **1**: 4–17.

Pagnamenta, A.T., Wing, K., Akha, E.S., *et al.* (2008). A 15q13.3 microdeletion segregating with autism. *European Journal of Human Genetics*, **17**: 687–692.

Peiffer, D.A., Le, J.M., Steemers, F.J., *et al.* (2006). High-resolution genomic profiling of chromosomal aberrations using Infinium whole-genome genotyping. *Genome Research*, **16**: 1136–1148.

Perry, G.H., Ben-Dor, A., Tsalenko, A., *et al.* (2008). The fine-scale and complex architecture of human copy-number variation. *American Journal of Human Genetics*, **82**: 685–695.

Persico, A.M., Bourgeron, T. (2006). Searching for ways out of the autism maze: genetic, epigenetic and environmental clues. *Trends in Neurosciences*, **29**: 349–358.

Persico, A.M., D'Agruma, L., Maiorano, N., *et al.* (2001). Reelin gene alleles and haplotypes as a factor predisposing to autistic disorder. *Molecular Psychiatry*, **6**: 150–159.

Persico, A.M., Pascucci, T., Puglisi-Allegra, S., *et al.* (2002). Serotonin transporter gene promoter variants do not explain the hyperserotoninemia in autistic children. *Molecular Psychiatry*, **7**: 795–800.

Persico, A.M., D'Agruma, L., Zelante, L., *et al.* (2004). Enhanced APOE2 transmission rates in families with autistic probands. *Psychiatric Genetics*, **14**: 73–82.

Philippe, A., Martinez, M., Guilloud-Bataille, M., *et al.* (1999). Genome-wide scan for autism susceptibility genes. Paris Autism Research International Sibpair Study. *Human Molecular Genetics*, **8**: 805–812.

Philippi, A., Roschmann, E., Tores, F., *et al.* (2005). Haplotypes in the gene encoding protein kinase c-beta (PRKCB1) on chromosome 16 are associated with autism. *Molecular Psychiatry*, **10**: 950–960.

Philippi, A., Tores, F., Carayol, J., *et al.* (2007). Association of autism with polymorphisms in the paired-like homeodomain transcription factor 1 (PITX1) on chromosome 5q31: a candidate gene analysis. *BMC Medical Genetics*, **8**: 74.

Piven, J., Tsai, G.C., Nehme, E., *et al.* (1991). Platelet serotonin, a possible marker for familial autism. *Journal of Autism and Developmental Disorders*, **21**: 51–59.

Ramoz, N., Reichert, J.G., Corwin, T.E., *et al.* (2006). Lack of evidence for association of the serotonin transporter gene SLC6A4 with autism. *Biological Psychiatry*, **60**: 186–191.

Ramoz, N., Cai, G., Reichert, J.G., Silverman, J.M., Buxbaum, J.D. (2008). An analysis of candidate autism loci on chromosome 2q24-q33: evidence for association to the STK39 gene. *American Journal of Medical Genetics Part B: Neuropsychiatric Genetics*, **147B**: 1152–1158.

Redon, R., Ishikawa, S., Fitch, K.R., *et al.* (2006). Global variation in copy number in the human genome. *Nature*, **444**: 444–454.

Rehnstrom, K., Ylisaukko-oja, T., Nummela, I., *et al.* (2009). Allelic variants in HTR3C show association with autism. *American Journal of Medical Genetics Part B: Neuropsychiatric Genetics*, **150B**: 741–746.

Risch, N. (1990). Linkage strategies for genetically complex traits. I. Multilocus models. *American Journal of Human Genetics*, **46**: 222–228.

Risch, N. (2001). Implications of multilocus inheritance for gene-disease association studies. *Theoretical Population Biology*, **60**: 215–220.

Risch, N., Merikangas, K. (1996). The future of genetic studies of complex human diseases. *Science*, **273**: 1516–1517.

Risch, N., Spiker, D., Lotspeich, L., *et al.* (1999). A genomic screen of autism: evidence for a multilocus etiology. *American Journal of Human Genetics*, **65**: 493–507.

Ritvo, E.R., Jorde, L.B., Mason-Brothers, A., *et al.* (1989). The UCLA-University of Utah epidemiologic survey of autism: recurrence risk estimates and genetic counseling. *American Journal of Psychiatry*, **146**: 1032–1036.

Robinson, P.D., Schutz, C.K., Macciardi, F., White, B.N., Holden, J.J. (2001). Genetically determined low maternal serum dopamine beta-hydroxylase levels and the etiology of autism spectrum disorders. *American Journal of Medical Genetics*, **100**: 30–36.

Rutter, M. (2000). Genetic studies of autism: from the 1970s into the millennium. *Journal of Abnormal Child Psychology*, **28**: 3–14.

Rutter, M. (2005). Aetiology of autism: findings and questions. *Journal of Intellectual Disability Research*, **49**: 231–238.

Salmon, B., Hallmayer, J., Rogers, T. (1999). Absence of linkage and linkage disequilibrium to chromosome 15q11-q13 markers in 139 multiplex families with autism. *American Journal of Medical Genetics*, **88**: 551–556.

Samaco, R.C., Nagarajan, R.P., Braunschweig, D., LaSalle, J.M. (2004). Multiple pathways regulate MeCP2 expression in normal brain development and exhibit defects in autism-spectrum disorders. *Human Molecular Genetics*, **13**: 629–639.

Samaco, R.C., Hogart, A., LaSalle, J.M. (2005). Epigenetic overlap in autism-spectrum neurodevelopmental disorders: MECP2 deficiency causes reduced expression of UBE3A and GABRB3. *Human Molecular Genetics*, **14**: 483–492.

Santangelo, S.L., Tsatsanis, K. (2005) What is known about autism: genes, brain and behavior. *American Journal of Pharmacogenetics*, **5**: 71–92.

Schanen, N.C. (2006). Epigenetics of autism spectrum disorders. *Human Molecular Genetics*, **15**: 138–150 (Special Issue).

Sebat, J., Lakshmi, B., Troge, J., *et al.* (2004). Large-scale copy number polymorphism in the human genome. *Science*, **305**: 525–528.

Sebat, J., Lakshmi, B, Malhotra, D., *et al.* (2007). Strong association of de novo copy number mutations with autism. *Science*, **316**: 445–449.

Segurado, R., Conroy, J., Meally, E., *et al.* (2005). Confirmation of association between autism and the mitochondrial aspartate/glutamate carrier SLC25A12 gene on chromosome 2q31. *American Journal of Psychiatry*, **162**: 2182–2184.

Seng, K.C., Seng, C.K. (2008). The success of the genome-wide association approach: a brief story of a long struggle. *European Journal of Human Genetics*, **16**: 554–564.

Serajee, F.J. Zhong, H., Nabi, R., Huq, A.H. (2003a). The metabotropic glutamate receptor 8 gene at 7q31: partial duplication and possible association with autism. *Journal of Medical Genetics*, **40**: e42.

Serajee, F.J., Nabi, R., Zhong, H., Mahbubul Huq, A.H. (2003b). Association of INPP1, PIK3CG, and TSC2 gene variants with autistic disorder: implications for phosphatidylinositol signalling in autism. *Journal of Medical Genetics*, **40**: e119.

Serajee, F.J., Nabi, R., Zhong, H., Huq, M. (2004). Polymorphisms in xenobiotic metabolism genes and autism. *Journal of Child Neurology*, **19**: 413–417.

Serajee, F.J., Zhong, H., Mahbubul Huq, A.H. (2006). Association of Reelin gene polymorphisms with autism. *Genomics*, **87**: 75–83.

Shao, Y., Wolpert, C.M., Raiford, K.L. (2002a). Genomic screen and follow-up analysis for autistic disorder. *American Journal of Medical Genetics*, **114**: 99–105.

Shao, Y., Raiford, K.L., Wolpert, C.M., *et al.* (2002b). Phenotypic homogeneity provides increased support for linkage on chromosome 2 in autistic disorder. *American Journal of Human Genetics*, **70**: 1058–1061.

Shao, Y., Cuccaro, M.L., Hauser, E.R. (2003). Fine mapping of autistic disorder to chromosome 15q11–q13 by use of phenotypic subtypes. *American Journal of Human Genetics*, **72**: 539–548.

Sharp, A.J., Locke, D.P., McGrath, S.D., *et al.* (2005). Segmental duplications and copy-number variation in the human genome. *American Journal of Human Genetics*, **77**: 78–88.

Sharp, A.J., Hansen, S., Selzer, R.R., *et al.* (2006). Discovery of previously unidentified genomic disorders from the duplication architecture of the human genome. *Nature Genetics*, **38**: 1038–1042.

Shibayama, A., Cook, E.H. Jr., Feng, J., *et al.* (2004). MECP2 structural and 3'-UTR variants in schizophrenia, autism and other psychiatric diseases: a possible association with autism. *American Journal of Medical Genetics Part B: Neuropsychiatric Genetics*, **128**: 50–53.

Shinawi, M., Schaaf, C.P., Bhatt, S.S., *et al.* (2009). A small recurrent deletion within 15q13.3 is associated with a range of neurodevelopmental phenotypes. *Nature Genetics*, **41**: 1269–1271.

Shuang, M., Liu, J., Jia, M.X., *et al.* (2004). Family-based association study between autism and glutamate receptor 6 gene in Chinese Han trios. *American Journal of Medical Genetics Part B: Neuropsychiatric Genetics*, **131**: 48–50.

Skaar, D.A., Shao, Y., Haines, J.L., *et al.* (2005). Analysis of the RELN gene as a genetic risk factor for autism. *Molecular Psychiatry*, **10**: 563–571.

Slater, H.R., Bruno, D.L., Ren, H., *et al.* (2003). Rapid, high throughput prenatal detection of aneuploidy using a novel quantitative method (MLPA). *Journal of Medical Genetics*, **40**: 907–912.

Sousa, I., Clark, T.G., Toma, C., *et al.* (2009). MET and autism susceptibility: family and case-control studies. *European Journal of Human Genetics*, **17**: 749–759.

Spielman, R.S., McGinnis, R.E., Ewens, W.J. (1993). Transmission test for linkage disequilibrium: the insulin gene region and insulin-dependent diabetes mellitus (IDDM). *American Journal of Human Genetics*, **52**: 506–516.

Splawski, I., Yoo, D.S., Stotz, S.C., *et al.* (2006). CACNA1H mutations in autism spectrum disorders. *Journal of Biological Chemistry*, **281**: 22085–22091.

Stefansson, H., Rujescu, D., Cichon, S., *et al.* (2008). Large recurrent microdeletions associated with schizophrenia. *Nature*, **455**: 232–236.

Steffenburg, S., Gillberg, C., Hellgren, L., *et al.* (1989). A twin study of autism in Denmark, Finland, Iceland, Norway and Sweden. *Journal of Child Psychology and Psychiatry*, **30**: 405–416.

Stoltenberg, S.F., Burmeister, M. (2000). Recent progress in psychiatric genetics – some hope but no hype. *Human Molecular Genetics*, **9**: 927–935.

Stone, J.L., Merriman, B., Cantor, R.M., *et al.* (2004). Evidence for sex-specific risk alleles in autism spectrum disorder. *American Journal of Human Genetics*, **75**: 1117–1123.

Stone, J.L., Merriman, B., Cantor, R.M., Gerschwind, D.H., Nelson, S.F. (2007). High density SNP association study of a major autism linkage region on chromosome 17. *Human Molecular Genetics*, **16**: 704–715.

Strachan, T., Read, A. (1996). *Human Molecular Genetics*. Oxford, UK: BIOS Scientific Publishers Ltd.

Strom, S.P., Stone, J.L., Ten Bosch, J.R., *et al.* (2009). High-density SNP association study of the 17q21 chromosomal region linked to autism identifies CACNA1G as a novel candidate gene. *Molecular Psychiatry*, Epub ahead of print doi: **10**.1038/mp.2009.41

Sutcliffe, J.S., Delahanty, R.J., Prasad, H.C., *et al.* (2005). Allelic heterogeneity at the serotonin transporter locus (SLC6A4) confers susceptibility to autism and rigid-compulsive behaviors. *American Journal of Human Genetics*, **77**: 265–279.

Sykes, N.H., Toma, C., Wilson, N., *et al.* (2009). Copy number variation and association analysis of SHANK3 as a candidate gene for autism in the IMGSAC collection. *European Journal of Human Genetics*, **17**: 1347–1353.

Szatmari, P., Jones, M.B., Zwaigenbaum, L., MacLean, J.E. (1998). Genetics of autism: overview and new directions. *Journal of Autism and Developmental Disorders*, **28**: 351–368.

Szatmari, P., Paterson, A.D., Zwaigenbaum, L., *et al.* (Autism Genome Project Consortium) (2007). Mapping autism risk loci using genetic linkage and chromosomal rearrangements. *Nature Genetics*, **39**: 319–328.

Talebizadeh, Z., Lam, D.Y., Theodoro, M.F., *et al.* (2006). Novel splice isoforms for NLGN3 and NLGN4 with possible implications in autism. *Journal of Medical Genetics*, **43**: e21.

The International HapMap Project. (2003). International HapMap Consortium. *Nature*, **426**: 789–796.

Tischfield, M.A., Bosley, T.M., Salih, M.A., *et al.* (2005). Homozygous HOXA1 mutations disrupt human brainstem, inner ear, cardiovascular and cognitive development. *Nature Genetics*, **37**: 1035–1037.

Tochigi, M., Kato, C., Koishi, S., *et al.* (2007). No evidence for significant association between GABA receptor genes in chromosome 15q11–q13 and autism in a Japanese population. *Journal of Human Genetics*, **52**: 985–989.

Tordjman, S., Gutknecht, L., Carlier, M., *et al.* (2001). Role of the serotonin transporter gene in the behavioral expression of autism. *Molecular Psychiatry*, **6**: 434–439.

Torres, A.R., Sweeten, T.L., Cutler, A., *et al.* (2006). The association and linkage of the HLA-A2 class I allele with autism. *Human Immunology*, **67**: 346–351.

Toyoda, T., Nakamura, K., Yamada, K., *et al.* (2007). SNP analyses of growth factor genes EGF, TGFbeta-1, and HGF reveal haplotypic association of EGF with autism. *Biochemical and Biophysical Research Communications*, **360**: 715–720.

Trikalinos, T.A., Karvouni, A., Zintzaras, E., *et al.* (2006). A heterogeneity-based genome search meta-analysis for autism-spectrum disorders. *Molecular Psychiatry*, **11**: 29–36.

Turunen, J.A., Rehnstrom, K., Kilpinen, H., *et al.* (2008). Mitochondrial aspartate/glutamate carrier SLC25A12 gene is associated with autism. *Autism Research*, **1**: 189–192.

Tuzun, E., Sharp, A.J., Bailey, J.A., *et al.* (2005). Fine-scale structural variation of the human genome. *Nature Genetics*, **37**: 727–732.

Van Vliet, J., Oates, N.A., Whitelaw, E. (2007). Epigenetic mechanisms in the context of complex diseases. *Cellular and Molecular Life Sciences*, **64**: 1531–1538.

Veenstra-VanderWeele, J., Cook, E.H. Jr. (2004). Molecular genetics of autism spectrum disorder. *Molecular Psychiatry*, **9**: 819–832.

Vincent, J.B., Konecki, D.S., Munstermann, E., *et al.* (1996). Point mutation analysis of the FMR-1 gene in autism. *Molecular Psychiatry*, **1**: 227–231.

Vincent, J.B., Kolozsvari, D., Roberts, W.S., *et al.* (2004). Mutation screening of X-chromosomal neuroligin genes: no mutations in 196 autism probands. *American Journal of Medical Genetics Part B: Neuropsychiatric Genetics*, **129**: 82–84.

Von Mering, C., Jensen, L.K., Kuhn, M. *et al.* (2007). STRING 7 – recent developments in the integration and prediction of protein interactions. *Nucleic Acids Research*, **35** (Database Issue): D358–362.

Vourc'h, P., Martin, I., Bonnet-Brilhault, F., *et al.* (2003). Mutation screening and association study of the UBE2H gene on chromosome 7q32 in autistic disorder. *Psychiatric Genetics*, **13**: 221–225.

Walsh, T., McClellan, J.M., McCarthy, S.E., *et al.* (2008). Rare structural variants disrupt multiple genes in neurodevelopmental pathways in schizophrenia. *Science*, **320**: 539–543.

Wang, K., Zhang, H., Ma, D., *et al.* (2009). Common genetic variants on 5p14.1 associate with autism spectrum disorders. *Nature*, **459**: 528–533.

Wang, L., Jia, M., Yue, W., *et al.* (2008). Association of the ENGRAILED 2 (EN2) gene with autism in Chinese Han population. *American Journal of Medical Genetics Part B: Neuropsychiatric Genetics*, **147B**: 434–438.

Warren, R.P., Odell, J.D., Warren, W.L., *et al.* (1996). Strong association of the third hypervariable region of HLA-DR beta 1 with autism. *Journal of Neuroimmunology*, **67**: 97–102.

Wassink, T.H., Piven, J., Vieland, V.J., *et al.* (2001). Evidence supporting WNT2 as an autism susceptibility gene. *American Journal of Medical Genetics*, **105**: 406–413.

Wassink, T.H., Piven, J., Vieland, V.J., *et al.* (2004). Examination of AVPR1a as an autism susceptibility gene. *Molecular Psychiatry*, **9**: 968–972.

Weiss, L.A., Shen, Y., Korn, J.M., *et al.* (2008). Association between microdeletion and microduplication at 16p11.2 and autism. *New England Journal of Medicine*, **358**: 667–675.

Weiss, L.A., Arking, D.E., Daly, M.J., Chakravarti, A. (2009). A genome-wide linkage and association scan reveals novel loci for autism. *Nature*, **461**: 802–808.

Wermter, A., Kamp-Becker, I., Strauch, K., Schulte-Korne, G., Remschmidt, H. (2008). No evidence for involvement of genetic variants in the X-linked neuroligins genes NLGN3 and NLGN4X in probands with autism spectrum disorder on high functioning level. *American Journal of Medical Genetics Part B: Neuropsychiatric Genetics*, **147**: 535–537.

Wu, S., Guo, Y., Jia, M., *et al.* (2005a). Lack of evidence for association between the serotonin transporter gene (SLC6A4) polymorphisms and autism in the Chinese trios. *Neuroscience Letters*, **381**: 1–5.

Wu, S., Jia, M., Ruan, Y., *et al.* (2005b). Positive association of the oxytocin receptor gene (OXTR) with autism in the Chinese Han population. *Biological Psychiatry*, **58**: 74–77.

Wu, S., Yue, W., Jia, M., *et al.* (2007). Association of the neuropilin-2 (NRP2) gene polymorphisms with autism in Chinese Han population. *American Journal of Medical Genetics Part B: Neuropsychiatric Genetics*, **144**: 492–495.

Yan, J., Oliveira, G., Coutinho, A., *et al.* (2005). Analysis of the neuroligin 3 and 4 genes in autism and other neuropsychiatric patients. *Molecular Psychiatry*, **10**: 329–332.

Yashin, A.I., Iachine, I.A. (1995). Genetic analysis of durations: correlated frailty model applied to survival of Danish twins. *Genetic Epidemiology*, **12**: 529–538.

Yirmiya, N., Pilowsky, T., Nemanov, L., *et al.* (2001). Evidence for an association with the serotonin transporter promoter region polymorphism and autism. *American Journal of Medical Genetics*, **105**: 381–386.

Yirmiya, N., Rosenberg, C., Levi, S., *et al.* (2006). Association between the arginine vasopressin 1a receptor (AVPR1a) gene and autism in a family-based study: mediation by socialization skills. *Molecular Psychiatry*, **11**: 488–494.

Ylisaukko-oja, T., Rehnstrom, K., Auranen, M., *et al.* (2005). Analysis of four neuroligin genes as candidates for autism. *European Journal of Human Genetics*, **13**: 1285–1292.

Yonan, A.L., Alarcon, M., Cheng, R., *et al.* (2003). A genomewide screen of 345 families for autism-susceptibility loci. *American Journal of Human Genetics*, **73**: 886–897.

Yoo, H.J., Cho, I.H., Park, M., *et al.* (2008): Association between PTGS2 polymorphism and autism spectrum disorders in Korean trios. *Neuroscience Research*, **62**: 66–69.

Yoo, H.J., Lee, S.K., Park, M., *et al.* (2009a): Family- and population-based association studies of monoamine oxidase A and autism spectrum disorders in Korean. *Neuroscience Research*, **63**: 172–176.

Yoo, H.K., Chung, S., Hong, J.P., Kim, B.N., Cho, S.C. (2009b). Microsatellite marker in gamma-aminobutyric acid-a receptor beta 3 subunit gene and autism spectrum disorders in Korean trios. *Yonsei Medical Journal*, **50**: 304–306.

Yrigollen, C.M., Han, S.S., Kochetkova, A., *et al.* (2008). Controlling affiliative behavior as candidate genes for autism. *Biological Psychiatry*, **63**: 911–916.

Zhang, H., Liu, X., Zhang, C., *et al.* (2002). Reelin gene alleles and susceptibility to autism spectrum disorders. *Molecular Psychiatry*, **7**: 1012–1017.

Zhao, X., Leotta, A., Kustanovich, V., *et al.* (2007). A unified genetic theory for sporadic and inherited autism. *Proceedings of the National Academy of Sciences USA*, **104**: 12831–12836.

Zhong, N., Ye, L., Ju, W., *et al.* (1999). 5-HTTLPR variants not associated with autistic spectrum disorders. *Neurogenetics*, **2**: 129–131.

Zhou, X.L., Giacobini, M., Anderlid, B.M., *et al.* (2007). Association of adenomatous polyposis coli (APC) gene polymorphisms with autism spectrum disorder (ASD). *American Journal of Medical Genetics Part B: Neuropsychiatric Genetics*, **144**: 351–354.

3

Brain imaging and the neuroanatomical correlates of autism

MICHAEL SPENCER, ANDREW STANFIELD AND EVE JOHNSTONE

Although brain structure in Autism Spectrum Disorders (ASD) has been extensively investigated using magnetic resonance imaging techniques, considerable heterogeneity across studies exists for findings at the level of individual brain structures and regions. An important theme to emerge, however, is of structural alterations within the neural circuit that has become known as the 'social brain' – including the amygdala, superior temporal sulcus, fusiform face area and orbito-frontal cortex. Evidence points also to altered structure in the caudate nucleus in association with restricted and repetitive behaviours. Diffusion tensor imaging studies suggest aberrant connectivity between social brain structures and also between these areas and other cortical regions. Important future roles for structural neuroimaging will include longitudinal studies to investigate developmental trajectories in ASD, and efforts to join together neuroimaging and genomic techniques and to relate these findings to neuropathological studies.

3.1 Background

The notion that mental illness is a somatic disorder of the brain was put forward in 1845 by Wilhelm Griesinger (Griesinger, 1845), first Professor of psychiatry and neurology in Berlin, and has been actively investigated ever since. The initial work was neuropathological as there existed no means of visualising the brain in life but clear cut results were obtained in some disorders (Alzheimer, 1897; Wernicke, 1881) and where no such findings could be demonstrated as in schizophrenia, work still continued (Dunlap, 1924; Klippel and Lhermitte, 1909).

Researching the Autism Spectrum: Contemporary Perspectives, ed. I. Roth and P. Rezaie. Published by Cambridge University Press.

The introduction of pneumoencephalography in 1919 – whereby the cerebrospinal fluid around the brain was replaced by a gas thus allowing images of the brain to be visualised on x-ray – allowed the brain to be examined in life and it was introduced into psychiatric research practice in the 1920s. Studies continued throughout the 1930s and to a lesser extent thereafter. There were technical difficulties with pneumoencephalography but the overriding problem was its association with unpleasant side-effects such as headache and vomiting and considerable risk, so that it was considered unethical to use. In 1973, Hounsfield devised structural imaging by the non-invasive method of computed tomography (CT) and it became possible to carry out controlled studies using this new technology (e.g. Johnstone *et al.* 1976). Although now CT scans are done very quickly, this was not the case shortly after the technique was introduced when a CT examination of the head could take over an hour. This involved significant amounts of radiation thereby limiting the application of CT scanning in research. In recent years, for psychiatric research purposes CT has essentially been superseded by structural magnetic resonance imaging (MRI) initially referred to as NMR or nuclear magnetic resonance. This term was used in 1946 by Bloch and Purcell to describe the physical phenomenon whereby under the influence of a strong magnetic field, protons within the nuclei of hydrogen atoms become aligned with the field. If a subsequent brief pulse of radio waves with a specific frequency is applied, altering the alignment of these protons, the termination of this radio pulse is accompanied by a realignment of these protons back to the magnetic field. This causes them to release a pulse of energy that can be detected indicating the presence of the particular tissue type that responds optimally to the applied radio frequency.

The application of this technique to man, with the ability to reconstruct the data to create an image was later developed with pioneering work being conducted by Mansfield and Maudsley (Mansfield and Maudsley, 1977), Lauterbur (Lauterbur, 1979) and Mallard and colleagues (Mallard *et al.* 1979). MRI is sensitive to subject movement which can cause difficulties but it is now the structural imaging modality of choice because of the absence of ionising radiation and its high spatial resolution, good soft tissue contrast and, in brain studies, separation of grey and white matter. The absence of ionising radiation is advantageous particularly in young subjects and in those where repeated examination is going to be required. The fact that it does not depend on x-rays means that there is no bone artefact which, with CT, obscures the posterior fossa.

The reporting of cerebral MRI data in clinical practice is most commonly performed by means of the direct visual inspection of film print-outs, typically providing a relatively small but representative range of axial and sagittal images of the brain. In recent years, the inspection by neuroradiologists of volume data presented on a computer screen has become increasingly widespread.

3.2 Important considerations relating to autism spectrum literature

3.2.1 *Heterogeneity of the autism spectrum*

Since its first description by Kanner (1943), the concept of autism has expanded such that it is now generally accepted that it represents not a discrete condition, but rather part of a spectrum of conditions. These conditions can vary dramatically in their clinical features and even within a diagnostic category there is a wide range of possible presentations. This heterogeneity between and within the various components of the autism spectrum has implications for the neurobiological study of autism spectrum disorders (ASD), as it is possible that different clinical presentations may reflect differences in underlying brain structure and function.

The effects of this heterogeneity can be minimised between research studies by the use of standardised diagnostic instruments. There are a number of such instruments, with the most widely used at present being a combination of the Autism Diagnostic Interview – Revised (ADI-R) (Lord *et al.* 1994) and the Autism Diagnostic Observational Schedule – Generic (ADOS-G) (Lord *et al.* 2000). However, not all studies use the same instrument or combination of instruments and even if the same diagnostic methods are used, the inclusion criteria for participants may still vary, with some studies recruiting only individuals with autism and others including those with disorders from across the spectrum. These differences in diagnostic methodology and inclusion criteria may account for some of the heterogeneity observed in the autism neuroimaging literature.

It should be noted that problems of heterogeneity in the neuroimaging literature are not confined to ASD. There is no biological marker for most disorders of mental health and diagnoses are made on the basis of the clinical picture and the course of the condition over time. Where diagnoses are made on this basis there are bound to be uncertainties, disagreements and illnesses which seem to lie across diagnostic borders. Reliability of diagnosis has been greatly enhanced by the introduction of operational definitions (e.g. those of the *Diagnostic and Statistical Manual of Mental Disorders, 4th Edition, Text Revised*/DSM-IV-TR) (American Psychiatric Association, 2000). In this context the operational criteria for schizophrenia and bipolar illness of DSM-IV-TR and indeed other systems of definition exclude cases due to a 'general medical condition' whereas those for autism and ASD do not. A variety of medical conditions such as epilepsy (see Section 3.2.2) can in themselves be associated with changes in brain structure detectable by neuroimaging and therefore these aspects of heterogeneity in imaging studies may well represent a greater problem in the study of ASD and autism than they would for example in schizophrenia or bipolar disorder research.

3.2.2 *Intellectual ability*

A high co-occurrence of intellectual disability and ASD has long been noted. Intellectual disability is defined by significant limitations in intellectual functioning, an intelligence quotient (IQ) of less than 70, and impaired adaptive behaviour, originating before eighteen years of age (American Association on Intellectual and Developmental Disabilities, 2010). Prevalence rates for intellectual disability among individuals with autism are usually quoted as around 70–80% (Fombonne, 2005), although studies which consider the whole range of ASD, as opposed to more tightly defined autism, tend to report much lower rates (Chakrabarti and Fombonne, 2005). The high prevalence of intellectual disability in autism poses a number of difficulties for neuroimaging studies of autism. This is particularly evident for studies examining individuals with low IQ where the choice of control group may be difficult. To enlist a control group without intellectual disability risks finding brain structural differences which are related to the IQ disparity (e.g. Spencer *et al.* 2005), in addition to those which are related to the expression of autistic features; conversely to control for IQ in this situation may lead to false negative findings due to the association between autism and intellectual impairment. If, however, a control group containing intellectually disabled individuals is to be chosen then the question arises as to whom exactly should be included – i.e. how does one select a control condition from among the multitude of conditions (known and unknown) which are associated with intellectual disability?

Another related consideration is that individuals with epilepsy, present in about 20–25% of individuals with moderate to severe intellectual disability (Lhatoo and Sander, 2001), and cerebral palsy, present in around 15–40% of individuals with severe intellectual disability (Fryers and Russell, 1997), are typically excluded from structural imaging studies. The exclusion of these individuals is principally due to the strong association between these conditions and structural abnormalities on neuroimaging (Bruggemann *et al.* 2009; Dabbs *et al.* 2009; Korzeniewski *et al.* 2008; Ong *et al.* 2009), and hence their potential role as confounding factors. In other words, if epilepsy were more prevalent in the subject group than in the control group of a study (such as a study of ASD), then the risk may arise that neuroimaging findings associated with epilepsy might be misattributed to ASD.

In fact, relatively few neuroimaging studies of autism have included subjects with intellectual disability. While this avoids the complications discussed above and has obvious practical advantages in terms of acceptability of the scanning procedure and the ability to administer cognitively relatively demanding functional MRI (fMRI) tasks, it does mean that the neuroimaging literature in autism cannot be considered as representative of the generality of the autistic population. This is particularly significant in the interpretation of any findings, as it cannot be assumed that intellectually impaired individuals will manifest the same brain-to-behaviour relationships as are seen in those with relatively high IQ.

3.2.3 *Gender*

Although there is an approximately 4:1 ratio of males to females with autism, this is not reflected in the structural neuroimaging literature, in which primarily males are considered. The gender disparity in the population prevalences of Asperger syndrome and non-specific pervasive developmental disorders, though less well characterised than for autism, is likely to be even more marked. While a number of recent studies have attempted to address this issue (see Section 3.7), the degree to which the overwhelming majority of the literature may be generalised beyond the male population is uncertain.

3.2.4 *The timing of brain development in ASD*

In recent years increasing interest has focused upon differences in the developmental time course of brain structures in ASD as compared to unaffected individuals. When cross-sectional studies from across the age range have been combined using meta-analytical methods, significant moderating effects of age have emerged for a range of brain regions (Redcay and Courchesne, 2005; Stanfield *et al.* 2008). Consequently, differences in brain anatomy between individuals with ASD and unaffected individuals may be evident at certain ages, but not at others. These developmental differences may provide clues as to the pathogenetic processes which lead to ASD and could aid in the development of future interventions. One important caveat is that the results to date are based upon relationships with age in cross-sectional studies and so must be assumed to be preliminary in nature. Longitudinal studies which follow up the same group of autistic individuals from infancy are required to confirm or refute these findings.

If, however, there are differences in the timing of brain development in ASD there are obvious implications for the interpretation of study results. Negative findings for a region do not necessarily exclude it from being important in ASD, as it is possible that structural differences would have been seen had the participants been scanned at a different age. The age of clinical diagnosis of autism is typically 3–4 years – however, the meta-analysis conducted by Redcay and Courchesne (2005) suggested a period of marked overgrowth and subsequent relative cessation of growth of the brain as occurring within the first 2–4 years of life. The authors therefore suggested that examining the neuroanatomy of participants older than this will inevitably result in the measuring of the outcome of a pathological process, rather than the actual pathology itself (Redcay and Courchesne, 2005). However, this is clearly not a reason to exclude older children and adults from neuroimaging studies – as knowledge of the process outcome is also important when determining structural differences. Rather, it points to the importance of considering the question to be addressed when planning a study, bearing in mind the possible confounding factors, and carefully choosing the appropriate sample for study.

3.3 Qualitative MRI findings

Naked eye inspection of MRI scans may reveal both *anomalies*, i.e., variations in structure of uncertain significance and *abnormalities*, i.e. variations in structure which would be regarded as outwith normal limits and could well be indicative of specific pathology. A broad range of qualitative anomalies of brain structure have been described in association with psychiatric disorders, such as white matter hyperintensities, dilatation of the lateral ventricles, thinning of the corpus callosum, cavum septi pellucidi (a separation of the septal laminae of the septum pellucidum) and dilated Virchow-Robin spaces. Figure 3.1 illustrates two such anomalies – thinning of the corpus callosum (Figure 3.1A–C) and lateral ventricular enlargement (Figure 3.1D–F). In routine clinical practice many of these anomalies are regarded as incidental findings on MRI scans, and the significance of their presence in the clinically well human – as well as the nature of their relationship with disease states – is poorly understood.

Qualitative abnormalities of brain structure, apparent on visual inspection by a neuroradiologist of a structural MRI scan, have been described in a range of neurodevelopmental conditions, most notably idiopathic intellectual disability (Decobert *et al.* 2005; Schaefer and Bodensteiner, 1999; Spencer *et al.* 2005) and schizophrenia (Degreef *et al.* 1992; Galderisi *et al.* 2000; Lubman *et al.* 2002; Nopoulos *et al.* 1997). A number of studies report such clear cut abnormalities of brain structure as occurring in association with autism. These abnormalities include defects of neuronal migration such as polymicrogyria, schizencephaly, macrogyria and focal pachygyria (Berthier *et al.* 1990; Piven *et al.* 1990; Schifter *et al.* 1994) and abnormalities of the septum pellucidum (Machado *et al.* 2003). Thinning and agenesis of the corpus callosum have been reported using qualitative assessment methods (Machado *et al.* 2003), while quantitative measurements of reduced corpus callosal volume have been reported within some studies (Egaas *et al.* 1995; Hardan *et al.* 2000; Manes *et al.* 1999; Piven *et al.* 1997) but not others (Elia *et al.* 2000; Gaffney *et al.* 1987b) (see Section 3.5.3). Enlarged Virchow-Robin spaces (Taber *et al.* 2004; Zeegers *et al.* 2006), arachnoid cysts (Zeegers *et al.* 2006) and Chiari I malformation (Zeegers *et al.* 2006) have also been reported in autism. For reasons mentioned earlier, it is not clear whether these abnormalities are related to autism *per se* or associated with co-morbidities such as epilepsy. It has been

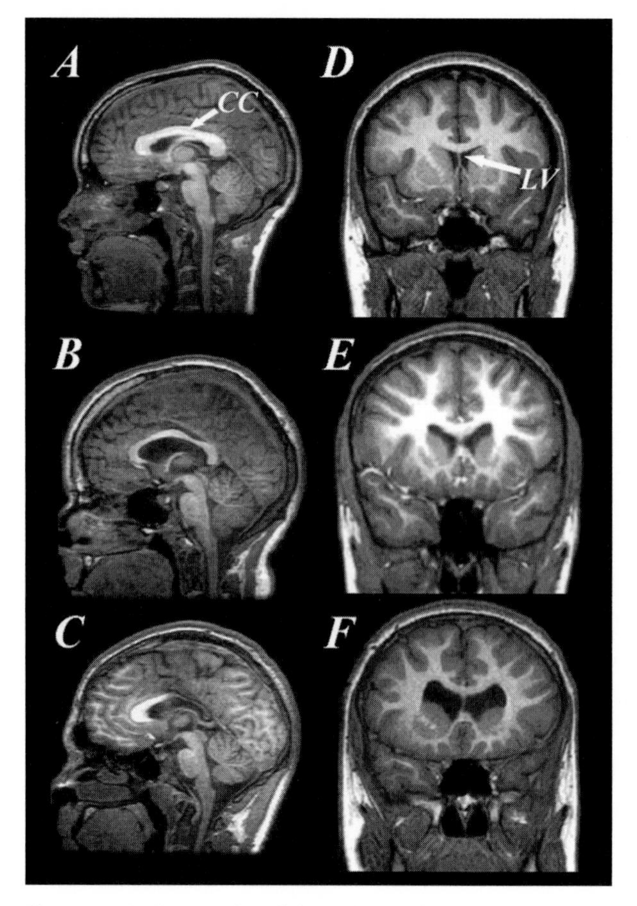

Figure 3.1 **A–C**, examples of absent (**A**), moderate (**B**) and marked (**C**) thinning of the corpus callosum (indicated as CC) on midsagittal section; **D–F**, examples of absent (**D**), moderate (**E**) and marked (**F**) enlargement of the frontal horns of the lateral ventricles (indicated as LV) on coronal section. Coronal images are displayed in neurological convention (i.e. left is left). (Adapted from Spencer, M.D., Gibson, R.J., Moorhead, T.W.J. *et al.* (2005). Qualitative assessment of brain anomalies in adolescents with intellectual disability. American Journal of Neuroradiology, 26: 2691–2697, with permission of the copyright holder, the American Society of Neuroradiology.)

reported, however, that the overall yield of qualitative anomalies in teenagers with special educational needs is related to the degree of intellectual impairment as measured using IQ (Spencer *et al.* 2005) – hence it seems likely that within an ASD sample such abnormalities would predominantly occur in those individuals with the greatest degree of intellectual disability.

In terms of volumes of ventricular spaces in autism, lateral ventricular enlargement has been reported in some studies (Balottin *et al.* 1989; Damasio *et al.* 1980;

3.4.3 *Other shape-based approaches*

Aside from the volume-based or tissue density-based techniques of region-of-interest and VBM, discussed above, there are a number of other possible approaches to deriving quantitative neuroanatomical information from MRI scans. These include manual and automated methods which aim to determine the shape of subcortical structures, the degree of cortical folding and the relative position of various major gyri and sulci (see 'Cerebral cortical folding' within Section 3.5.2). Various factors are thought to affect the pattern of cortical convolutions including brain growth, the balance of local and long range connectivity and the mechanical properties of the cerebral cortical layers (Toro and Burnod, 2005). In turn, these factors are likely to be determined by genes, the environment and their interaction. The examination of cortical folding may therefore provide information regarding the nature and timing of pathogenetic processes. In addition, sulco-gyral shape and even position are thought to change with age, therefore differences between groups may also relate to processes which are ongoing throughout life (Blanton *et al.* 2001; Kochunov *et al.* 2005; Magnotta *et al.* 1999).

3.4.4 *Diffusion tensor imaging*

A relatively recent development in magnetic resonance technology which is becoming increasingly important in the field of autism research is diffusion tensor imaging (DTI) – an MRI modality that allows the direction of flow of water molecules within brain tissue to be estimated. In white matter, the direction of tracts is strongly related to the principal diffusion direction of water protons. As described by Basser *et al.* (1994), the anisotropic diffusion of water – which reflects the diffusion of water molecules along axons within white matter tracts – can be measured, providing information as to the directionality and integrity of white matter structures within the brain. When axons in white matter are tightly packed, run in the same direction and/or are well myelinated the level of anisotropy (expressed as fractional anisotropy (FA)) will be high. The use of DTI therefore allows researchers to make inferences about white matter microstructure *in vivo*. A further development in DTI methodology, DTI tractography, enables the three-dimensional characterisation of white matter pathways within the brain (see Conturo *et al.* 1999). DTI tractography allows the reconstruction of fibre bundles and enhances our ability to study the structural connectivity of distinct brain regions. Given the view that autism may be a disorder of brain connectivity (Frith, 2004) it is evident that the ability of DTI to study anatomical connectivity *in vivo* is of particular relevance and potentially holds great promise for the future study of the condition.

3.5 Quantitative structural MRI imaging findings, grouped by brain region

3.5.1 *Whole brain*

Although not identified by all studies, increased mean brain volume of individuals with ASD as compared to controls is one of the most consistent neuroimaging findings in autism research (Aylward *et al.* 2002; Courchesne, 2002; Hardan *et al.* 2001b; Piven *et al.* 1995). Studies of infant head circumference, which is strongly correlated with brain size in very young children, have identified greater growth in the first year of life in infants who later develop ASD (Courchesne *et al.* 2003; Dawson *et al.* 2007; Mraz *et al.* 2007). It is less clear, however, whether this persists throughout life, or whether the rate of brain growth in autistic children then falls behind that seen in typically developing children, leading to a gradual normalisation in size. It has been reported that brain weight is heavier in children with autism than controls but lighter in adults with autism than controls (Bauman and Kemper, 1997). MRI studies of young children do appear to show greater enlargements than are seen in older individuals (Courchesne *et al.* 2001; Sparks *et al.* 2002), however, increased brain volume has also been reported in some adults with ASD (Piven *et al.* 1995). A meta-analysis which combined post-mortem head circumference and MRI data concluded that there is a period of early overgrowth followed by a reduction in growth rates and a subsequent normalisation in volume (Redcay and Courchesne, 2005). However, it is important to note that most of the existing studies examining this issue have used cross-sectional designs and the results may not be directly applicable to the study of longitudinal changes to brain structure. A preliminary longitudinal study investigated children aged 8–12 years measuring brain volume and cortical thickness at baseline and at follow-up after a 30-month interval and found evidence of greater reductions over time in grey matter volume and cortical thickness in individuals with ASD than in controls – with the changes in cortical thickness being related to higher ratings on ADI-R subdomains (Hardan *et al.* 2009a). In this study no differences in brain volume between individuals with ASD and controls were found to occur at either time-point – possibly reflecting the fact that these children were all older than the 2–4-year-olds within whom brain enlargement has previously been reported as occurring (Courchesne *et al.* 2001). The conduct of longitudinal imaging studies to definitively determine the timing of brain enlargement in ASD is clearly a priority.

The causes underlying enlarged brain volumes in autism remain unknown at present. Little work to determine these has as yet been conducted and there are no well replicated findings. It may be that differential trajectories of total brain volume exist for different subgroups of individuals with ASD. One study investigated brain volumes in subgroups of people with ASD and reported increased grey matter volume in adolescents with autism but not Asperger syndrome as compared to controls (Lotspeich *et al.* 2004). It has been reported in one study that there is a relationship between increased brain volume and a low activity genetic variant of monoamine oxidase A (Davis *et al.* 2008) which is an enzyme responsible for the breakdown of catecholamines in the brain. This would indicate the involvement of factors which are genetically controlled. The involvement of issues relating to monoamine oxidase A has been reported in a variety of mental health disorders over the years. A tantalising link between ASD genetics and brain volume involves the *PTEN* (Phosphatase and tensin homologue on chromosome ten) gene – mutations in which have been reported in individuals with ASD and macrocephaly (Butler *et al.* 2005). *Pten* mutant mice demonstrate neuronal hypertrophy, macrocephaly and abnormalities of social interaction with some parallels to certain aspects of the ASD phenotype (Kwon *et al.* 2006). An important caveat is that, even if replicated, such genetic findings do not indicate cause as such but rather a vulnerability which acting together with other factors – genetic and otherwise – may push an individual towards developing a condition.

Not only is the cause of brain enlargement and the evident abnormality of brain growth in ASD unclear but it is not known whether the same processes drive brain growth in ASD as in typically developing children. This raises the question as to whether the increase in brain size reported to occur in ASD represents an increase in normal growth processes or whether it is the product of some alternative process of abnormal neurodevelopment.

3.5.2 *Cerebral hemispheres*

Grey / white matter and lobar volumes

Overall the cerebrum is reported to be enlarged in ASD (Stanfield *et al.* 2008). What is less clear is the timing of the enlargement, whether it occurs to the same degree across all lobes and whether it is localised to one particular tissue compartment (grey matter or white matter).

Although there are few studies which have examined the relationship between age and cerebral volume, given that the cerebrum makes up approximately 90% of the total brain volume it is difficult to envisage a situation in which age would affect whole brain size and not total cerebral volume. There is, however, evidence that not all lobes of the cerebrum are affected equally. The vast majority of studies have found enlargements of either the grey or white matter compartments in the frontal, temporal and parietal lobes in individuals with ASD, although the evidence for the latter is less strong (Carper and Courchesne, 2000; Carper *et al.* 2002; Hazlett *et al.* 2005; 2006; Palmen *et al.* 2004; 2005). In contrast, there appears to be relative sparing of the occipital lobe with none of the aforementioned studies finding significant increases in either total occipital grey or white matter volume, although some did report trends towards significance (Hazlett *et al.* 2005; Palmen *et al.* 2004; 2005).

Although there is some inconsistency within the literature, increases in both the grey and the white matter compartments of the cerebrum have been reported to occur in ASD. Studies which have examined cortical (grey matter) thickness have found increases to occur in individuals with autism, which may account for the increased grey matter volume (Chung *et al.* 2005; Hardan *et al.* 2006c). An increase in the thickness of grey matter is consistent with post-mortem studies of autism and may be related to an increase in cell number or size (Bailey *et al.* 1998). As regards white matter, one study has suggested that regional differences may occur within an enlarged white matter compartment (Herbert *et al.* 2004). In this study the authors found an increase in volume in superficial (mainly lobar) white matter which was not seen in deeper white matter, including the corpus callosum and internal capsule. Myelination occurs in superficial white matter later and for longer than it does in deeper white matter, where it is usually complete by birth. The authors speculate that interference with myelination occurring post-natally, with a sparing of the process *in utero*, may have led to their results (Herbert *et al.* 2004), raising interesting questions about the timing of the insult.

It should be noted that in individuals who are not affected by autism, cerebral growth is dependent upon both region and tissue compartment, rather than proceeding in a uniform fashion throughout the brain (Giedd *et al.* 1999). This raises the possibility that in individuals with ASD the pattern of relative lobar and grey/white matter enlargement may depend on the age of the participants, with different lobes and compartments of the brain appearing enlarged at different times throughout development.

Frontal lobe sub-regions

The frontal lobe is considered to be the seat of executive function, which has frequently been found to be impaired in ASD (Hill, 2004). In addition, it is home to Broca's area, the main brain region involved in expressive language, and is involved in social cognition through connections with limbic regions. There is therefore good reason to suspect that individuals with ASD will show frontal lobe neuroanatomical differences in comparison with typically developing individuals. Indeed, VBM studies provide evidence of structural abnormality of frontal lobe structures in ASD – although conflicting findings are reported. These include reports of reductions (Abell *et al.* 1999) as well as increases (Rojas *et al.* 2006; Waiter *et al.* 2004) in grey matter and reduced white matter (Schmitz *et al.* 2008; Waiter *et al.* 2005) in frontal lobe regions.

A reversal of asymmetry of Broca's area has been found in two studies, such that the right side is greater in size than the left (De Fossé *et al.* 2004; Herbert *et al.* 2002), suggesting that an insult to the process of cerebral lateralisation may be important in autism. This finding gains indirect support from studies which have shown an increase in non-right handedness among individuals with ASD (Dane and Balci, 2007; Escalante-Mead *et al.* 2003). There is also some evidence that an increase in the size of the orbitofrontal cortex may be related to a greater degree of restricted and repetitive behaviours in individuals with ASD (Hardan *et al.* 2006b). This would be consistent with the rich connectivity between this region and the caudate nucleus, which is also found to be enlarged in ASD and associated with repetitive behaviours (Hollander *et al.* 2005; Rojas *et al.* 2006).

Cingulate cortex

The cingulate cortex is located on the medial surface of the human brain and runs parasagitally curving around the corpus callosum. In 1937, James Papez proposed that the cingulate cortex was critical to the subjective experience of emotions (Papez, 1937). The anterior cingulate cortex (ACC) has been extensively studied through electrophysiological, neuropathological and neuroimaging studies, and is believed to regulate a range of functions related to emotion, including autonomic functions such as blood pressure and heart rate, and cognitive functions such as reward and decision making (Bush *et al.* 2002). Recent reports suggest abnormal activation in the ACC in individuals with ASD in reward related fMRI paradigms (Schmitz *et al.* 2008) and emotion processing fMRI paradigms. In addition Chiu *et al.* (2008a) proposed that changes in anterior cingulate gyrus function were particularly associated with a dysfunction in self-referential processing.

Structural differences in the anterior cingulate cortex have been described in ASD. Haznedar and colleagues (Haznedar *et al.* 1997) divided the anterior cingulate cortex into three parts and found the dorsorostral region to be decreased in size whereas the dorsoventral region was increased in size in adults with ASD. Reductions in glucose metabolism in the dorsorostral region were also seen indicating a reduction in the activity of this region. Chiu and colleagues (Chiu *et al.* 2008b) found no difference in anterior cingulate volume in children with ASD but did not subdivide the structure so these findings may disguise the sub-regional differences described by Haznedar and colleagues (Haznedar *et al.* 1997). Several VBM studies have reported structural abnormalities of the cingulate gyrus (particularly the ACC) in ASD – including reports of reduced grey matter density (Kwon *et al.* 2004), increased grey matter volume (Waiter *et al.* 2004) and reduced white matter volume (Ke *et al.* 2008).

Lateral temporal lobe sub-regions

The fusiform face area (FFA) is located on the ventral surface of the temporal lobe and is involved in the processing of facial stimuli (Kanwisher *et al.* 1997). Impairments in facial affect recognition are well established in ASD and the FFA has been found to show altered activations when individuals with ASD view facial stimuli (Dalton *et al.* 2005; Deeley *et al.* 2007). Although there is some debate as to the nature of these functional differences in the FFA, VBM studies provide evidence of neuroanatomical abnormalities in the fusiform gyrus in ASD (Kwon *et al.* 2004; Waiter *et al.* 2004).

The superior temporal sulcus (STS) divides the superior and the middle temporal gyri (STG, MTG respectively). This region of the brain has long been known to be associated with auditory perception but more recently has been suggested to be important in the perception and initial analysis of more complex social stimuli, particularly those with a temporal component (Zilbovicius *et al.* 2006). Consistent with this idea, functional imaging studies have reported activation differences in the superior temporal sulcus region during emotion processing tasks in individuals with ASD (Freitag *et al.* 2008; Gervais *et al.* 2004; Hadjikhani *et al.* 2007; Herrington *et al.* 2007; Pelphrey *et al.* 2005).

From a structural perspective, a decrease in cortical thickness has been reported to occur around the superior temporal sulcus in individuals with autism, the degree of which was associated with the severity of the expressed autistic features (Hadjikhani *et al.* 2006). Anterior shifting of the relative position of the superior temporal sulcus within the brain has also been reported (Levitt *et al.* 2003). A number of VBM studies have reported structural abnormalities of superior temporal sulcal structures – including the STG and MTG – in ASD. These include findings of reduced (Boddaert *et al.* 2004) as well as increased STS grey matter (Waiter *et al.* 2004), reduced (McAlonan *et al.* 2005) as well as increased STG grey matter (Waiter *et al.* 2004), reduced (Brieber *et al.* 2007) as well as increased MTG grey matter (Abell *et al.* 1999), increased STG white matter (Spencer *et al.* 2006) and reduced MTG white matter (Waiter *et al.* 2005). Wernicke's area is a poorly defined region located at the posterior end of the superior temporal gyrus which is involved in receptive language functions. Some studies have identified a change to the asymmetry of the structures which make up Wernicke's area; however, conflicting findings as to the direction of this change are reported (Herbert *et al.* 2002; Rojas *et al.* 2002; 2005).

Parietal sub-regions

One study has reported grey matter deficits occurring in a network of cortical sites, including the medial parietal lobe bilaterally (McAlonan *et al.* 2005).

Increased grey matter within the left inferior parietal of individuals with ASD as compared to controls has been described (Brieber *et al.* 2007), in common with similar findings in individuals with attention deficit hyperactivity disorder (ADHD) as compared to controls as reported within the same study.

Occipital sub-regions

Two VBM studies of brain structure in ASD report conflicting findings of decreased (Abell *et al.* 1999) as opposed to increased (Waiter *et al.* 2004) grey matter density in the region of the left inferior occipital lobe and occipito-temporal junction. It may be that age-related effects account for this apparent difference, as participants in the study showing reduced grey matter density were a mean of approximately 12 years older than those in whom increased grey matter density was found.

Cerebral cortical folding

Anterior and superior shifting of a number of major frontal and temporal lobe sulci has been reported which authors have interpreted as representing an immature pattern of cortical development (Levitt *et al.* 2003). Another study found an increase in the depth of the frontal operculum in higher IQ individuals with autism, parietal operculum in those with lower IQ and intraparietal sulcus in those with Asperger syndrome (Nordahl *et al.* 2007). In addition, the depth of the intraparietal sulcus was positively correlated with the degree of repetitive behaviours in those with Asperger syndrome. A further study reported an increase in the left prefrontal gyrification index (i.e. greater cortical folding) in children and adolescents with autism relative to normal controls (Hardan *et al.* 2004). The same relationship was not seen in adults. Differences were also seen in the relationship between gyrification index and age with a negative association occurring in the controls but not in participants with autism, a finding consistent with the idea that the autistic brain continues to develop differently post-natally.

3.5.3 *Subcortical regions*

Amygdala and other medial temporal lobe findings

The amygdala is a collection of nuclei which lies in the medial temporal lobe, sitting just anterior to the hippocampus. It is known to play an important role in social cognition including the mediation of fear and arousal and the attribution of emotional valence to stimuli. There is evidence from functional neuroimaging studies that amygdala function is disturbed in individuals with autism, particularly with respect to emotion processing (Ashwin *et al.* 2007; Dalton *et al.* 2005; Pinkham *et al.* 2008; Williams *et al.* 2006).

Table 3.1 *Region of interest studies comparing amygdala volume between individuals with ASD and controls*

	ASD participants				Controls			
Study (year)	Diagnoses	N (M:F)	Age	IQ	N (M:F)	Age	IQ	Findings in ASD group
Sparks *et al.* (2002)	Autism	29 (26:3)	3.9	–	26 (18:8)	4.0	–	Enlarged in autism but not in PDD-NOS
	PDD-NOS	16 (12:4)	4.1	–				
Schumann *et al.* (2004)	LFA	18 (18:0)	13.1	56	22 (22:0)	13.1	115	Enlarged in 7.5–12.5-year-olds with HFA or LFA; no difference in 12.5–18.5-year-olds with HFA or LFA; non-significant enlargements in Asp
	HFA	21 (21:0)	12.7	91				
	Asp	24 (24:0)	13.0	106				
Nacewicz *et al.* (2006) Study ii*	Autism / Asp / PDD-NOS	16 (16:0), comprising 11 autism and 5 Asp/PDD-NOS	14.3	97	14 (14:0)	13.7	122	No difference in 8–12.5-year-olds; reduced in 12.5–21-year-olds
Nacewicz (2006) Study i*	Autism	12 (12:0)	16.8	–	12 (12:0)	17.0	–	No difference
Aylward *et al.* (1999)	Autism	14 (14:0)	20.5	106	14 (14:0)	20.3	109	Reduced
Boucher *et al.* (2005)	Autism	10 (10:0)	23.9	–	10 (10:0)	24.3	–	Enlarged
Haznedar *et al.* (2000)	Autism	17 (15:2)	27.7	55–125	17 (15:2)	28.8	88–136	No difference
Pierce *et al.* (2001)	Autism	7 (7:0)	29.5	84	8 (8:0)	28.3	–	Reduced
Rojas *et al.* (2004)	Autism	15 (13:2)	30.3	98	17 (8:9)	43.6	122	Reduced

Age and IQ given as means.

PDD-NOS –pervasive developmental disorder not otherwise specified; LFA – low functioning autism; HFA – high functioning autism; Asp – Asperger syndrome.

* Presented in the same paper.

–, data not provided.

As with structural neuroimaging findings for whole brain volume there is evidence to suggest that amygdala development may proceed differently in people with autism than it does in those with typical development. ROI findings concerning amygdala volume are summarised in Table 3.1.

The findings of most studies suggest that larger amygdalae are confined to younger people with autism, with older individuals showing no difference or even a reduction in volume as compared to controls (Schumann *et al.* 2004; Stanfield *et al.* 2008). Increased grey matter density in medial temporal lobe structures including the amygdala and the hippocampus may be associated with more severe parentally rated autistic symptomatology in children with ASD (Salmond *et al.* 2005). Early amygdala damage has been found to be associated with difficulties in aspects of social cognition whereas later damage has not (Shaw *et al.* 2004), suggesting that this early amygdala overgrowth may be important in the development of ASD. Furthermore, amygdala enlargement in young children has been reported to be correlated with impairments in social interaction (Schumann *et al.* 2009) and joint attention (Mosconi *et al.* 2009). It has been proposed that an enlarged amygdala in early life in people with ASD leads to chronic feelings of fear and a heightened stress response, which in turn cause damage to the amygdala and a subsequent reduction in size (Schumann and Amaral, 2006). The association between amygdala enlargement and anxiety in children with ASD (Juranek *et al.* 2006) adds weight to this hypothesis. In addition to demonstrating reduced amygdala volume in older but not younger children as compared to controls, Nacewicz and colleagues (2006) demonstrated correlations between reductions in amygdala volume and increased gaze avoidance and greater social impairment as measured by ADI-R subdomains. Related evidence for a central role of the amygdala in ASD comes from a gaze-tracking fMRI study which found that activation of the amygdala during face-processing tasks in ASD was strongly correlated with the time that the participant spent fixating the eye-regions of the stimuli (Dalton *et al.* 2005). This finding requires replication but nonetheless suggests that eye-fixation in ASD is highly emotionally salient and possibly aversive and that this may contribute to the impairment in eye contact frequently observed in ASD. Another potential link between amygdala structure and behavioural impairments in autism is suggested by a recent case report which documented a lack of inter-personal distance awareness in an individual with bilateral amygdala damage (Kennedy *et al.* 2009), which is particularly interesting given the fact that individuals with ASD often appear to display impaired judgement and/or modulation of inter-personal space.

Primarily involved in memory, the hippocampus has been variously shown to be enlarged, reduced or not different in size in ASD. However, in contrast to the amygdala, no significant effect of age has been found on the results and when the existing ROI studies were combined using meta-analytical techniques, no

Table 3.2 *Region of interest studies comparing corpus callosum size between individuals with ASD and controls*

	ASD participants				Controls			
Study (year)	Diagnoses	N (M:F)	Age	IQ	N (M:F)	Age	IQ	Findings in ASD group
Boger-Megiddo *et al.* (2006)	Autism	29 (26:3)	3.9	–	26 (18:8)	4.0	–	Reductions in anterior, middle and posterior regions in autism group, no difference for PDD-NOS
	PDD-NOS	16 (12:4)	4.1	–				
Vidal *et al.* (2006)	Autism	24 (24:0)	10.0	96	26 (26:0)	11.0	105	Reduction in anterior third
Elia *et al.* (2000)	Autism	22 (22:0)	10.9	'Mental age' 1.7 years	11 (11:0)	10.9	–	No difference
Gaffney *et al.* (1987a)	Autism	13 (10:3)	11.3	84.9	35 (21:14)	12.0	–	No difference
Manes *et al.* (1999)	Autism	27 (22:5)	14.3	'Mental age' 4.6 years	17 (11:6)	11.8	'Mental age' 4.5 years	General reductions throughout callosum
Kilian *et al.* (2008)	NC autism	28 (28:0)	14.6	97	20 (20:0) NC	13.6	102	Smaller anterior regions in NC autism; larger middle regions in MC regardless of autism status
	MC autism	13 (13:0)	12.6	114	8 (8:0) MC	12.4	122	
Egaas *et al.* (1995)	Autism	51 (45:6)	15.5	–	51 (45:6)	15.5	–	Reduction in posterior regions
Piven *et al.* (1997)	Autism	35 (26:9)	18.0	91	36 (20:16)	20.2	102	Reduction in middle and posterior regions
Hardan *et al.* (2000)	Autism	22 (22:0)	22.4	100	22 (22:0)	22.4	101	Reduction in anterior regions
Hardan *et al.* (2009b)	Autism/ PDD-NOS	22 (22:0)	10.7	95.1	23 (23:0)	10.5	116	Reduction overall and in several subdivisions, particularly posteriorly

Age and IQ given as means.
PDD-NOS – pervasive developmental disorder not otherwise specified; NC – normocephalic; MC – macrocephalic.
–, data not provided.

significant difference in hippocampal volume was identified between people with autism and controls (Stanfield *et al.* 2008). VBM studies have reported increased grey matter volume in the hippocampus in individuals with ASD (Rojas *et al.* 2006), and these differences may be related to increased autistic symptomatology (Salmond *et al.* 2005).

In contrast to the interest in the amygdala and hippocampus the parahippocampal gyrus has been considered in only one ROI study of 10 participants and has been found to be reduced in volume (Boucher *et al.* 2005). This finding gains support from VBM studies which have identified reduced grey matter volume in this structure (Ke *et al.* 2008). However, such results require replication before they can be considered to be reliable.

Corpus callosum findings

The corpus callosum (see Figures 3.1 and 3.2) is the largest white matter tract in the human brain and serves interhemispheric communication between homologous cortical areas. Its fibres are mainly myelinated and are topographically organised such that the different sub-regions contain axons from different areas of the cortex (Witelson, 1989). Reductions in the size of the corpus callosum may therefore represent a specific reduction in interhemispheric connectivity, a more generalised reduction in the size of the cerebral areas from which the fibres originate and/or reductions in the degree of myelination of the callosal axons.

ROI studies, summarised in Table 3.2, have consistently found the total corpus callosum to be reduced in cross-sectional area in autism (Stanfield *et al.* 2008), although whether these reductions are confined to specific callosal sub-regions is less clear (Egaas *et al.* 1995; Manes *et al.* 1999; Piven *et al.* 1997; Vidal *et al.* 2006). Using VBM Chung and colleagues (Chung *et al.* 2004) found reduced white matter concentration in both the anterior and posterior callosum, while Waiter and colleagues (Waiter *et al.* 2005) found white matter volume deficits in similar areas. Recent studies have demonstrated associations between corpus callosum volume reductions and social impairments, repetitive behaviours, sensory deficits and impaired performance on executive function tasks (Hardan *et al.* 2009b; Keary *et al.* 2009).

Thalamus findings

The thalamus is widely recognised as a key structure in many neural pathways and is of particular relevance to the study of autistic features, given its central role in information processing within the brain. There are a number of recent reports of reduced thalamic volume in individuals with ASD, including VBM findings of reduced grey matter (Spencer *et al.* 2006; Waiter *et al.* 2004) as

Table 3.3 *Region of interest studies comparing caudate size between individuals with ASD and controls*

	ASD participants				Controls			
Study (year)	Diagnoses	N (M:F)	Age	IQ	N (M:F)	Age	IQ	Findings in ASD group
Aylward *et al.* (1999)	Autism	11 (11:0)	29	–	25 (19:6)	32	–	No difference
Hardan *et al.* (2003)	Autism	40 (38:2)	19.3	103	41 (39:2)	18.6	104	No difference
Hollander *et al.* (2005)	Autism/Asp/ PDD-NOS	17 (15:2)	28.4	97	17 (15:2)	29.4	112	Increased
McAlonan *et al.* (2002)	Asp	21 (19:2)	32	96	24 (22:2)	33	114	No difference
Sears *et al.* (1999) Study i*	Autism	35 (26:9)	18.0	91	36 (20:16)	20.2	102	Increased
Sears (1999) Study ii*	Autism	13 (13:0)	–	–	25 (25:0)	–	–	Increased
Haznedar *et al.* (2006)	Autism/Asp	17 (15:2)	27.7	97	17 (15:2)	28.8	112	Increased right caudate in autism; no difference in Asp
Langen *et al.* (2007) Study i**	Autism/Asp	21 (21:0)	11.1	107	21 (21:0)	10.4	103	Increased
Langen (2007) Study ii**	Autism/Asp	21 (19:2)	20.1	115	21 (20:1)	17.3	113	Increased

Age and IQ given as means.

PDD-NOS – pervasive developmental disorder not otherwise specified; Asp – Asperger syndrome.

*,**Presented in the same paper.

–, data not provided.

illustrated in Figure 3.3, and reduced thalamic volume using manual tracing techniques (Tsatsanis *et al.* 2003).

Several studies have identified a lack of the normal positive relationship between brain size and thalamus volume in ASD (Hardan *et al.* 2006a; Hardan *et al.* 2008; Tsatsanis *et al.* 2003), suggesting that the increase in cortical volume in ASD may not be paralleled by an increase in cortico-subcortical connectivity, as would be expected in typically developing individuals.

Basal ganglia findings

There is a general consensus that the caudate is increased in volume in people with ASD (Brambilla *et al.* 2003; Stanfield *et al.* 2008) and findings are summarised in Table 3.3.

As mentioned earlier, the caudate and the oribitofrontal cortex are richly connected and enlargements of both have been found to be positively associated with the degree of restricted and repetitive behaviours in ASD (Hardan *et al.* 2006b; Hollander *et al.* 2005; Rojas *et al.* 2006) suggesting that an abnormality in the structure of this circuit may underlie the development of such behaviours. This is reminiscent of the fronto-striatial dysfunction reported to occur in obsessive-compulsive disorder (van den Heuvel *et al.* 2005). It should be noted that Rojas and colleagues (Rojas *et al.* 2006) also reported that caudate size was positively related to the degree of social impairment and communication indicating that the effects of its dysfunction may not be confined solely to repetitive patterns of behaviour.

Results for other sub-regions of the basal ganglia are less consistent – with one study (Hollander *et al.* 2005) but not others (Hardan *et al.* 2003; Herbert *et al.* 2003) reporting an increase in putamen volume.

3.5.4 *Cerebellar findings*

The contribution of the cerebellum to non-motor processes has been increasingly recognised in recent years. The cerebellum is extensively connected to many non-motor areas of the brain and a detailed characterisation of cognitive features in patients with cerebellar lesions reported a range of deficits including impaired executive function, impaired visual–spatial memory and language impairments. These effects appeared to amount to 'a general lowering of intellectual function' (Schmahmann and Sherman, 1998).

Post-mortem studies of the cerebellum have consistently identified a loss of Purkinje cells in the cerebellar hemispheres in autism (Bauman and Kemper, 2005) and a reduction in the midsagittal area of the neocerebellar vermis was one of the first quantitative neuroanatomical abnormalities reported in ASD (Courchesne *et al.* 1988). This finding has been replicated (Hashimoto *et al.* 1995), however, it has been argued that vermal reductions may reflect differences in IQ between cases and controls as opposed to being associated with autism *per se*. Investigations of cerebellar vermis volume in ASD have revealed often conflicting findings and opposing directions of volume changes in different lobule areas within the vermis. However, combining existing reported findings together suggests that younger individuals with ASD show reductions in the cerebellar vermis which are not seen in older individuals (Stanfield *et al.* 2008), a pattern opposite in direction to that suggested for the whole brain. Although this may seem paradoxical it is consistent with the finding that the frontal lobe and the neocerebellar vermis show a reciprocal relationship with respect to size (Carper and Courchesne, 2000). In contrast to the vermis, studies of the cerebellar hemispheres tend to show an increase in volume, despite the post-mortem evidence of reduced cell number; whether it shows the same pattern of growth that is suggested for the whole brain volume is unknown (Hardan *et al.* 2001a; Herbert *et al.* 2003; Sparks *et al.* 2002).

Unsurprisingly, the cerebellum is an area within which structural abnormalities have been reported in a number of VBM studies of ASD. Several studies report increased grey matter within the cerebellum (Abell *et al.* 1999) and some studies also report reductions in grey matter (McAlonan *et al.* 2002; Rojas *et al.* 2006) and reductions in cerebellar white matter volume (Boddaert *et al.* 2004; McAlonan *et al.* 2005). It has furthermore been reported that reduced cerebellar grey matter volume is associated with increased repetitive and stereotyped behaviours in autism (Rojas *et al.* 2006). There is evidence that grey matter volume in the cerebellum may be differentially affected in ASD according to the level of intellectual functioning. Salmond and colleagues (Salmond *et al.* 2007) found that while individuals with ASD of below average intellectual functioning demonstrated reduced cerebellar grey matter density, increased grey matter density was evident in those of higher intellectual functioning.

These cerebellar findings are consistent with reports within the functional MRI literature which document differences in cerebellar function in individuals with autism during motor (Allen and Courchesne, 2003; Allen *et al.* 2004) and emotion processing tasks (Critchley *et al.* 2000).

3.5.5 *Brainstem findings*

The brainstem is made up primarily of three regions: the medulla, pons and midbrain. Although these brain regions received significant early interest they have been little considered in recent neuroimaging studies of ASD. Reductions in the size of these regions have been found in some studies, although these mainly concerned cross-sectional areas and findings are heterogeneous (Stanfield *et al.* 2008) and therefore ought to be interpreted with caution. Findings of one recent study suggest that reductions in total brainstem grey matter are correlated with greater oral sensory symptom severity in children with ASD (Jou *et al.* 2009), possibly reflecting the sensory involvement of brainstem structures such as the nuclei of the vagus nerve, the innervations of which are widespread and include the palate, pharynx and larynx.

3.6 Diffusion tensor imaging studies

Recent years have seen a considerable expansion in the investigation of white matter structure and connectivity in ASD using DTI. Findings to date suggest that this technique holds promise in identifying disrupted connectivity between brain areas subserving cognitive domains that are particularly central to the ASD phenotype, and in demonstrating correlations between DTI findings and clinical symptomatology.

The DTI investigation of structural connectivity between areas subserving social intelligence finds reports of reduced fractional anisotropy (FA) in the proximity of the superior temporal sulcus, temporal stem and amygdala (Barnea-Goraly *et al.* 2004; Lee *et al.* 2007), as well differences in limbic tract volume in ASD as compared to controls (Pugliese *et al.* 2009). Furthermore, Conturo and colleagues (Conturo *et al.* 2008) identified reduced diffusivity in the right hippocampal-fusiform pathway and demonstrated that this abnormality was related to important behavioural measures – namely impaired face recognition and block design object processing.

A number of studies have investigated the relationship between altered connectivity in ASD and the severity of clinical symptoms – such as repetitive behaviours and social impairment – as measured by the ADI-R. In this way it has been reported that higher ADI-R ratings of repetitive behaviours are associated with reduced FA in the right anterior cingulate cortex (Thakkar *et al.* 2008) as well as a range of more posterior brain regions including the splenium of the corpus callosum, the temporo-parietal lobe and the cerebellum (Cheung *et al.* 2009). ADI-R ratings of impaired social interaction have been related to reduced FA in the left superior cerebellar peduncle (Catani *et al.* 2008), which the authors hypothesised as possibly reflecting impaired feedback from the cerebellum and hence a reduction in the ability of such inputs from the cerebellum to modify social behaviour. This finding is concordant with other reports of reduced FA in the left superior cerebellar puduncle in ASD (Brito *et al.* 2009). Impaired social interaction and abnormalities in communication, as measured by the ADI-R, have also been related to reduced FA within fronto-striatal and posterior corpus callosal regions (Cheung *et al.* 2009).

Studies have reported reduced FA in the region of the corpus callosum (Alexander *et al.* 2007; Brito *et al.* 2009; Keller *et al.* 2007), with these findings being related to reduced cognitive performance on measures of performance IQ. Further studies have reported abnormal frontal fibre connectivity (Sundaram *et al.* 2008; Sahyoun *et al.* 2010), as well as suggesting abnormal trajectories of white matter maturation in young children with ASD – particularly within left frontal regions – comprising accelerated age-related increases in FA (Ben-Bashat *et al.* 2007).

This structural evidence for dysconnectivity in ASD finds further support from functional imaging studies which have identified a mixture of under- and over-connectivity between brain regions in ASD – such as the finding of reduced functional connectivity between the fusiform gyrus and frontal regions during face-processing tasks (Koshino *et al.* 2008). Functional dysconnectivity involving the fusiform gyrus in terms of reduced connectivity with the left amygdala and increased connectivity with the right inferior frontal gyrus during face-processing tasks has also been reported to be correlated with greater degrees of social impairment (Kleinhans *et al.* 2008).

3.7 Neuroanatomical findings in females with ASD

There are only two studies to date which have specifically examined the neuroanatomy of women with ASD. Both have found broadly similar findings to those in males (Bloss and Courchesne, 2007; Craig *et al.* 2007); however, Bloss and Courchesne identified more extensive temporal and cerebellar abnormalities in the female group, suggesting that a greater degree of disruption to brain structure may be associated with the expression of ASD in women than in men. If replicated, these findings may represent a neuroanatomical reflection of the hypothesis that females with autism are affected by a greater degree of 'genetic loading' than males with autism (Tsai *et al.* 1981; Tsai and Beisler, 1983).

There is an established gender related dimorphism of brain structure and development in typically developing individuals (Allen *et al.* 2003; Giedd, 2004; Giedd *et al.* 1999; Goldstein *et al.* 2001; Gur *et al.* 1999; Haier *et al.* 2005; Im *et al.* 2006; Nopoulos *et al.* 2000), therefore it is important that future studies examine further the effects of gender on brain structure in groups with ASD. Given the proposal that autism may represent an extreme form of male intelligence (Asperger, 1944; Baron-Cohen *et al.* 2005) the identification of gender specific brain structural differences in individuals with ASD may well provide information regarding important aetiological and pathogenetic processes across the autism spectrum.

3.8 'Low-functioning' autism, 'high-functioning' autism, Asperger syndrome and non-specific pervasive developmental disorders

Until this point no distinction has been made between the disorders which are considered to make up the autism spectrum. In the main this is reflective of the original research in which disorders from across the spectrum are often combined as a uniform group. Given that even distinguishing between individuals with ASD and unaffected individuals can at times be difficult, and that there is likely to be significant heterogeneity even within each diagnostic category, the validity of defining different components of the autism spectrum is unclear. The boundary between autism and Asperger syndrome can be clinically difficult to establish and the place of non-specific pervasive developmental disorders (PDD-NOS) on the spectrum is even less clear. Finally, as alluded to earlier, the picture is further complicated by the issue of IQ, with some groups distinguishing 'low'- and 'high'-functioning autism on the basis of the generally held IQ cut-off for intellectual disability (i.e. IQ less than 70). Although several groups, as described below, have attempted to address these difficulties in classification using structural neuroimaging, more research is required before any firm conclusions can be drawn.

One group has published a series of studies examining a population of children and adolescent males with either 'low-functioning' autism (LFA), 'high-functioning' autism (HFA) or Asperger syndrome. The LFA and HFA groups were found to have significantly more cortical grey matter than controls, with individuals with Asperger syndrome showing non-significant enlargements relative to controls (Lotspeich *et al.* 2004). In addition, the relationship between performance IQ and cortical grey matter volume was found to differ significantly between the HFA and the Asperger syndrome groups (Lotspeich *et al.* 2004). A similar pattern was also found for hippocampal volumes across the whole age range of this group, whereas for the amygdala it was only seen in the younger participants (Schumann *et al.* 2004). The LFA, HFA and Asperger syndrome groups were also found to show differences in sulcal depth compared to controls; notably these differences were not seen in the same sulci. Finally, VBM was used in a subset of these participants to compare individuals with HFA and Asperger syndrome with the former showing greater grey matter density in the cingulate gyrus compared to the latter (Kwon *et al.* 2004).

Other groups have compared brain structure between the different components of the autism spectrum disorders and have also identified similarities and differences between such groups. Sparks and colleagues (Sparks *et al.* 2002) found that the amygdala was enlarged in young children with autism as compared to those with PDD-NOS, but did not identify any difference in cerebral, cerebellar or hippocampal volumes – results which partially replicate but generally contrast with those described above. Salmond and colleagues (2007) compared LFA and HFA using VBM and found that while both groups shared differences in parts of the cerebellum, fusiform gyrus and frontal cortex as compared to controls, when they were directly compared to each other they demonstrated differences in other parts of the cerebellum, dorsolateral prefrontal cortex and post-central gyrus.

3.9 Conclusions and future directions

Perhaps the most striking feature of the ASD neuroimaging literature is the heterogeneity of the findings to date (Stanfield *et al.* 2008). As discussed earlier, there are a number of factors inherent to ASD that are likely to lead to this variability including the descriptive nature of the diagnosis, the co-morbidity with intellectual disability and with other neurological disorders and possible gender related differences in brain structure. In addition, some studies have examined relatively small populations thus also tending to increase the heterogeneity of findings. Future studies should deal with these difficulties through the examination of large populations, probably recruited through multi-centre collaborations (Belmonte *et al.* 2008). The UK Medical Research Council Autism Imaging Multi-Centre Study (MRC-AIMS) – involving the Institute of Psychiatry, London and the Universities of Cambridge and Oxford – is the first UK multi-centre imaging collaboration in autism research and is currently underway. Such multi-centre collaborations will be increasingly important in the future, particularly with the advent of imaging genetics and consequently the greater importance of large sample sizes. The use of tightly defined clinical cohorts will also help to reduce heterogeneity, facilitate comparisons between studies and allow for the accurate examination of the structural underpinnings of specific autistic traits. This approach may be particularly fruitful given recent suggestions that the features which make up the autistic triad may not be as tightly associated as was originally thought (Happé *et al.* 2006). Studies which directly compare the different conditions which make up the autism spectrum are also required as are studies to determine the boundaries of the spectrum in relation to other related conditions. In addition, further studies of females with ASD and of individuals with ASD and low IQ are required so that the literature becomes more representative of the generality of the autistic population. The selection of an appropriate control group for the study of individuals with ASD and low IQ is imperative. Perhaps the closest to a 'perfect' situation will be the concurrent use of two control groups – one matched to the main subject group for IQ and one containing typically developing individuals.

Most groups exclude individuals with a history of epilepsy or cerebral palsy and, in view of the difficulties in the interpretation of imaging findings (highlighted above) raised by these potential confounding factors, this exclusion seems justified. The decision as to whether to exclude participants with other co-morbid conditions such as attention deficit hyperactivity disorder (ADHD) – which one study employing structured assessments within a population-derived sample found to occur in 28% of participants with ASD (Simonoff *et al.* 2008) – is more difficult. On the one hand structural brain abnormalities are well documented in ADHD (Castellanos *et al.* 2002; Sowell *et al.* 2003) – hence the potential role of ADHD as a confounding factor in neuroimaging studies. However, the suggestion that shared biological pathways may exist between autistic and ADHD traits (Ronald *et al.* 2010) would support a view that participants with co-morbid ADHD and ASD should be studied in order to elucidate potentially important pathways in the aetiology of ASD. The issue of the composition of participant groups with respect to co-morbidity is a challenging one and ought to be the subject of continuing debate.

Bearing in mind these difficulties, there are a number of themes that can be drawn from the existing structural neuroimaging literature on ASD. Increasingly the evidence points to the presence of structural abnormalities in areas of the social brain including the amygdala, superior temporal sulcus, fusiform face area and the orbitofrontal cortex. Structural change to the caudate nucleus has also been consistently identified and may be related to the development of the characteristic patterns of restricted and repetitive behaviours seen in ASD, possibly through its relationship with the orbitofrontal cortex. In addition to the differences identified within specific brain regions, the findings from recent DTI studies suggest that the effects of aberrant connectivity between distributed areas of the brain are also likely to be important. Finally, although the evidence at present comes overwhelmingly from cross-sectional studies, there is an increasing consensus that individuals with ASD show differences in longitudinal brain development compared to those which occur in typically developing individuals.

In addition to addressing the difficulties mentioned above, future studies of ASD should aim to confirm and build upon existing findings. It is clear that longitudinal studies, some of which are already underway (Hazlett *et al.* 2005), are needed to either confirm or refute the suggestion that individuals with ASD show a different developmental trajectory to typically developing individuals. A longitudinal neuroimaging study of very young infants at high risk of developing ASD could be of particular benefit. Such studies are likely to be ethically and practically difficult; however, given their success in the examination of other conditions (Johnstone *et al.* 2005; Pantelis *et al.* 2003), they could prove to play a key role in unravelling the pathophysiological processes which lead to the development of ASD.

Furthermore, attempts to link brain structure to proposed aetiological factors are required. As new putative risk factors for ASD are identified through genomic techniques such as whole genome analysis for the detection of single nucleotide polymorphisms and copy number variations, neuroanatomical data will continue to be central to assessing the aetiological significance of these genetic factors. The search for specific gene-to-structure associates holds great promise of yielding new insight into the aetiology of ASD, including risk factors associated with the condition and the neuroanatomical associates of possible endophenotypes and extended phenotypes of ASD.

Finally, although recent years have brought significant technological advances, there remain limitations to the inferences that can be drawn from neuroimaging data. While it is possible to say that a structure differs in size, shape or density, one can often only speculate as to the actual changes to brain microstructure which underlie these differences. The development of DTI is a welcome step towards the *in vivo* determination of underlying microstructural abnormalities; however, the technology must advance considerably before it will allow firm conclusions to be drawn based upon neuroimaging findings alone. There is no prospect at present that technical advances in imaging will provide definition at a cellular level in the living subject. It is perhaps instructive to bear in mind that even with the promise that modern imaging technology has brought to the study of ASD, we must still turn to post-mortem tissue examination to establish the cellular and molecular basis of structural changes identified using brain imaging techniques.

3.10 Final remarks

The use of magnetic resonance imaging has led to significant advances in the understanding of the brain anatomy which underlies ASD. The prospect of future discoveries, relating to methodological and technological advances, makes this an exciting area of study to be involved in from a scientific perspective. At the last, however, it is important to remember why this research is conducted – for the benefit of affected individuals and their families. A greater understanding of the brain structures which underlie neurodevelopmental conditions such as ASD is vital in order to enable the focused study of their neurobiological underpinnings, and is therefore likely to form an important part of the journey towards eventually making real and measurable differences to the lives of individuals affected by these disorders.

3.11 Acknowledgements

MDS is funded by a Clinician Scientist Fellowship from the Medical Research Council, and ACS is funded by a Research Training Fellowship from the Wellcome Trust.

3.12 References

Abell, F., Krams, M., Ashburner, J., *et al.* (1999). The neuroanatomy of autism: a voxel-based whole brain analysis of structural scans. *Neuroreport*, **10**: 1647–1651.

Alexander, A.L., Lee, J.E., Lazar, M., *et al.* (2007). Diffusion tensor imaging of the corpus callosum in autism. *Neuroimage*, **34**: 61–73.

Allen, G., Courchesne, E. (2003). Differential effects of developmental cerebellar abnormality on cognitive and motor functions in the cerebellum: an fMRI study of autism. *American Journal of Psychiatry*, **160**: 262–273.

Allen, G., Muller, R.A., Courchesne, E. (2004). Cerebellar function in autism: functional magnetic resonance image activation during a simple motor task. *Biological Psychiatry*, **56**: 269–278.

Allen, J.S., Damasio, H., Grabowski, T.J., Bruss, J., Zhang, W. (2003). Sexual dimorphism and asymmetries in the gray-white composition of the human cerebrum. *Neuroimage*, **18**: 880–894.

Alzheimer, A. (1897). Beitrage zur pathologischen anatomie der hirnrinde und zur anatoischen grundlage der psychosen. *Monatsschrift für Psychiatrie und Neurologie*, **2**: 82–120.

American Association on Intellectual and Developmental Disabilities. (2010). *Intellectual Disability: Definition, Classification, and Systems Of Supports*, 11th edn. Washington: AAIDD.

American Psychiatric Association. (2000). *Diagnostic and Statistical Manual of Mental Disorders, 4th edn, Text Revised (DSM-IV TR)*. Washington, DC: American Psychiatric Association.

Ashburner, J., Friston, K.J. (2000). Voxel-based morphometry – the methods. *Neuroimage*, **11**: 805–821.

Ashwin, C., Baron-Cohen, S., Wheelwright, S., O'Riordan, M., Bullmore, E.T. (2007). Differential activation of the amygdala and the 'social brain' during fearful face-processing in Asperger Syndrome. *Neuropsychologia*, **45**: 2–14.

Asperger, H. (1944). Die 'Autistichen Psychopathen' im Kindersalter. *Archive für Psychiatrie und Nervenkrankheiten*, **117**: 76–136.

Aylward, E.H., Schwartz, J., Machlin, S., Pearlson, G. (1991). Bicaudate ratio as a measure of caudate volume on MR images. *American Journal of Neuroradiology*, **12**: 1217–1222.

Aylward, E.H., Minshew, N.J., Goldstein, G., *et al.* (1999). MRI volumes of amygdala and hippocampus in non-mentally retarded autistic adolescents and adults. *Neurology*, **53**: 2145–2150.

Aylward, E.H., Minshew, N.J., Field, K., Sparks, B.F., Singh, N. (2002). Effects of age on brain volume and head circumference in autism. *Neurology*, **59**: 175–183.

Bailey, A., Luthert, P., Dean, A., *et al.* (1998). A clinicopathological study of autism. *Brain*, **121**: 889–905.

Balottin, U., Bejor, M., Cecchini, A., *et al.* (1989). Infantile autism and computerized tomography brain-scan findings: specific versus nonspecific abnormalities. *Journal of Autism and Developmental Disorders*, **19**: 109–117.

Barnea-Goraly, N., Kwon, H., Menon, V., *et al.* (2004). White matter structure in autism: preliminary evidence from diffusion tensor imaging. *Biological Psychiatry*, **55**: 323–326.

Baron-Cohen, S., Knickmeyer, R.C., Belmonte, M.K. (2005). Sex differences in the brain: implications for explaining autism. *Science*, **310**: 819–823.

Basser, P.J., Mattiello, J., LeBihan, D. (1994). MR diffusion tensor spectroscopy and imaging. *Biophysical Journal*, **66**: 259–267.

Battaglia, A., Carey, J.C. (2006). Etiologic yield of autistic spectrum disorders: A prospective study. *American Journal of Medical Genetics Part C: Seminars in Medical Genetics*, **142**: 3–7.

Bauman, M.L., Kemper, T.L. (1997). Is autism a progressive process? *Neurology*, **48** (Suppl.): 285.

Bauman, M.L., Kemper, T.L. (2005). Neuroanatomic observations of the brain in autism: a review and future directions. *International Journal of Developmental Neuroscience*, **23**: 183–187.

Belmonte, M.K., Mazziotta, J.C., Minshew, N.J., *et al.* (2008). Offering to share: how to put heads together in autism neuroimaging. *Journal of Autism and Developmental Disorders*, **38**: 2–13.

Ben-Bashat, D., Kronfeld-Duenias, V., Zachor, D.A., *et al.* (2007). Accelerated maturation of white matter in young children with autism: a high b value DWI study. *Neuroimage*, **37**: 40–47.

Berthier, M.L., Starkstein, S.E., Leiguarda, R. (1990). Developmental cortical anomalies in Asperger's syndrome: neuroradiological findings in two patients. *Journal of Neuropsychiatry and Clinical Neurosciences*, **2**: 197–201.

Blanton, R.E., Levitt, J.G., Thompson, P.M., *et al.* (2001). Mapping cortical asymmetry and complexity patterns in normal children. *Psychiatry Research*, **107**: 29–43.

Bloss, C.S., Courchesne, E. (2007). MRI neuroanatomy in young girls with autism: a preliminary study. *Journal of the American Academy of Child and Adolescent Psychiatry*, **46**: 515–523.

Boddaert, N., Chabane, N., Gervais, H., *et al.* (2004). Superior temporal sulcus anatomical abnormalities in childhood autism: a voxel-based morphometry MRI study. *Neuroimage*, **23**: 364–369.

Boger-Megiddo, I., Shaw, D.W., Friedman, S.D., *et al.* (2006). Corpus callosum morphometrics in young children with autism spectrum disorder. *Journal of Autism and Developmental Disorders*, **36**: 733–739.

Boucher, J., Cowell, P., Howard, M., *et al.* (2005). A combined clinical, neuropsychological, and neuroanatomical study of adults with high functioning autism. *Cognitive Neuropsychiatry*, **10**: 165–213.

Brambilla, P., Hardan, A., di Nemi, S.U., *et al.* (2003). Brain anatomy and development in autism: review of structural MRI studies. *Brain Research Bulletin*, **61**: 557–569.

Brieber, S., Neufang, S., Bruning, N., *et al.* (2007). Structural brain abnormalities in adolescents with autism spectrum disorder and patients with attention deficit/hyperactivity disorder. *Journal of Child Psychology and Psychiatry*, **48**: 1251–1258.

Brierley, B., Shaw, P., David, A.S. (2002). The human amygdala: a systematic review and meta-analysis of volumetric magnetic resonance imaging. *Brain Research Reviews*, **39**: 84–105.

Brito, A.R., Vasconcelos, M.M., Domingues, R.C., *et al.* (2009). Diffusion tensor imaging findings in school-aged autistic children. *Journal of Neuroimaging*, **19**: 337–343.

Bruggemann, J.M., Wilke, M., Som, S.S., *et al.* (2009). Voxel-based morphometry in the detection of dysplasia and neoplasia in childhood epilepsy: limitations of grey matter analysis. *Journal of Clinical Neuroscience*, **16**: 780–785.

Bush, G., Vogt, B.A., Holmes, J., *et al.* (2002). Dorsal anterior cingulate cortex: a role in reward-based decision making. *Proceedings of the National Academy of Sciences USA*, **99**: 523–528.

Butler, M.G., Dasouki, M.J., Zhou, X.P., *et al.* (2005). Subset of individuals with autism spectrum disorders and extreme macrocephaly associated with germline PTEN tumour suppressor gene mutations. *Journal of Medical Genetics*, **42**: 318–321.

Carper, R.A., Courchesne, E. (2000). Inverse correlation between frontal lobe and cerebellum sizes in children with autism. *Brain*, **123**: 836–844.

Carper, R.A., Moses, P., Tigue, Z.D., Courchesne, E. (2002). Cerebral lobes in autism: early hyperplasia and abnormal age effects. *Neuroimage*, **16**: 1038–1051.

Castellanos, F.X., Lee, P.P., Sharp, W., *et al.* (2002).Developmental trajectories of brain volume abnormalities in children and adolescents with attention-deficit/hyperactivity disorder. *Journal of the American Medical Association*, **288**: 1740–1748.

Catani, M., Jones, D.K., Daly, E., *et al.* (2008). Altered cerebellar feedback projections in Asperger syndrome. *Neuroimage*, **41**: 1184–1191.

Chakrabarti, S., Fombonne, E. (2005). Pervasive developmental disorders in preschool children: confirmation of high prevalence. *American Journal of Psychiatry*, **162**: 1133–1141.

Cheung, C., Chua, S.E., Cheung, V., *et al.* (2009). White matter fractional anisotrophy differences and correlates of diagnostic symptoms in autism. *Journal of Child Psychology and Psychiatry*, **50**: 1102–1112.

Chiu, P.H., Kayali, M.A., Kishida, K.T., *et al.* (2008a). Self responses along cingulate cortex reveal quantitative neural phenotype for high-functioning autism. *Neuron*, **57**: 463–473.

Chiu, S., Widjaja, F., Bates, M.E., *et al.* (2008b). Anterior cingulate volume in pediatric bipolar disorder and autism. *Journal of Affective Disorders*, **105**: 93–99.

Chung, M.K., Dalton, K.M., Alexander, A.L., Davidson, R.J. (2004). Less white matter concentration in autism: 2D voxel-based morphometry. *Neuroimage*, **23**: 242–251.

Chung, M.K., Robbins, S.M., Dalton, K.M., *et al.* (2005). Cortical thickness analysis in autism with heat kernel smoothing. *Neuroimage*, **25**: 1256–1265.

Conturo, T.E., Lori, N.F., Cull, T.S., *et al.* (1999). Tracking neuronal fiber pathways in the living human brain. *Proceedings of the National Academy of Sciences USA*, **96**: 10422–10427.

Conturo, T.E., Williams, D.L., Smith, C.D., *et al.* (2008). Neuronal fiber pathway abnormalities in autism: an initial MRI diffusion tensor tracking study of hippocampo-fusiform and amygdalo-fusiform pathways. *Journal of the International Neuropsychological Society*, **14**: 933–946.

Courchesne, E. (2002). Abnormal early brain development in autism. *Molecular Psychiatry*, **7** (Suppl. 2): S21-S23.

Courchesne, E., Yeung-Courchesne, R., Press, G.A., Hesselink, J.R., Jernigan, T.L. (1988). Hypoplasia of cerebellar vermal lobules VI and VII in autism. *New England Journal of Medicine*, **318**: 1349–1354.

Courchesne, E., Karns, C.M., Davis, H.R., *et al.* (2001). Unusual brain growth patterns in early life in patients with autistic disorder: an MRI study. *Neurology*, **57**: 245–254.

Courchesne, E., Carper, R., Akshoomoff, N. (2003). Evidence of brain overgrowth in the first year of life in autism. *Journal of the American Medical Association*, **290**: 337–344.

Craig, M.C., Zaman, S.H., Daly, E.M., *et al.* (2007). Women with autistic-spectrum disorder: magnetic resonance imaging study of brain anatomy. *British Journal of Psychiatry*, **191**: 224–228.

Critchley, H.D., Daly, E.M., Bullmore, E.T., *et al.* (2000). The functional neuroanatomy of social behaviour: changes in cerebral blood flow when people with autistic disorder process facial expressions. *Brain*, **123**: 2203–2212.

Dabbs, K., Jones, J., Seidenberg, M., Hermann, B. (2009). Neuroanatomical correlates of cognitive phenotypes in temporal lobe epilepsy. *Epilepsy and Behavior*, **15**: 445–451.

Dalton, K.M., Nacewicz, B.M., Johnstone, T., *et al.* (2005). Gaze fixation and the neural circuitry of face processing in autism. *Nature Neuroscience*, **8**: 519–526.

Damasio, H., Maurer, R.G., Damasio, A.R., Chui, H.C. (1980). Computerized tomographic scan findings in patients with autistic behavior. *Archives of Neurology*, **37**: 504–510.

Dane, S., Balci, N. (2007). Handedness, eyedness and nasal cycle in children with autism. *International Journal of Developmental Neuroscience*, **25**: 223–226.

Davis, L.K., Hazlett, H.C., Librant, A.L., *et al.* (2008). Cortical enlargement in autism is associated with a functional VNTR in the monoamine oxidase A gene. *American Journal of Medical Genetics Part B: Neuropsychiatric Genetics*, **147B**: 1145–1151.

Dawson, G., Munson, J., Webb, S.J., *et al.* (2007). Rate of head growth decelerates and symptoms worsen in the second year of life in autism. *Biological Psychiatry*, **61**: 458–464.

De Fossé, L., Hodge, S.M., Makris, N., *et al.* (2004). Language-association cortex asymmetry in autism and specific language impairment. *Annals of Neurology*, **56**: 757–766.

Decobert, F., Grabar, S., Merzoug, V., *et al.* (2005). Unexplained mental retardation: is brain MRI useful? *Pediatric Radiology*, **35**: 587–596.

Deeley, Q., Daly, E.M., Surguladze, S., *et al.* (2007). An event related functional magnetic resonance imaging study of facial emotion processing in Asperger syndrome. *Biological Psychiatry*, **62**: 207–217.

Degreef, G., Bogerts, B., Falkai, P., *et al.* (1992). Increased prevalence of the cavum septum pellucidum in magnetic resonance scans and post-mortem brains of schizophrenic patients. *Psychiatry Research*, **45**: 1–13.

Dunlap, C.B. (1924). Dementia praecox: some preliminary observations on brains from carefully selected cases and a consideration of certain sources of error. *American Journal of Psychiatry*, **80**: 403–421.

Egaas, B., Courchesne, E., Saitoh, O. (1995). Reduced size of corpus callosum in autism. *Archives of Neurology*, **52**: 794–801.

Elia, M., Ferri, R., Musumeci, S.A., *et al.* (2000). Clinical correlates of brain morphometric features of subjects with low-functioning autistic disorder. *Journal of Child Neurology*, **15**: 504–508.

Escalante-Mead, P.R., Minshew, N.J., Sweeney, J.A. (2003). Abnormal brain lateralization in high-functioning autism. *Journal of Autism and Developmental Disorders*, **33**: 539–543.

Fombonne, E. (2005). The changing epidemiology of autism. *Journal of Applied Research in Intellectual Disabilities*, **18**: 281–284.

Freitag, C.M., Konrad, C., Haberlen, M., *et al.* (2008). Perception of biological motion in autism spectrum disorders. *Neuropsychologia*, **46**: 1480–1494.

Frith, C. (2004). Is autism a disconnection disorder? *Lancet Neurology*, **3**: 577.

Fryers, T., Russell, O. (1997). Applied epidemiology. In *Seminars in the Psychiatry of Learning Disability*. London: Gaskell pp. 31–47.

Gaffney, G.R., Kuperman, S., Tsai, L.Y., Minchin, S., Hassanein, K.M. (1987a). Midsagittal magnetic resonance imaging of autism. *British Journal of Psychiatry*, **151**: 831–833.

Gaffney, G.R., Tsai, L.Y., Kuperman, S., Minchin, S. (1987b). Cerebellar structure in autism. *American Journal of Diseases of Children*, **141**: 1330–1332.

Galderisi, S., Vita, A., Rossi, A., *et al.* (2000). Qualitative MRI findings in patients with schizophrenia: a controlled study. *Psychiatry Research*, **98**: 117–126.

Garber, H.J., Ritvo, E.R., Chiu, L.C., *et al.* (1989). A magnetic resonance imaging study of autism: normal fourth ventricle size and absence of pathology. *American Journal of Psychiatry*, **146**: 532–534.

Gervais, H., Belin, P., Boddaert, N., *et al.* (2004). Abnormal cortical voice processing in autism. *Nature Neuroscience*, **7**: 801–802.

Giedd, J.N. (2004). Structural magnetic resonance imaging of the adolescent brain. *Annals of the New York Academy of Sciences*, **1021**: 77–85.

Giedd, J.N., Blumenthal, J., Jeffries, N.O., *et al.* (1999). Brain development during childhood and adolescence: a longitudinal MRI study. *Nature Neuroscience*, **2**: 861–863.

Goldstein, J.M., Seidman, L.J., Horton, N.J., *et al.* (2001). Normal sexual dimorphism of the adult human brain assessed by in vivo magnetic resonance imaging. *Cerebral Cortex*, **11**: 490–497.

Griesinger, W. (1845). *Die Pathologie und Therapie der Psychischen Krankheiten für Aerzte und Studirende*. Stuttgart: Adolph Krabbe (2nd revised edition published in 1861).

Gur, R.C., Turetsky, B.I., Matsui, M., *et al.* (1999). Sex differences in brain gray and white matter in healthy young adults: correlations with cognitive performance. *Journal of Neuroscience*, **19**: 4065–4072.

Hadjikhani, N., Joseph, R.M., Snyder, J., Tager-Flusberg, H. (2006). Anatomical differences in the mirror neuron system and social cognition network in autism. *Cerebral Cortex*, **16**: 1276–1282.

Hadjikhani, N., Joseph, R.M., Snyder, J., Tager-Flusberg, H. (2007). Abnormal activation of the social brain during face perception in autism. *Human Brain Mapping*, **28**: 441–449.

Haier, R.J., Jung, R.E., Yeo, R.A., Head, K., Alkire, M.T. (2005). The neuroanatomy of general intelligence: sex matters. *Neuroimage*, **25**: 320–327.

Happé, F., Ronald, A., Plomin, R. (2006). Time to give up on a single explanation for autism. *Nature Neuroscience*, **9**: 1218–1220.

Hardan, A.Y., Minshew, N.J., Keshavan, M.S. (2000). Corpus callosum size in autism. *Neurology*, **55**: 1033–1036.

Hardan, A.Y., Minshew, N.J., Harenski, K., Keshavan, M.S. (2001a). Posterior fossa magnetic resonance imaging in autism. *Journal of the American Academy of Child and Adolescent Psychiatry*, **40**: 666–672.

Hardan, A.Y., Minshew, N.J., Mallikarjuhn, M., Keshavan, M.S. (2001b). Brain volume in autism. *Journal of Child Neurology*, **16**: 421–424.

Hardan, A.Y., Kilpatrick, M., Keshavan, M.S., Minshew, N.J. (2003). Motor performance and anatomic magnetic resonance imaging (MRI) of the basal ganglia in autism. *Journal of Child Neurology*, **18**: 317–324.

Hardan, A.Y., Jou, R.J., Keshavan, M.S., Varma, R., Minshew, N.J. (2004). Increased frontal cortical folding in autism: a preliminary MRI study. *Psychiatry Research*, **131**: 263–268.

Hardan, A.Y., Girgis, R.R., Adams, J., *et al.* (2006a). Abnormal brain size effect on the thalamus in autism. *Psychiatry Research*, **147**: 145–151.

Hardan, A.Y., Girgis, R.R., Lacerda, A.L., *et al.* (2006b). Magnetic resonance imaging study of the orbitofrontal cortex in autism. *Journal of Child Neurology*, **21**: 866–871.

Hardan, A.Y., Muddasani, S., Vemulapalli, M., Keshavan, M.S., Minshew, N.J. (2006c). An MRI study of increased cortical thickness in autism. *American Journal of Psychiatry*, **163**: 1290–1292.

Hardan, A.Y., Girgis, R.R., Adams, J., *et al.* (2008). Brief report: abnormal association between the thalamus and brain size in Asperger's disorder. *Journal of Autism and Developmental Disorders*, **38**: 390–394.

Hardan, A.Y., Libove, R.A., Keshavan, M.S., Melhem, N.M., Minshew, N.J. (2009a). A preliminary longitudinal magnetic resonance imaging study of brain volume and cortical thickness in autism. *Biological Psychiatry*, **66**: 320–326.

Hardan, A.Y., Pabalan, M., Gupta, N., *et al.* (2009b). Corpus callosum volume in children with autism. *Psychiatry Research*, **174**: 57–61.

Hashimoto, T., Tayama, M., Miyazaki, M., Murakawa, K., Kuroda, Y. (1993). Brainstem and cerebellar vermis involvement in autistic children. *Journal of Child Neurology*, **8**: 149–153.

Hashimoto, T., Tayama, M., Murakawa, K., *et al.* (1995). Development of the brainstem and cerebellum in autistic patients. *Journal of Autism and Developmental Disorders*, **25**: 1–18.

Hazlett, H.C., Poe, M., Gerig, G., *et al.* (2005). Magnetic resonance imaging and head circumference study of brain size in autism: birth through age 2 years. *Archives of General Psychiatry*, **62**: 1366–1376.

Hazlett, H.C., Poe, M.D., Gerig, G., Smith, R.G., Piven, J. (2006). Cortical gray and white brain tissue volume in adolescents and adults with autism. *Biological Psychiatry*, **59**: 1–6.

Haznedar, M.M., Buchsbaum, M.S., Metzger, M., *et al.* (1997). Anterior cingulate gyrus volume and glucose metabolism in autistic disorder. *American Journal of Psychiatry*, **154**: 1047–1050.

Haznedar, M.M., Buchsbaum, M.S., Wei, T.C., *et al.* (2000). Limbic circuitry in patients with autism spectrum disorders studied with positron emission tomography and magnetic resonance imaging. *American Journal of Psychiatry*, **157**: 1994–2001.

Haznedar, M.M., Buchsbaum, M.S., Hazlett, E.A., *et al.* (2006). Volumetric analysis and three-dimensional glucose metabolic mapping of the striatum and thalamus in patients with autism spectrum disorders. *American Journal of Psychiatry*, **163**: 1252–1263.

Herbert, M.R., Harris, G.J., Adrien, K.T., *et al.* (2002). Abnormal asymmetry in language association cortex in autism. *Annals of Neurology*, **52**: 588–596.

Herbert, M.R., Ziegler, D.A., Deutsch, C.K., *et al.* (2003). Dissociations of cerebral cortex, subcortical and cerebral white matter volumes in autistic boys. *Brain*, **126**: 1182–1192.

Herbert, M.R., Ziegler, D.A., Makris, N., *et al.* (2004). Localization of white matter volume increase in autism and developmental language disorder. *Annals of Neurology*, **55**: 530–540.

Herrington, J.D., Baron-Cohen, S., Wheelwright, S.J., *et al.* (2007). The role of MT+/V5 during biological motion perception in Asperger Syndrome: An fMRI study. *Research in Autism Spectrum Disorders*, **1**: 14–27.

Hill, E.L. (2004). Executive dysfunction in autism. *Trends in Cognitive Science*, **8**: 26–32.

Hollander, E., Anagnostou, E., Chaplin, W., *et al.* (2005). Striatal volume on magnetic resonance imaging and repetitive behaviors in autism. *Biological Psychiatry*, **58**: 226–232.

Holttum, J.R., Minshew, N.J., Sanders, R.S., Phillips, N.E. (1992). Magnetic resonance imaging of the posterior fossa in autism. *Biological Psychiatry*, **32**: 1091–1101.

Im, K., Lee, J.M., Lee, J., *et al.* (2006). Gender difference analysis of cortical thickness in healthy young adults with surface-based methods. *Neuroimage*, **31**: 31–38.

Johnstone, E.C., Crow, T.J., Frith, C.D., Husband, J., Kreel, L. (1976). Cerebral ventricular size and cognitive impairment in chronic schizophrenia. *Lancet*, **2**: 924–926.

Johnstone, E.C., Ebmeier, K.P., Miller, P., Owens, D.G., Lawrie, S.M. (2005). Predicting schizophrenia: findings from the Edinburgh High-Risk Study. *British Journal of Psychiatry*, **186**: 18–25.

Jou, R.J., Minshew, N.J., Nelhem, N.M., *et al.* (2009). Brainstem volumetric alterations in children with autism. *Psychological Medicine*, **39**: 1347–1354.

Juranek, J., Filipek, P.A., Berenji, G.R., *et al.* (2006). Association between amygdala volume and anxiety level: magnetic resonance imaging (MRI) study in autistic children. *Journal of Child Neurology*, **21**: 1051–1058.

Kanner, L. (1943). Autistic disturbances of affective contact. *Nervous Child*, **2**: 217–250.

Kanwisher, N., McDermott, J., Chun, M.M. (1997). The fusiform face area: a module in human extrastriate cortex specialized for face perception. *Journal of Neuroscience*, **17**: 4302–4311.

Ke, X., Hong, S., Tang, T., *et al.* (2008). Voxel-based morphometry study on brain structure in children with high-functioning autism. *Neuroreport*, **19**: 921–925.

Keary, C.J., Minshew, N.J., Bansal, R., *et al.* (2009). Corpus callosum volume and neurocognition in autism. *Journal of Autism and Developmental Disorders*, **39**: 834–841.

Keller, T.A., Kana, R.K., Just, M.A. (2007). A developmental study of the structural integrity of white matter in autism. *Neuroreport*, **18**: 23–27.

Kennedy, D.P., Glascher, J., Tyszka, J.M., Adolphs, R. (2009). Personal space regulation by the human amygdala. *Nature Neuroscience*, **12**: 1226–1227.

Kilian, S., Brown, W.S., Hallam, B.J., *et al.* (2008). Regional callosal morphology in autism and macrocephaly. *Developmental Neuropsychology*, **33**: 74–99.

Kleinhans, N.M., Richards, T., Sterling, L. *et al.* (2008). Abnormal functional connectivity in autism spectrum disorders during face processing. *Brain*, **131**: 1000–1012.

Klippel, M., Lhermitte, J. (1909). Un cas de demence precoce a type catatonique, avec autopsie. *Revue Neurologique*, **17**: 157–158.

Kochunov, P., Mangin, J.F., Coyle, T. *et al.* (2005). Age-related morphology trends of cortical sulci. *Human Brain Mapping*, **26**: 210–220.

Korzeniewski, S.J., Birbeck, G., DeLano, M.C., Potchen, M.J., Paneth, N. (2008). A systematic review of neuroimaging for cerebral palsy. *Journal of Child Neurology*, **23**: 216–227.

Koshino, H., Kana, R.K., Keller, T.A. *et al.* (2008). fMRI investigation of working memory for faces in autism: visual coding and underconnectivity with frontal areas. *Cerebral Cortex*, **18**: 289–300.

Krug, D.A., Arick, J.R., Almond, P.J. (1993). *Autism Screening Instrument for Educational Planning: an Assessment and Educational Planning System for Autism and Developmental Disabilities*, 2nd edn. Austin: Pro-ed.

Kwon, H., Ow, A.W., Pedatella, K.E., Lotspeich, L.J., Reiss, A.L. (2004). Voxel-based morphometry elucidates structural neuroanatomy of high-functioning autism and Asperger syndrome. *Developmental Medicine and Child Neurology*, **46**: 760–764.

Kwon, C.H., Luikart, B.W., Powell, C.M., *et al.* (2006). Pten regulates neuronal arborization and social interaction in mice. *Neuron*, **50**: 377–388.

Lagae, L. (2000). Cortical malformations: a frequent cause of epilepsy in children. *European Journal of Pediatrics*, **159**: 555–562.

Langen, M., Durston, S., Staal, W.G., Palmen, S.J., van Engeland, H. (2007). Caudate nucleus is enlarged in high-functioning medication-naive subjects with autism. *Biological Psychiatry*, **62**: 262–266.

Lauterbur, P.C. (1979). Medical imaging by nuclear magnetic-resonance zeugmatography. *IEEE Transactions on Nuclear Science*, **26**: 2808–2811.

Lee, J.E., Bigler, E.D., Alexander, A.L., *et al.* (2007). Diffusion tensor imaging of white matter in the superior temporal gyrus and temporal stem in autism. *Neuroscience Letters*, **424**: 127–132.

Levitt, J.G., Blanton, R.E., Smalley, S., *et al.* (2003). Cortical sulcal maps in autism. *Cerebral Cortex*, **13**: 728–735.

Lhatoo, S.D., Sander, J.W. (2001). The epidemiology of epilepsy and learning disability. *Epilepsia*, **42** (Suppl 1): 6–9.

Lord, C., Rutter, M., Le Couteur, A. (1994). Autism Diagnostic Interview-Revised: a revised version of a diagnostic interview for caregivers of individuals with possible pervasive developmental disorders. *Journal of Autism and Developmental Disorders*, **24**: 659–685.

Lord, C., Risi, S., Lambrecht, L., *et al.* (2000). The autism diagnostic observation schedule-generic: a standard measure of social and communication deficits associated with the spectrum of autism. *Journal of Autism and Developmental Disorders*, **30**: 205–223.

Lotspeich, L.J., Kwon, H., Schumann, C.M., *et al.* (2004). Investigation of neuroanatomical differences between autism and Asperger syndrome. *Archives of General Psychiatry*, **61**: 291–298.

Lubman, D.I., Velakoulis, D., McGorry, P.D., *et al.* (2002). Incidental radiological findings on brain magnetic resonance imaging in first-episode psychosis and chronic schizophrenia. *Acta Psychiatrica Scandinavica*, **106**: 331–336.

Machado, M.G., Oliveira, H.A., Cipolotti, R., *et al.* (2003) [Anatomical and functional abnormalities of central nervous system in autistic disorder: an MRI and SPECT study]. *Arquivos de Neuro-Psiquiatria*, **61**: 957–961.

Magnotta, V.A., Andreasen, N.C., Schultz, S.K., *et al.* (1999). Quantitative in vivo measurement of gyrification in the human brain: changes associated with aging. *Cerebral Cortex*, **9**: 151–160.

Mallard, J., Hutchison, J.M.S., Edelstein, W., Ling, R., Foster, M. (1979). Imaging by nuclear magnetic-resonance and its biomedical implications. *Journal of Biomedical Engineering*, **1**: 153–160.

Manes, F., Piven, J., Vrancic, D., *et al.* (1999). An MRI study of the corpus callosum and cerebellum in mentally retarded autistic individuals. *Journal of Neuropsychiatry and Clinical Neurosciences*, **11**: 470–474.

Mansfield, P., Maudsley, A.A. (1977). Medical imaging by NMR. *British Journal of Radiology*, **50**: 188–194.

McAlonan, G.M., Cheung, V., Cheung, C., *et al.* (2005). Mapping the brain in autism: A voxel-based MRI study of volumetric differences and intercorrelations in autism. *Brain*, **128**: 268–276.

McAlonan, G.M., Daly, E., Kumari, V., *et al.* (2002). Brain anatomy and sensorimotor gating in Asperger's syndrome. *Brain*, **125**: 1594–1606.

Mosconi, M.W., Cody-Hazlett, H., Poe, M.D., *et al.* (2009). Longitudinal study of amygdala volume and joint attention in 2- to 4-year-old children with autism. *Archives of General Psychiatry*, **66**: 509–516.

Mraz, K.D., Green, J., Dumont-Mathieu, T., Makin, S., Fein, D. (2007). Correlates of head circumference growth in infants later diagnosed with autism spectrum disorders. *Journal of Child Neurology*, **22**: 700–713.

Nacewicz, B.M., Dalton, K.M., Johnstone, T., *et al.* (2006). Amygdala volume and nonverbal social impairment in adolescent and adult males with autism. *Archives of General Psychiatry*, **63**: 1417–1428.

Nopoulos, P., Swayze, V., Flaum, M., *et al.* (1997). Cavum septi pellucidi in normals and patients with schizophrenia as detected by magnetic resonance imaging. *Biological Psychiatry*, **41**: 1102–1108.

Nopoulos, P., Flaum, M., O'Leary, D., Andreasen, N.C. (2000). Sexual dimorphism in the human brain: evaluation of tissue volume, tissue composition and surface anatomy using magnetic resonance imaging. *Psychiatry Research*, **98**: 1–13.

Nordahl, C.W., Dierker, D., Mostafavi, I., *et al.* (2007). Cortical folding abnormalities in autism revealed by surface-based morphometry. *Journal of Neuroscience*, **27**: 11725–11735.

Ong, B., Bergin, P., Heffernan, T., Stuckey, S. (2009). Transient seizure-related MRI abnormalities. *Journal of Neuroimaging*, **19**: 301–310.

Palmen, S.J., Hulshoff Pol, H.E., Kemner, C., *et al.* (2004). Larger brains in medication naive high-functioning subjects with pervasive developmental disorder. *Journal of Autism and Developmental Disorders*, **34**: 603–613.

Palmen, S.J., Hulshoff Pol, H.E., Kemner, C., *et al.* (2005). Increased gray-matter volume in medication-naive high-functioning children with autism spectrum disorder. *Psychological Medicine*, **35**: 561–570.

Pantelis, C., Velakoulis, D., McGorry, P.D., *et al.* (2003). Neuroanatomical abnormalities before and after onset of psychosis: a cross-sectional and longitudinal MRI comparison. *Lancet*, **361**: 281–288.

Papez, J.W. (1937). A proposed mechanism of emotion. *Archives of Neurology and Psychiatry*, **38**: 725–743.

Pelphrey, K.A., Morris, J.P., McCarthy, G. (2005). Neural basis of eye gaze processing deficits in autism. *Brain*, **128**: 1038–1048.

Pierce, K., Muller, R.A., Ambrose, J., Allen, G., Courchesne, E. (2001). Face processing occurs outside the fusiform 'face area' in autism: evidence from functional MRI. *Brain*, **124**: 2059–2073.

Pinkham, A.E., Hopfinger, J.B., Pelphrey, K.A., Piven, J., Penn, D.L. (2008). Neural bases for impaired social cognition in schizophrenia and autism spectrum disorders. *Schizophrenia Research*, **99**: 164–175.

Piven, J., Berthier, M.L., Starkstein, S.E., *et al.* (1990). Magnetic resonance imaging evidence for a defect of cerebral cortical development in autism. *American Journal of Psychiatry*, **147**: 734–739.

Piven, J., Arndt, S., Bailey, J. *et al.* (1995). An MRI study of brain size in autism. *American Journal of Psychiatry*, **152**: 1145–1149.

Piven, J., Bailey, J., Ranson, B.J., Arndt, S. (1997). An MRI study of the corpus callosum in autism. *American Journal of Psychiatry*, **154**: 1051–1056.

Pugliese, L., Catani, M., Ameis, S., *et al.* (2009). The anatomy of extended limbic pathways in Asperger syndrome: a preliminary diffusion tensor imaging tractography study. *Neuroimage*, **47**: 427–434.

Redcay, E., Courchesne, E. (2005). When is the brain enlarged in autism? A meta-analysis of all brain size reports. *Biological Psychiatry*, **58**: 1–9.

Rojas, D.C., Bawn, S.D., Benkers, T.L., Reite, M.L., Rogers, S.J. (2002). Smaller left hemisphere planum temporale in adults with autistic disorder. *Neuroscience Letters*, **328**: 237–240.

Rojas, D.C., Smith, J.A., Benkers, T.L., *et al.* (2004). Hippocampus and amygdala volumes in parents of children with autistic disorder. *American Journal of Psychiatry*, **161**: 2038–2044.

Rojas, D.C., Camou, S.L., Reite, M.L., Rogers, S.J. (2005). Planum temporale volume in children and adolescents with autism. *Journal of Autism and Developmental Disorders*, **35**: 479–486.

Rojas, D.C., Peterson, E., Winterrowd, E., *et al.* (2006). Regional gray matter volumetric changes in autism associated with social and repetitive behavior symptoms. *BMC Psychiatry*, **6**: 56.

Ronald, A., Edelson, L.R., Asherson, P., Saudino, K.J. (2010). Exploring the relationship between autistic-like traits and ADHD behaviors in early childhood: findings from a community twin study of 2-year-olds. *Journal of Abnormal Child Psychology*, **38**: 185–196.

Salmond, C.H., Ashburner, J., Connelly, A., *et al.* (2005). The role of the medial temporal lobe in autistic spectrum disorders. *European Journal of Neuroscience*, **22**: 764–772.

Salmond, C.H., Vargha-Khadem, F., Gadian, D.G., de Haan, M., Baldeweg, T. (2007). Heterogeneity in the patterns of neural abnormality in autistic spectrum disorders: evidence from ERP and MRI. *Cortex*, **43**: 686–699.

Schaefer, G.B., Bodensteiner, J.B. (1999). Developmental anomalies of the brain in mental retardation. *International Review of Psychiatry*, **11**: 47–55.

Schifter, T., Hoffman, J.M., Hatten, H.P. Jr., *et al.* (1994). Neuroimaging in infantile autism. *Journal of Child Neurology*, **9**: 155–161.

Schmahmann, J.D., Sherman, J.C. (1998). The cerebellar cognitive affective syndrome. *Brain*, **121**: 561–579.

Schmitz, N., Rubia, K., van Amelsvoort, T., *et al.* (2008). Neural correlates of reward in autism. *British Journal of Psychiatry*, **192**: 19–24.

Schumann, C.M., Amaral, D.G. (2006). Stereological analysis of amygdala neuron number in autism. *Journal of Neuroscience*, **26**: 7674–7679.

Schumann, C.M., Hamstra, J., Goodlin-Jones, B.L., *et al.* (2004). The amygdala is enlarged in children but not adolescents with autism; the hippocampus is enlarged at all ages. *Journal of Neuroscience*, **24**: 6392–6401.

Schumann, C.M., Barnes, C.C., Lord, C., Courchesne, E. (2009). Amygdala enlargement in toddlers with autism related to severity of social and communication impairments. *Biological Psychiatry*, **66**: 942–949.

Sears, L.L., Vest, C., Mohamed, S., *et al.* (1999). An MRI study of the basal ganglia in autism. *Progress in Neuropsychopharmacology and Biological Psychiatry*, **23**: 613–624.

Shaw, P., Lawrence, E.J., Radbourne, C., *et al.* (2004). The impact of early and late damage to the human amygdala on 'theory of mind' reasoning. *Brain*, **127**: 1535–1548.

Simonoff, E., Pickles, A., Charman, T., *et al.* (2008). Psychiatric disorders in children with autism spectrum disorders: prevalence, comorbidity, and associated factors in a population-derived sample. *Journal of the American Academy of Child and Adolescent Psychiatry*, **47**: 921–929.

Sowell, E.R., Thompson, P.M., Welcome, S.E., *et al.* (2003). Cortical abnormalities in children and adolescents with attention-deficit hyperactivity disorder. *Lancet*, **362**: 1699–1707.

Sparks, B.F., Friedman, S.D., Shaw, D.W., *et al.* (2002). Brain structural abnormalities in young children with autism spectrum disorder. *Neurology*, **59**: 184–192.

Spencer, M.D., Gibson, R.J., Moorhead, T.W.J., *et al.* (2005). Qualitative assessment of brain anomalies in adolescents with mental retardation. *American Journal of Neuroradiology*, **26**: 2691–2697.

Spencer, M.D., Moorhead, T.W.J., Lymer, G.K.S., *et al.* (2006). Structural correlates of intellectual impairment and autistic features in adolescents. *Neuroimage*, **33**: 1136–1144.

Stanfield, A.C., McIntosh, A.M., Spencer, M.D., *et al.* (2008). Towards a neuroanatomy of autism: A systematic review and meta-analysis of structural magnetic resonance imaging studies. *European Journal of Psychiatry*, **23**: 289–299.

Sundaram, S.K., Kumar, A., Makki, M.I., *et al.* (2008). Diffusion tensor imaging of frontal lobe in autism spectrum disorder. *Cerebral Cortex*, **18**: 2659–2665.

Taber, K.H., Shaw, J.B., Loveland, K.A., *et al.* (2004). Accentuated Virchow-Robin spaces in the centrum semiovale in children with autistic disorder. *Journal of Computer Assisted Tomography*, **28**: 263–268.

Thakkar, K.N., Polli, F.E., Joseph, R.M., *et al.* (2008). Response monitoring, repetitive behaviour and anterior cingulate abnormalities in autism spectrum disorders (ASD). *Brain*, **131**: 2464–2478.

Toro, R., Burnod, Y. (2005). A morphogenetic model for the development of cortical convolutions. *Cerebral Cortex*, **15**: 1900–1913.

Tsai, L.Y., Beisler, J.M. (1983). The development of sex differences in infantile autism. *British Journal of Psychiatry*, **142**: 373–378.

Tsai, L., Stewart, M.A., August, G. (1981). Implication of sex differences in the familial transmission of infantile autism. *Journal of Autism and Developmental Disorders*, **11**: 165–173.

Tsatsanis, K.D., Rourke, B.P., Klin, A., *et al.* (2003). Reduced thalamic volume in high-functioning individuals with autism. *Biological Psychiatry*, **53**: 121–129.

van den Heuvel, O.A., Veltman, D.J., Groenewegen, H.J., *et al.* (2005). Frontal-striatal dysfunction during planning in obsessive-compulsive disorder. *Archives of General Psychiatry*, **62**: 301–309.

van Karnebeek, C.D., Jansweijer, M.C., Leenders, A.G., Offringa, M., Hennekam, R.C. (2005). Diagnostic investigations in individuals with mental retardation: a systematic literature review of their usefulness. *European Journal of Human Genetics*, **13**: 6–25.

Vidal, C.N., **Nicolson, R.**, **DeVito, T.J.**, *et al.* (2006). Mapping corpus callosum deficits in autism: an index of aberrant cortical connectivity. *Biological Psychiatry*, **60**: 218–225.

Waiter, G.D., **Williams, J.H.**, **Murray, A.D.**, *et al.* (2004). A voxel-based investigation of brain structure in male adolescents with autistic spectrum disorder. *Neuroimage*, **22**: 619–625.

Waiter, G.D., **Williams, J.H.**, **Murray, A.D.**, *et al.* (2005). Structural white matter deficits in high-functioning individuals with autistic spectrum disorder: a voxel-based investigation. *Neuroimage*, **24**: 455–461.

Wernicke, C. (1881). *Lehrbuch der Gehirnkrankheiten*. Kassel, Germany: Theodore Fischer.

Williams, J.H., **Waiter, G.D.**, **Gilchrist, A.**, *et al.* (2006). Neural mechanisms of imitation and 'mirror neuron' functioning in autistic spectrum disorder. *Neuropsychologia*, **44**: 610–621.

Witelson, S.F. (1989). Hand and sex differences in the isthmus and genu of the human corpus callosum. A postmortem morphological study. *Brain*, **112**: 799–835.

Zeegers, M., **Van Der Grond, J.**, **Durston, S.**, *et al.* (2006). Radiological findings in autistic and developmentally delayed children. *Brain and Development*, **28**: 495–499.

Zilbovicius, M., **Meresse, I.**, **Chabane, N.**, *et al.* (2006). Autism, the superior temporal sulcus and social perception. *Trends in Neuroscience*, **29**: 359–366.

4

Magnetoencephalography (MEG) as a tool to investigate the neurophysiology of autism

SVEN BRAEUTIGAM, STEPHEN SWITHENBY AND ANTHONY BAILEY

This chapter introduces a modern functional neuroimaging method, magnetoencephalography (MEG), and addresses how this technique is being applied to study dynamic brain activity and neural processing in autism. An outline will be given of relevant technical and analytical approaches, before discussing functional systems and presenting important findings associated with autism, using MEG. The focus is directed at aspects of neural processing that are affected in individuals on the autism spectrum, including auditory processing, semantic processing, face processing and theory-of-mind (progressed through study of imitation-related processes linked to activity within the 'mirror neuron' system). While MEG is a relatively new tool, the studies available to date lend some support to the notion that autism involves altered cognitive strategies as opposed to cognitive impairments or deficits. In addition, the research on this subject is reviewed, which suggests that MEG may help define and further characterise subclinical epilepsy and epileptiform activity (seizures) in individuals with autism spectrum disorders.

4.1 Instrumentation and measurements

Magnetoencephalography (MEG) is one of a range of functional neuroimaging methods that may be applied to the study of autism. It is of interest because it allows changes in activity to be followed dynamically with millisecond resolution, and thus provides direct information on the evolution of processing along neural pathways.

Researching the Autism Spectrum: Contemporary Perspectives, ed. I. Roth and P. Rezaie. Published by Cambridge University Press.

By far the most common method of imaging brain activity is functional magnetic resonance imaging (fMRI). At the heart of this technique is the weak dependence of the magnetic resonance signal on the oxygenation level of the blood, which in turn depends on brain activity. fMRI is capable of providing millimetre-scale functional images of the level of activity in the brain but with time resolution limited to the rate at which the oxygenation level changes, i.e. of the order of seconds. The technique has been used extensively to study autism (see Seyffert and Castellanos, 2005 and Sanders *et al.* 2008 for general reviews). Functional neuroimaging of face processing in autism is addressed by Dekowska *et al.* (2008) and Jemel *et al.* (2006). Issues concerning autism specificity (of putative impairments) are discussed by these authors. Semantic processing has been addressed by Wang *et al.* (2006) with a particular emphasis on abnormal laterality of activation in autism. These references should be regarded as entry points to the literature, as a more complete discussion of fMRI and imaging techniques other than MEG in the context of autism research is beyond the scope of the present chapter.

MEG is based on the detection of magnetic fields that are generated by currents flowing in neurons. MEG is preferentially sensitive to magnetic fields generated in the cerebral cortex, but modern, whole-head systems employing multiple sensor configurations can detect activity in sub-cortical regions. Typically, neural field changes are extremely small – ranging from $\sim 10^{-12}$ T (T: tesla) during interictal epileptic spikes to $\sim 10^{-14}$ T or less for evoked fields. By comparison, the Earth's magnetic field is about 10^{-4} T, urban noise is about 10^{-7} T and a typical fMRI scanner operates at 1.5 T. Thus the Earth's field, albeit small by technical standards, is some 10 billion times stronger than a brain response. The only practical individual detectors capable of recording such small field changes are superconducting loops that are coupled into Superconducting Quantum Interference Devices that respond to the *changes* in magnetic flux through the loops (Hämäläinen *et al.* 1993; Vrba, 1999). A loop may be configured as a small simple planar coil, in which case the detector measures the magnetic field perpendicular to the plane, or as a more complex shape such as a figure of eight, in which case the detector measures the magnetic field gradient. It would be more accurate to state these sensitivities in terms of magnetic flux but the distinction is not important within the context of this discussion.

A typical MEG imaging system has several hundred sensors (or measurement channels) surrounding a head-shaped recess in a liquid helium filled dewar (Figure 4.1). Typically the head to detector distance is 2–3 cm. The whole instrument is housed in a magnetically screened room that is required to reduce the ambient magnetic field noise, which may be as high as $\sim 10^{-7}$ T. The best instruments achieve noise levels approaching 10^{-15} T per square root of the bandwidth over which the signals are recorded, easily sufficient to detect the signals from the brain.

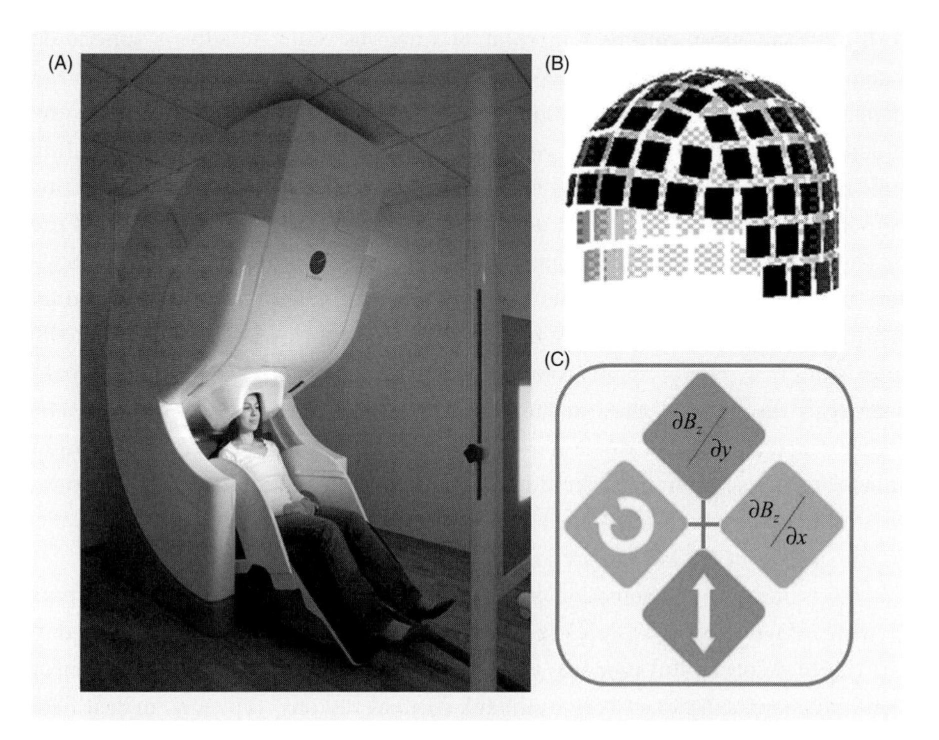

Figure 4.1 The MEG scanner at the Oxford Centre for Human Brain Activity. The scanner itself is shown in (**A**). The system features a helmet-shaped array of 102 detectors (black plates, totalling 306 sensors) covering the whole head (**B**). Each detector consists of one magnetometer (grey loop) which measures the magnetic field, and two first-order planar gradiometers (diamonds) which measure magnetic field gradients along orthogonal directions (**C**). The outputs of the latter are most sensitive to the tangential current flow in the region directly below the detectors. The root-mean-square signal summed over the two readings is a measure of current strength. Comparing the head to a globe, $\partial B_Z/\partial y$ gradiometers measure the variation of the magnetic field (more precisely its z-component perpendicular to the head) along longitudinal directions, and $\partial B_Z/\partial x$ gradiometers measure along latitudinal directions. See plate section for colour version.

There are some subtleties associated with the sources that are detected in MEG. Externally detectable field changes require large numbers (> a few thousand) of neighbouring cells to carry aligned currents of suitable strength and duration to allow for spatial and temporal integration. It is generally assumed that these conditions are met through post-synaptic currents rather than currents associated with action potentials. Modelling the sources underlying MEG signals ('source localisation'; see also next section) necessitates not only assumptions to be made about geometry and electrical properties of the source space (brain/head) but also about the potential source configurations. Information extracted from other brain imaging techniques can inform source models, where, perhaps most commonly, structural MR information is used to define and restrict source volumes. Often, a spherical conductor is assumed restricting the MEG analysis to tangential sources, the strongest of which are typically currents flowing along pyramidal cells within cortical sulci (Hämäläinen *et al.* 1993).

Although technically demanding, MEG has some significant advantages. It is a passive measurement that is completely non-invasive and makes very few demands on the subject. The instrument is silent in its operation. The MEG detector simply records the brain activity continuously as the subject carries out whatever task the investigator requires. Longitudinal studies are ethically possible and acceptable to subjects. Finally and most importantly, the detectors are sensitive to field changes occurring over timescales of milliseconds to seconds, thus complementing fMRI which is sensitive to longer term changes.

4.2 Analytical approaches

The primary outputs provided by any magnetoencephalographic scanner are readings of the variation in time of the magnetic fields (or their spatial gradients) produced by electrical activity in the brain and detected over defined positions on the head. It is these 'raw' signals which are pre-processed, analysed in various ways, correlated with experimental conditions and, possibly, with findings obtained from other imaging modalities and, ultimately, are interpreted within the framework of a given scientific investigation. Ever since the inception of MEG, a plethora of analytical techniques to extract information from the signals has been developed. New methods often emerge at a staggering rate. The analytical approaches range from straightforward topographical maps of signals to complex source estimation procedures typically involving anatomical information as well as sophisticated time-frequency and other abstract state–space representations of the data. The abundance of approaches implies that there is currently an absence of rigorous standard protocols for MEG analysis; however, certain approaches have crystallised that are used fairly consistently across studies. In this short account, three of the most relevant approaches to investigation and analysis will be described. These are not alternatives but well-documented practice for those striving for insight into autism.

The most direct and easily understood approach involves developing protocols that yield event-related fields (ERFs), the direct analogue of the more familiar event-related potentials (ERPs). Event-related approaches are commonly used to analyse electrophysiological data obtained from readings outside the brain itself. Typically, within a chosen experimental setting, a stimulus is presented to a subject repeatedly. The appearance of a stimulus marks a point in time, usually denoted as *stimulus-onset*, with respect to which an epoch of data is defined which includes both pre- and post-stimulus intervals. The signal observed in the post-stimulus interval is often assumed to be independent of stimulus repetition but to be contaminated by random noise. This assumption may have limited validity, particularly in studies of higher order function.

Within the assumption of independence against repetition, the neural response can be recovered from the measured signal by averaging the response data (or trials) with respect to stimulus-onset. For random noise, this reduces the noise variance proportionally to the number of stimuli. The resultant waveform is usually called an ERP/ERF or simply an evoked response. Although the process of averaging may be applied at the levels of individual channels of measurement and individual subjects, it may be extended over several subjects to yield grand mean waveforms (Gevins and Remond, 1987). Typically, peaks in the evoked waveforms are correlated with the experimental parameters to map the temporal sequence of neuronal processing stages. The stimulus and subject dependence of the responses allows some insight into their functional significance.

The second approach, often undertaken after an initial ERF analysis, involves source estimation, the identification of the brain areas generating a given signal recorded by EEG or MEG. Such a signal will often be an average evoked response but single trials can be analysed as well. Every source estimation procedure has to face the so-called inverse problem, the mathematical transformation that uses the data as input and outputs the sources of the data. Here there is a problem that is shared with many algorithmic procedures – the inverse problem in MEG is deeply mathematically ambiguous. No matter how many detectors one uses and how high quality the data, there can always be silent currents (sources) in the brain that are not recorded by any of the detectors. These may be neurophysiologically relevant. Moreover, some sources leave only a very weak record – identifying them is difficult. The MEG inverse problem has been researched extensively (see, for example, Lin *et al.* 2006) and is solved pragmatically by simplifying the description of the sources or by adding additional physiologically reasonable assumptions.

The most basic and, until recently, most commonly used source estimation technique is that of equivalent current dipoles (ECDs). Formally, the use of equivalent current dipoles is equivalent to assuming that the electric and magnetic fields that are measured originate from discrete source regions, the spatial extent of which is small compared with the distances to the detectors. In this approximation, the dipole can be viewed as the spatial average of all source (or impressed) currents within that area. The impressed currents are due to the electromotive forces associated with biological (mainly synaptic) activity in neural tissue (Jackson, 1962; Katila, 1983).

In the last few years, source estimation techniques have developed to embrace distributed images of current sources. These may be generated by several distinct but in many cases related algorithms (Lin *et al.* 2006). They yield images that are broadly consistent and robust and may, in favourable circumstances, offer meaningful insights into functional anatomy at the centimetre level. Interpretation of such images should include consideration of the nature of the underlying algorithm.

The third investigative approach that will be highlighted is time-frequency analysis. This includes a wide range of mathematical algorithms that analyse neurophysiological signals in terms of oscillations that vary in frequency and time. There is a long history of studying fundamental brain rhythms such as theta (4–7 Hz) or alpha (8–13 Hz) waves that, under certain conditions, can be detected by visual inspection of the data and may indicate general states of the brain, e.g. increased alpha is often seen when subjects close their eyes.

Modern approaches have formalised and extended the analysis of oscillatory activity. In many cases, transient oscillatory brain activity is now considered in conjunction with well-defined stimuli, and is identified as either an evoked oscillatory response appearing at the same latency and phase in each single trial which is detectable in the averaged field, or an induced oscillatory response appearing with a jitter in latency from one trial to another, and therefore not observable in the averaged data (Tallon-Baudry and Bertrand, 1999). Both types of response provide information about brain dynamics beyond the understanding that can be extracted from the traditional evoked response which is broadband in nature, i.e. includes all frequencies. In particular, oscillations at higher frequency ($>$ 20 Hz) in the so-called gamma-band have received much attention in recent years. Experimental data reveal that synchronisation of gamma-band activity is involved in processes such as working memory, perceptual awareness, semantic processing and sensory–motor integration and that synchronisation may be altered in pathological brain states (Uhlhaas and Singer, 2006). Theoretical considerations suggest that synchrony of oscillations is a fundamental property of neural systems. It appears to facilitate the coordinated interactions of large neuronal populations distributed within and across distinct regions of the brain; an interaction deemed necessary for most cognitive processes. The precise mechanisms underlying synchronisation through gamma oscillations are still unknown; however, interneuron networks are believed to play an important role (Bartos *et al.* 2007; Engel *et al.* 2001).

4.3 MEG studies of autism spectrum disorders (ASD)

Starting in the late 1990s, magnetoencephalography has been used increasingly as an investigative tool to study the neurophysiological basis of autism, mirroring a more general trend of intensified usage of neuroimaging technologies in developmental disorders and paediatrics (Paetvu, 2002; Rumsey and Ernst, 2000). Many peer-reviewed papers utilising MEG have been published on cognitive anomalies considered to be characteristic of autism spectrum disorders adding to the established literature involving behavioural tests. To date, essentially all relevant MEG studies have focused on affected, often high-functioning, individuals with ASD. However, the first MEG based investigations of parents of children with autism are beginning to emerge, reflecting an ever-growing interest in the broader phenotype of autism. The remainder of this chapter provides a brief overview of recent findings of studies of autism made using MEG.

4.3.1 *Epileptiform activity*

The contribution of subclinical epilepsy to autism spectrum and developmental and acquired language disorders is commonly considered as one of the most important issues in developmental neurosciences. This importance derives from the observation that mute or dysfluent children with Landau-Keffler syndrome (LKS; acquired aphasia), autism or developmental language disorders, who show common features in their ability to decode speech, are at higher risk for epilepsy than children with the fluent, albeit aberrant, language of verbal children with autism (Kanner, 2000; Neville, 1999; Rapin, 2006). Although MEG is gaining widespread momentum as a clinical tool for seizure disorders, there appear to be only two MEG studies into epileptiform activity in individuals with autism.

Initially, researchers at the University of Utah studied electrophysiological responses during stage III sleep in 50 children with regressive ASD with onset between 20 and 36 months of age (16 with autism, 34 with PDD-NOS; 15 out of 50 with a clinical seizure disorder) and 6 children with Landau-Kleffner syndrome (5 with complex seizures). The MEG data demonstrated epileptiform activity during slow wave sleep in 82% of the children with ASD independent of the presence or absence of clinically relevant seizures. Using equivalent current dipoles to model abnormal activity, the authors found similar periSylvian generators (foci of electrical discharge) in both groups of patients (Lewine *et al.* 1999). It is generally agreed that this study has provided evidence that MEG has greater yield than traditional EEG sleep recordings and that this appears to be related to electrical characteristics of epileptiform discharges arising in the Sylvian fissure. However, the study has been strongly criticised on grounds of referral bias, methodological shortcomings and conflating regressive autism and LKS (Kallen, 2001; Neville, 1999).

More recently, a group of researchers at the Universitat Autònoma de Barcelona studied spontaneous neural activity under wakefulness in 36 children with early onset autism spectrum disorders (22 with autism, 9 with Asperger syndrome, and

5 with PDD-NOS) using MEG. An ECD model was employed to calculate the location of the neural generators underlying epileptiform activity. In about 86% of all children with ASD, the MEG data revealed specific abnormalities in the form of low amplitude monophasic and biphasic spikes as well as acute waves, predominately distributed in the perisylvian areas. A right-lateralisation of epileptiform spikes was only observed in patients with Asperger syndrome (Muñoz-Yunta *et al.* 2008). This study, to some extent, replicates the prior investigation by the Utah group, and provides further evidence that subclinical epilepsy can be detected in many children with ASD. Unfortunately, further conclusions could not be drawn as comparable typically developing children were not investigated.

4.3.2 *Auditory processing*

Arguably, the dominant approach to understanding the neurobiological basis of language impairment in autism has been the study of abnormalities in low-level, early auditory processing. Many researchers have concentrated on the event-related M100 field in response to simple pure tones. The M100 or its electric counterpart N100 can be viewed as the brain's first strong response to tones generated in primary auditory cortices and is readily detected by MEG (Roberts and Poeppel, 1996). Note that these components typically peak at around 100 ms after stimulus onset, hence M100 (N100). In the case of electrical (EEG) readings, this peak is negative (N) with respect to reference sites commonly used. For MEG, components are simply prefixed with 'M' as magnetic fields are reference free.

Past and present research has included studies of: the frequency dependence of M100 latency; the developmental trajectory of the M100 latency; and the hemispherical asymmetry of the M100 generators. The latency data seem to imply that individuals with autism show a normal pattern of responses in that M100 onset decreases with both tone frequency and age. However, reduced variation with respect to frequency changes and overall longer M100 latency clearly distinguish patients from typically developing controls. Much of this work has been reviewed very recently by researchers at the Children's Hospital of Philadelphia who are also major contributors to this area of autism research (Roberts *et al.* 2008). In their view, MEG's strength lies in examining primary and secondary auditory processes and providing independent electrophysiological markers of autism spectrum disorders.

In line with experiments based on pure tones, a group of researchers at the Neuromagnetic Imaging Center of the University of Colorado have investigated the 40 Hz oscillatory response elicited by simple tones (Wilson *et al.* 2007). When very short tones (clicks of $\leq$ 2 ms duration) are presented 40 times a second, the human brain generates a strong steady-state gamma-band response of the same frequency of 40 Hz as the stimuli. This steady state response activity is thought to be correlated with intra-regional and short-range inter-regional processing, or local connectivity in more general.

Magnetic field data were obtained in 10 boys and male adolescents with autism and 10 male, age-matched typically developing individuals. Both groups listened passively to monaurally presented acoustic trains consisting of short tone pulses and 40 Hz gamma-band power was estimated over the contralateral hemisphere. The main finding was a significantly reduced left hemisphere steady state response in the children with autism. There was no significant inter-hemisphere difference in the control group. The authors noted the unexpected hemispheric asymmetry in their data and interpreted their data as indicating that, in individuals with autism, certain brain areas might be impaired in generating the high frequency oscillations that are likely to be involved in the synchronisation of short-range neural interactions.

The group have followed up on the 40 Hz oscillatory response study by measuring the magnetic field responses of 16 parents of children with autism and comparing the data with responses obtained in 11 adults with autism and 16 typically developing adult controls. This time, the authors analysed the 40 Hz induced and stimulus (phase)-locked oscillations with a standard evoked response paradigm, where subjects passively listened to 1 kHz sinusoidal tones presented for 200 ms repeated every 4 s. Independent of hemisphere, significantly higher induced gamma-power was observed in parents and individuals with autism compared to controls, while evoked gamma power was significantly highest in controls. Hemispheric asymmetry was observed for neuronal generators of the 40 Hz induced oscillations, with equivalent current dipoles (at M100 latency) located more anterior in the right than the left hemisphere. This was true for all three groups, but the asymmetry was strongest (and significant) in control subjects, weaker in parents and almost absent in individuals with ASD (Rojas *et al.* 2008). As this is effectively the first (MEG) study of its kind, the authors are aware that no strong conclusion can be drawn at present. However, it is reasonable to assert that gamma-band oscillations might be potentially useful endophenotypes for autism, given recent insight into the molecular and synaptic mechanisms underlying the generation of such macroscopic signals.

Turning to more naturalistic sounds, researchers at the University of Tokyo have employed vowel stimuli to elicit a mismatch negativity (MMN) in 9 adults with autism and 19 matched typically developing volunteers. The MMN is an event-related potential or field peaked at 100–200 ms after the onset of a physically deviant auditory stimulus in identical and repeated sequence. The response is commonly considered an index of the neural mechanisms of automatic detection of acoustic change (Näätänen, 2001).

Interestingly, significant group differences were observed in the across-phoneme condition eliciting mismatch negativities in response to deviant (Japanese) vowels /o/ in a sequences of vowels /a/. Compared to controls, the left-hemispherical MMN was significantly delayed in participants with autism and this latency delay was positively correlated with symptom severity (using the childhood autistic rating scale – Tokyo version, CARS-TV). No between-group differences were observed for mismatch negativity responses to tone- or vowel-duration changes (Kasai *et al.* 2005). This work is broadly consistent with pure tone studies: it provides evidence for delayed processing of change in speech sound.

4.3.3 *Semantic processing*

It is generally accepted that subtle abnormalities in semantic processing are always present in autism spectrum disorders, although linguistic ability can vary significantly across the spectrum, from severe language impairment to normal or even partially superior language skills. A recurring clinical observation in autism is a deficit in interpreting language in context, and studies of reading suggest that high-functioning children and adults with autism do not use sentence context fully under normal reading conditions (Happé, 1997; Walenski *et al.* 2006).

Commonly, the electrophysiological correlates of semantic processing in autism have been investigated by studying the N400 event-related potentials, which are robust markers of contextual integration. Although the N400, observed about 400 ms after stimulus onset (negative deflection in EEG; MEG equivalent M400 but often referred to simply as N4 or N400), is strongest in response to semantic violations, it is not simply an index of anomaly, but rather reflects the extent to which an individual word is expected on the basis of word, sentence or larger scale context (Kutas and Federmeier, 2000). Apart from the N400, other context-sensitive evoked responses exist. For example, at longer latency, so-called late positive components (LPCs) are observed at about 700–800 ms after stimulus onset. Such components are thought to reflect the formation of novel semantic representations and associations (Salmon and Pratt, 2002).

The only published MEG study of N400 responses in autism was performed by the authors of this chapter (Braeutigam *et al.* 2008). This work attempted to map out in detail N400, and stimulus-locked gamma-band neural responses recorded in 11 able adults with autism spectrum disorders (nine individuals had a clinical diagnosis of autism and two a clinical diagnosis of Asperger syndrome) and 11 typically developing controls (matched for age, gender and handedness with comparable but not strictly matched IQ scores) reading meaningful sentences and sentences ending with a semantically incongruous word (e.g. '*The blankets were in a plate*'). The MEG data, which revealed spatially extended evoked N400 and LPC

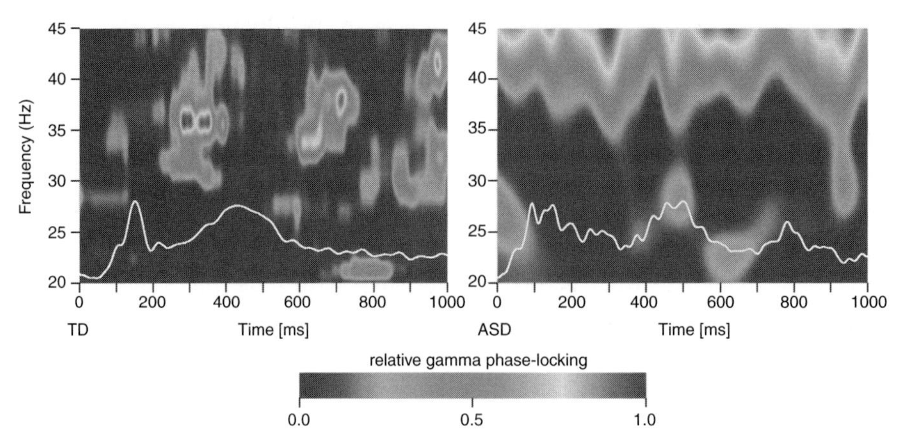

Figure 4.2 This figure shows time-frequency plane (t-f plane) representations of the phase-locked gamma-responses following incongruous words. The planes take into account the data from all typically developing individuals (left) and all individuals with ASD (right) studied in Braeutigam *et al.* (2008). For each plane, the corresponding root-mean-square signals (evoked power = total brain activation) have been superimposed for reference. Remarkably, in individuals with autism spectrum disorders, gamma phase-locking to incongruous words is observed within a very long interval independent of evoked power. (The effects here are significant, but the underlying statistical argument is beyond the scope of this chapter.) See plate section for colour version.

responses, as well as synchronised gamma-oscillations, provided clear evidence for specific neuronal processes sensitive to sentence context that differed in individuals with autism compared to controls. In particular, the N400 responses following incongruous words were weaker over left temporal cortices, whereas LPC responses to incongruous words and long-latency gamma-oscillations following congruous words were stronger over central and prefrontal regions in individuals with autism compared to the control group. Strikingly, incongruous words elicited long-lasting gamma-oscillations above 40 Hz in the clinical group, but not in typically developing subjects (Figure 4.2). In conclusion, these findings might indicate that appreciation of sentence context in individuals with ASD involves both more and different neural stages. However, it is unclear whether such neuronal stages reflect genuinely anomalous pathways (i.e. pathways that are never utilised in typically developing individuals).

4.3.4 *Face processing*

Face processing is one of the most active areas of investigation of autism. Those with ASD show clear behavioural differences that are established from infancy, including speed of processing, as well as a range of impairments that are face linked, e.g. in patterns of eye contact (Dawson *et al.* 2005). Schultz has made the provocative suggestion that the deficit in face processing may cascade out via perception to generate the social and communicative deficits seen later in those with autism (Schultz, 2005).

During subsequent development, autism is manifest in reduced memory for faces and a deficit in recognizing facially expressed emotion. However, autism is also associated with an enhanced ability to recognise upside down faces and to extract information from some face features compared to typically developing individuals. Such observations underlie the suggestion that people with autism do not process faces as a whole but attend to individual features (Elgar *et al.* 2002). This is an example of the more general observation that people with autism use different strategies to accomplish familiar and important tasks.

There are many published neuroimaging studies of face processing in both the normal and the autistic population (Dekowska *et al.* 2008; Jemel *et al.* 2006). Within the normal population, it has been found that viewing faces activates selectively the ventral occipito-temporal cortex particularly, though not exclusively, in the right hemisphere. The area involved is sometimes termed the fusiform face area or 'FFA'. This observation is consistent with previous behavioural studies in which prosopagnosia is linked with fusiform abnormality and event related potential ERP observations of an N170 component (negative deflection in EEG; MEG equivalent M170) that is elicited by viewing faces and which is located in the fusiform gyrus (see, for example, Seeck and Grüsser, 1992). Considerable effort has been expended in identifying the nature of the face specificity with the suggestion that it is predominantly associated with the nature of the visual stimulus rather than the details of the task or the expertise involved (Carmel and Bentin, 2002). Face linked activity is not confined to the FFA but has also been reported in the superior temporal sulcus and other regions (Dekowska *et al.* 2008). The functional roles of these activations are not clear but they have been associated with judgements of emotion and identity as well as pre-processing and examination of gaze, facial detail, movement, etc.

Much of the neuroimaging literature on face processing in autistic subjects has concentrated on the FFA with a general consensus that there is atypical activation (Hadjikhani *et al.* 2007; Jemel *et al.* 2006; O'Connor *et al.* 2005; Schultz *et al.* 2000). Although the earlier literature emphasised FFA hypoactivation there is now some debate as to whether this is intrinsic or is connected with the details of the task (e.g. the degree of engagement, see Dalton *et al.* 2005; Schultz, 2005). Jemel *et al.* (2006) have reviewed these issues.

There have been just two published MEG studies of face processing in autistic subjects, both by the authors of this article and their collaborators (Bailey *et al.* 2005; Kylliäinen *et al.* 2006a; 2006b). These build on their MEG studies of face

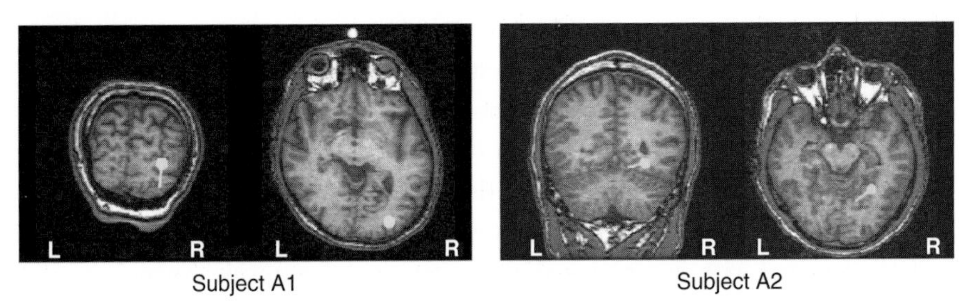

Figure 4.3 The images show the equivalent-current-dipole locations (orange dots) for responses to statically presented images of faces at about 150 ms after stimulus in two subjects with autism spectrum disorders. The dipoles have been superimposed on individual structural (MRI) scans. These figures (adapted from Bailey *et al.* 2005) illustrate that the generator of the N170 response might locate more towards the medial aspects of the (inferior) temporal lobe and more towards striate cortex than in typically developing subjects. There is little consistency in dipole orientation (orange line), which suggests a greater-than-normal heterogeneity in individuals with ASD. See plate section for colour version.

processing in normal subjects that replicated previous observations of a reduced N170 component in the FFA though with reduced latency (Swithenby *et al.* 1998) as well as reports by other authors detailing the dependence of the response on the details of the stimulus (Halgren *et al.* 2000). Perhaps the most relevant MEG study of face processing in normal subjects is by Kylliäinen *et al.* (2006a) who studied the responses of 10 boys (ages 8–11) and 10 adult males to photographs of faces (eyes open, shut, and with averted gaze) and motorbikes. The results for adults in the study replicated previous findings, including the inferior occipito-temporal cortex N170 response. The activity in the children at the same latency was less prominent, not lateralised and was evoked similarly by faces and motorbikes. Averted gaze stimuli produced longer latency right-lateralised activity in children only. These findings indicate that, even in middle childhood, the neural mechanisms underlying face processing are less specialised than in adults.

Bailey *et al.* (2005) studied 12 able adults with autism spectrum disorders (ASD) and 22 adult controls as they performed image categorisation and image identification tasks (same matching criteria as in Braeutigam *et al.* 2008). Those with ASD generated responses to images of faces in right extrastriate cortices at ~145 ms after stimulus onset that were significantly weaker, less lateralised and less affected by stimulus repetition (Figure 4.3). Early latency (30–60 ms) responses to face images over right anterior temporal regions were different for the two groups in the image identification task. Overall the study suggests that those with ASD develop differently located and functionally different extra-striate processing pathways. These pathways are functionally competent for some aspects of face processing. However, it is currently unresolved whether such processing routes may provide advantage in socially linked cognition.

The most recent MEG study of face processing in those with ASD was carried out by Kylliäinen *et al.* (2006b) on 10 children with ASD and 10 mental age and gender matched children who were typically developing boys aged 7–12 years. The task was the same as that used previously (Bailey *et al.* 2005). Overall, the study demonstrated that the response differences between the two groups of children were less marked than between the adult groups and between children and adults. Both groups showed similarity in immaturity of face processing though there were subtle differences with, apparently, greater recruitment of extrastriate cortex in processing non-face (motorbike) stimuli and a less face-specific response. Together these findings suggest that there is divergence between the developing face and object processing systems. An interesting though as yet inconclusive observation was differences in longer latency responses to averted and direct gaze images with those with ASD responding more strongly to direct gaze. The authors speculate that this may be linked to an amygdala modulated face-processing system as described previously (Schultz, 2005).

4.3.5 *Mirror neuron system*

The term 'mirror neuron system' referred initially to a class of neurons in the monkey's pre-motor cortex that responds both when an action is performed by the animal and when the same kind of action is observed. Since discovery, findings obtained from a large number of investigations suggest that mirror neurons may form a generic cortical system involved in matching observation and execution of goal-related motor actions not only in non-human primate brains but also in humans. Moreover, theoretical considerations propose that the function of mirror neurons might be part of, or a necessary precursor to, a human ability to assign and understand goals, intentions and beliefs of other people under normal conditions. In other words, over and above being responsible for aspects of motor learning and imitation, the mirror neurons might underlie our normal 'mind-reading' ability or theory-of-mind (Gallese and Goldman, 1998; Rizzolatti *et al.* 2001). This putative link between mirror systems and mind-reading ability is of particular interest to autism researchers as affected individuals often show clinically recognised signs of impaired recognition and interpretation of other peoples' intentions, or, more generally, state of mind.

Although studies have been published addressing the broader issue of social cognition in autism (e.g. Domes *et al.* 2008; Iacoboni, 2009), so far only researchers at the Brain Research Unit of Helsinki University of Technology have employed

MEG to study the neural basis of imitation related processes. Initially, the group studied the neuronal response in four adult individuals with Asperger syndrome, one individual with autism and eight typically developing controls all of whom viewed passively and actively mirrored hand actions presented visually. Focusing on the 20 Hz oscillatory neuronal response generated in primary motor cortex, the authors found similar patterns of activity in both ASD and control groups in the passive hand-action viewing condition (Avikainen *et al.* 1999). Pointing to the limitation imposed by a rather small sample size, the authors concluded that impaired mind-reading and imitation skills found in ASD could not be explained in terms of a dysfunction of the motor cortex part of the action observation and execution system.

More recently, the group recorded the neural responses in subjects imitating oro-facial gestures presented as static images of human faces showing various lip forms typically associated with facial expressions. Eight adult individuals with Asperger syndrome and ten typically developing age-matched adults were studied. Here, the data analysis focused on the 40 Hz oscillatory response modelled as equivalent-current-dipoles at various latencies following imitation inducing stimuli. In the control subjects, the authors found a characteristic sequence of cortical activation rapidly progressing from occipital cortices to the superior temporal sulcus, to the inferior parietal lobe, to the inferior frontal lobe and, finally, to the primary motor cortex of both hemispheres. In affected subjects, a broadly similar pattern was found. However, activity in inferior frontal areas was both delayed and weaker, and activity in primary motor cortex was weaker in affected individuals compared to typically developing subjects (Nishitani *et al.* 2004). Noting that the clinical group showed normal task performance, the authors concluded that the observed abnormal imitation related cortical activity might be indicative of a more general mirror neuron dysfunction which, in turn, could account in part for imitation and social impairments.

4.4 Discussion

Magnetoencephalograpy has become more important for autism researchers over the past decade. Overall, the MEG data are broadly consistent with but build on results obtained from EEG or other functional neuroimaging studies addressing comparable issues. Interestingly, the data available to date often point to subtle anomalies in the brain response in individuals with autism. One example of this is the observation that the early auditory responses such as the M100 are clearly present but are characterised by different-from-normal dynamical range or generator location. Another is that the extra-striate cortices appear to be involved in differentiation between face and other objects as in typically developing subjects, but the activity is anomalous with respect to the strength and location of the source(s), and the task condition. Clearly, context sensitive responses are seen in autism, but the activation exhibits abnormal lateralisation or strength. In the case of the mirror system as well, abnormalities in activation appear to be characterised by delay and reduction in strength rather than absence.

The current research findings appear, to some extent, to support models describing autism in terms of anomalous cognitive strategies rather than cognitive impairments or deficits *per se* (Happé, 1999). The long term goal for autism researchers across the discipline is to synthesise an overarching biological and psychological theory of autism (Baron-Cohen and Belmonte, 2005). The contribution that MEG is beginning to make is to provide insight into 'connectivity' at a local and wider scale as evidenced by both event related field and gamma-band analyses. Thus, one tries to understand how synchronisation and connectivity in functional neural networks may represent local to global relationships at the level of behaviour (Just *et al.* 2004; Rippon *et al.* 2007; Rubenstein and Merzenich, 2003). The MEG work to date tends to support the psychological theory of weak central coherence (WCC), which suggests a relative shift from global to local processing in individuals with autism (Frith, 1989; see Pellicano, Chapter 7 of this volume).

The present contributions of MEG to this debate are limited. However, it is clear that, in order to develop neurophysiological theories of autism spectrum disorders, it will be necessary to resolve: (a) the role of neuroanatomical (neuronal tracts) and functional (activation pathways) contributions to long-range connectivity; and (b) the extent to which behaviourally local and global processes are represented by independent neural entities (Dakin and Frith, 2005) and large scale, coordinated neuronal networks, respectively.

In conclusion, given the current rapid development, it appears safe to claim that MEG will contribute to autism research for many years to come. This is not to deny that there are obvious limitations. So far, studies are rather fragmented in terms of experimental design and scientific objectives, sample sizes are typically low, subject matching criteria vary substantially from one investigation to the next, and comparisons are often limited to ASD and typically developing populations rather than pathologies exhibiting some overlap with the autistic spectrum.

The research into autism, based on MEG as well as other techniques, faces important challenges as to whether the observed electrophysiological anomalies are indeed specific to autism, or merely indicative of a wider class of abnormal conditions. More work is needed to establish precisely how the altered brain responses relate to higher order behavioural, communication and language deficits. Only time will tell how the current research can contribute to a better understanding of heterogeneity of the autistic spectrum, its diagnosis and long-term treatment.

4.5 References

Avikainen, S., Kulomäki, T., Hari, R. (1999). Normal movement reading in Asperger subjects. *Neuroreport*, **10**: 3467–3470.

Bailey, A.J., Braeutigam, S., Jousmäki, V., Swithenby, S.J. (2005). Abnormal activation of face processing systems at early and intermediate latency in individuals with autism spectrum disorder: a magnetoencephalographic study. *European Journal of Neuroscience*, **21**: 2575–2585.

Baron-Cohen, S., Belmonte, M.K. (2005). Autism: a window onto the development of the social and analytic brain. *Annual Review of Neuroscience*, **28**: 109–126.

Bartos, M., Vida, I., Jonas, P. (2007). Synaptic mechanisms of synchronized gamma oscillations in inhibitory interneuron networks. *Nature Reviews Neuroscience*, **8**: 45–56.

Bolton, P.F., Griffiths, P.D. (1997). Association of tuberous sclerosis of temporal lobes with autism and atypical autism. *Lancet*, **349**: 392–395.

Braeutigam, S., Swithenby, S.J., Bailey, A.J. (2008). Contextual integration the unusual way: a magnetoencephalographic study of responses to semantic violation in individuals with autism spectrum disorders. *European Journal of Neuroscience*, **27**: 1026–1036.

Carmel, D., Bentin, S. (2002). Domain specificity versus expertise: factors influencing distinct processing of faces. *Cognition*, **83**: 1–29.

Chez, M.G., Chang, M., Krasne, V., *et al.* (2006). Frequency of epileptiform EEG abnormalities in a sequential screening of autistic patients with no known clinical epilepsy from 1996 to 2005. *Epilepsy and Behavior*, **8**: 267–271.

Dakin, S., Frith, U. (2005). Vagaries of visual perception in autism. *Neuron*, **48**: 497–507.

Dalton, K.M., Nacewicz, B.M., Johnstone, T., *et al.* (2005). Gaze fixation and the neural circuitry of face processing in autism. *Nature Neuroscience*, **8**: 519–526.

Dawson, G., Webb, S.J., McPartland, J. (2005). Understanding the nature of face processing impairment in autism: insights from behavioural and electrophysiological studies. *Developmental Neuropsychology*, **27**: 403–424.

Dekowska, M., Kuniecki, M., Jaśkowski, P. (2008). Facing facts: Neuronal mechanisms of face perception. *Acta Neurobiologiae Experimentalis*, **68**: 229–252.

Domes, G., Kumbier, E., Herpertz-Dahlmann, B., Herpertz, S.C. (2008). Social cognition in autism: A survey of functional imaging studies. *Nervenarzt*, **79**: 261–272.

Elgar, K., Campbell, R, Skuse, D. (2002). Are you looking at me? Accuracy in processing line-of-sight in Turner syndrome. *Proceedings of the Royal Society B – Biological Sciences*, **269**: 2415–2422.

Engel, A.K., Fries, P., Singer, W. (2001). Dynamic predictions: oscillations and synchrony in top-down processing. *Nature Reviews Neuroscience*, **2**: 704–716.

Frith, U. (1989). *Autism: Explaining the Enigma*. Oxford: Blackwell.

Gallese, V., Goldman, A. (1998). Mirror neurons and the simulation theory of mind-reading. *Trends in Cognitive Sciences*, **2**: 493–501.

Gevins, A.S., Remond, A. (1987). *Handbook of Electroencephalography and Clinical Neurophysiology*. Amsterdam: Elsevier.

Hadjikhani, N., Joseph, R.M., Snyder, J., Tager-Flusberg, H. (2007). Abnormal activation of the social brain during face perception in autism. *Human Brain Mapping*, **28**: 441–444.

Halgren, E., Raij, T., Marinkovic, K., Jousmäki, V., Hari, R. (2000). Cognitive response profile of the human fusiform face area as determined by MEG. *Cerebral Cortex*, **10**: 69–81.

Hämäläinen, M., Hari, R., Ilmoniemi, R.J., Knuutila, J., Lounasmaa, O.V. (1993). Magnetoencephalography – theory, instrumentation and applications to non-invasive studies of the human brain. *Reviews of Modern Physics*, **65**: 413–497.

Happé, F.G. (1997). Central coherence and theory of mind in autism: reading homographs in context. *British Journal of Developmental Psychology*, **15**: 1–12.

Happé, F.G. (1999). Autism: cognitive deficit or cognitive style? *Trends in Cognitive Sciences*, **3**: 216–222.

Iacoboni, M. (2009). Imitation, empathy, and mirror neurons. *Annual Review of Psychology*, **60**: 653–670.

Jackson, J.D. (1962). *Classical Electrodynamics*. New York: John Wiley.

Jemel, B., Mottron, L., Dawson, M. (2006). Impaired face processing in autism: fact or artifact? *Journal of Autism and Developmental Disorders*, **36**: 91–106.

Just, M.A., Cherkassky, V.L., Keller, T.A., Minshew, N.J. (2004). Cortical activation and synchronization during sentence comprehension in high-functioning autism: evidence of underconnectivity. *Brain*, **127**: 1811–1821.

Kallen, R.J. (2001). A long letter and an even longer reply about autism magnetoencephalography and electroencephalography. *Pediatrics*, **107**: 1232–1235.

Kanner, A.M. (2000). Commentary: The treatment of seizure disorders and EEG abnormalities in children with autism spectrum disorders: are we getting ahead of ourselves? *Journal of Autism and Developmental Disorders*, **30**: 491–495.

Kasai, K., Hashimoto, O., Kawakubo, Y., *et al.* (2005). Delayed automatic detection of change in speech sounds in adults with autism: a magnetoencephalographic study. *Clinical Neurophysiology*, **116**: 1655–1664.

Katila, T. (1983). On the current multipole presentation of the primary current distribution. *Nuovo Cimento*, **2**: 660–664.

Kutas, M., Federmeier, K.D. (2000). Electrophysiology reveals semantic memory use in language comprehension. *Trends in Cognitive Sciences*, **4**: 463–470.

Kylliäinen, A., Braeutigam, S., Hietanen, J.K., Swithenby, S.J., Bailey, A.J. (2006a). Face and gaze processing in normally developing children: a magnetoencephalographic study. *European Journal of Neuroscience*, **23**: 801–810.

Kylliäinen, A., Braeutigam, S., Hietanen, J.K., Swithenby, S.J., Bailey, A.J. (2006b). Face- and gaze-sensitive neural responses in children with autism: a magnetoencephalographic study. *European Journal of Neuroscience*, **24**: 2679–2690.

Lewine, J.D., Andrews, R., Chez, M., *et al.* (1999). Magnetoencephalographic patterns of epileptiform activity in children with regressive autism spectrum disorders. *Pediatrics*, **104**: 405–418.

Lin, F.H., Witzel, T., Ahlfors, S.P., *et al.* (2006). Assessing and improving the spatial accuracy in MEG source localization by depth-weighted minimum-norm estimates. *Neuroimage*, **31**: 160–171.

Muñoz-Yunta, J.A., Ortiz, T., Palau-Baduell, M., *et al.* (2008). Magnetoencephalographic pattern of epileptiform activity in children with early-onset autism spectrum disorders. *Clinical Neurophysiology*, **119**: 626–634.

Näätänen, R. (2001). The perception of speech sounds by the human brain as reflected by the mismatch negativity (MMN) and its magnetic equivalent (MMNm). *Psychophysiology*, **38**: 1–21.

Neville, B.G. (1999). Magnetoencephalographic patterns of epileptiform activity in children with regressive autism spectrum disorders – commentary. *Pediatrics*, **104**: 558–559.

Nishitani, N., Avikainen, S., Hari, R. (2004). Abnormal imitation-related cortical activation sequences in Asperger's syndrome. *Annals of Neurology*, **55**: 558–562.

O'Connor, K., Hamm, J.P., Kirk, I.J. (2005). The neurophysiological correlates of face processing in adults and children with Asperger's syndrome. *Brain and Cognition*, **59**: 82–95.

Paetvu, R. (2002). Magnetoencephalography on pediatric neuroimaging. *Developmental Science*, **5**: 361–370.

Rapin, I. (2006). Language heterogeneity and regression in the autism spectrum disorders – overlaps with other childhood language regression syndromes. *Clinical Neuroscience Research*, **6**: 209–218.

Rippon, G., Brock, J., Brown, C., Boucher, J. (2007). Disordered connectivity in the autistic brain: challenges for the 'new psychophysiology'. *International Journal of Psychophysiology*, **63**: 164–172.

Rizzolatti, R., Fogassi, L., Gallese, V. (2001). Neurophysiological mechanisms underlying the understanding and imitation of action. *Nature Reviews Neuroscience*, **22**: 661–670.

Roberts, T.P., Poeppel, D. (1996). Latency of auditory evoked M100 as a function of tone frequency. *Neuroreport*, **7**: 1138–1140.

Roberts, T.P., Schmidt, G.L., Egeth, M., *et al.* (2008). Electrophysiological signatures: magnetoencephalographic studies of the neural correlates of language impairment in autism spectrum disorders. *International Journal of Psychophysiology*, **68**: 149–160.

Rojas, D.C., Maharajh, K., Teale, P., Rogers, S.J. (2008). Reduced neural synchronization of gamma-band MEG oscillations in first-degree relatives of children with autism. *BMC Psychiatry*, **8**: 1–9.

Rubenstein, J.L., Merzenich, M.M. (2003). Models of autism: increased ratio of excitation/inhibition in key neural systems. *Genes Brain and Behavior*, **2**: 255–267.

Rumsey, J.M., Ernst, M. (2000). Functional neuroimaging of autistic disorders. *Mental Retardation and Developmental Disabilities Research Reviews*, **6**: 171–179.

Salmon, N., Pratt, H. (2002). A comparison of sentence- and discourse-level semantic processing: an ERP study. *Brain and Language*, **83**: 367–383.

Sanders, J., Johnson, K.A., Garavan, H., Gill, M., Gallagher, L. (2008). A review of neuropsychological and neuroimaging research in autistic spectrum disorders: Attention, inhibition and cognitive flexibility. *Research in Autism Spectrum Disorders*, **2**: 1–16.

Schultz, R.T. (2005). Developmental deficits in social perception in autism: the role of the amygdala and fusiform face area. *International Journal of Developmental Neuroscience*, **23**: 125–141.

Schultz, R.T., Gauthier, I., Klin, A., *et al.* (2000). Abnormal ventral temporal cortical activity during face discrimination among individuals with autism and Asperger syndrome. *Archives of General Psychiatry*, **57**: 331–340.

Seeck, M., Grüsser, O.J. (1992). Category related components in visual evoked potentials: photographs of faces, persons, flowers and tools as stimuli. *Experimental Brain Research*, **92**: 338–349.

Seyffert, M., Castellanos, F.X. (2005). Functional MRI in pediatric neurobehavioral disorders. *International Review of Neurobiology*, **67**: 239–284.

Swithenby, S.J., Bailey, A.J., Braeutigam, S. (1998). Neural processing of human faces: a magnetoencephalographic study. *Experimental Brain Research*, **118**: 501–510.

Tallon-Baudry, C., Bertrand, O. (1999). Oscillatory gamma activity in humans and its role in object representation. *Trends in Cognitive Sciences*, **3**: 151–162.

Uhlhaas, P.J., Singer, W. (2006). Neural synchrony in brain disorders: relevance for cognitive dysfunctions and pathophysiology. *Neuron*, **52**: 155–168.

Vrba, J. (1999). Multichannel squid biomagnetic systems. *Conference of the NATO-Advanced-Study-Institute on Applications of Superconductivity. Series E: Applied Sciences*, **365**: 61–138.

Walenski, M., Tager-Flusberg, H., Ullman, M.T. (2006). Language in autism. In Moldin, S.O. and Rubenstein, J.L.R. (eds) *Understanding Autism: from Basic Neuroscience to Treatment*, Ch 9. Boca Raton, Florida: CRC Press, Taylor and Francis Group.

Wang, A.T., Lee, S.S., Sigman, M., Dapretto, M. (2006). Neural basis of irony comprehension in children with autism: the role of prosody and context. *Brain*, **129**: 932–943.

Wilson, T.W., Rojas, D.C., Reite, M.L., Teale, P.D., Rogers, S.J. (2007). Children and adolescents with autism exhibit reduced MEG steady-state gamma responses. *Biological Psychiatry*, **62**: 192–197.

5

Autism and epilepsy

CHRISTOPHER GILLBERG AND BRIAN NEVILLE

Epilepsy, autism and cognitive impairment are over-represented in all studies that take one of these major categories as the starting point. The rates of epilepsy and autism are related to the severity of cognitive impairment. Those with primary or early regressive autism show a steadily rising rate of epilepsy with age reaching 30–50% in some adult studies but without evidence of causative relationship. Seizures of all types occur with complex partial attacks being prominent but we have no convincing explanation for this relationship. However, in several particularly early onset epilepsies, autism and cognitive impairment develop with the epilepsy suggesting causation (i.e. an epileptic encephalopathy). This process seems to preferentially involve the temporal neocortex and medical or surgical treatment of the epilepsy may cause remission of autistic symptoms in these cases.

5.1 Introduction

In 1943, Kanner described 11 children with his then new 'autistic disturbances of affective contact' (Kanner, 1943). One of these 11 suffered from epilepsy. In 1971, Kanner reported on a follow-up of the 11 patients; by now, two patients – 18% of his original series – were suffering from epilepsy (Kanner, 1971). Thus, in this seminal report, which defined autism, the patients already formed a clinically heterogeneous group – those with and those without seizures.

What has become clear over the years since Kanner's writings is that patients with autism are, in fact, at greater risk of seizures than are children with other types of developmental problems, such as developmental dysphasia or Down

Researching the Autism Spectrum: Contemporary Perspectives, ed. I. Roth and P. Rezaie. Published by Cambridge University Press.

syndrome (Wong, 1993). The frequency of epilepsy in autism, regardless of IQ, is higher than in 'non-autism' severe mental retardation (Gillberg *et al.* 1986), even though a population of individuals with severe mental retardation is likely to include a group with autism often with an additional diagnosable genetic syndrome.

Medical specialities may approach the same conditions from quite different perspectives, for reasons of referral bias or through the way that their discipline has come to recognise the condition. Autism and epilepsy are both good examples of this phenomenon and therefore when patients have both conditions this may lead to the assumption that one condition is primary and the other is a 'co-morbidity'. Since cognitive impairment is so common in those who have autism and epilepsy we have in effect three disorders which need disinterested handling and have been somewhat artificially separated for the convenience of medical study. The literature and our research designs may reflect this bias of different starting points.

We will therefore review the evidence from the starting points of primary developmental autism including those who show regression in the second year; specific early onset epilepsy syndromes and epilepsy more generally. We will then develop these strands into an overall hypothesis.

There is an important potential interaction between the three domains of autism, cognitive impairment and epilepsy and that is the phenomenon referred to as epileptic encephalopathy. This is the hypothesis that some aspect of the epilepsy, particularly subclinical epileptic activity in sleep, is the cause of the additional impairments including cognitive decline and autism (Engel, 2001). In some specific situations which will be quoted, the circumstantial evidence for such a process is strong but in others is weaker or lacking. Specifically there is no strong evidence to support the notion that in general, or rather 'in the average case' (if such a case exists), autism should be construed as an epileptic encephalopathy.

5.2 Prevalence aspects

If one looks at studies of individuals with autism, the percentage of those with epilepsy varies greatly. The prevalence of epilepsy in the general population is 0.5%; the published figures on epilepsy in autism range from 4% to 47% (Carod *et al.* 1995). There appear to be at least two reasons for this rather large variation. One is the fact that each group of patients with autism contains a different mixture of disease entities within the whole, some of which have seizures and some of which do not. Second, the frequency of epilepsy varies with the length of the follow-up period, rising as the follow-up period lengthens. Although epilepsy in children with autism often appears during the first three years of life (Ritvo, 1990), new cases emerge through childhood, adolescence and into adult life (Danielsson *et al.* 2005). The rate of epilepsy in autism tends to be highest in general population samples of cases with autism followed from childhood into adult life, and lowest in child and adolescent psychiatric clinic patients with autism looked at cross-sectionally at any time under 18 years of age.

Also, individuals with 'classic' autism usually have varying degrees of intellectual disability, and the rate of epilepsy is higher in those with lower IQ. Thus, if one considers the rate of epilepsy only in those with classic autism, the percentage is about 35% (Billstedt *et al.* 2005). In those with other types of autism 'spectrum' disorders, including Asperger syndrome, the rate is considerably lower, probably in the order of 5–15%. Thus, if one were to suggest an epilepsy prevalence rate for all the autisms (including cases with mental retardation and cases with low normal, normal or above average IQ), it would probably be in the range of 10–20%.

An epidemiological study of infantile autism conducted in a county in Norway found that 9 (32%) had epilepsy out of 28 individuals with autism (Herder, 1993). In a Spanish series of 62 children with autism (Carod *et al.* 1995), 47% had some kind of epileptic syndrome, including two children with brain tumors – which is an unusual finding in any autism series. Danielsson *et al.* (2005) and Billstedt *et al.* (2005), in their Swedish general population cohort of 120 individuals with classic autism ($N = 87$) and atypical autism ($N = 33$), found that 40% had developed epilepsy in early adult life. Gillberg *et al.* (2010), reporting from the same cohort, found that mortality was very high in autism (8% had died between ages 10 and 40 years), and that much of the increased mortality rate was attributable to epilepsy (including several cases of sudden unexplained death in epilepsy).

5.3 Gender aspects

Thirty years ago, Wing (1981) suggested that girls diagnosed with autism have more severe indices of brain damage than boys, this being one of the reasons that they are not as under-represented at very low IQ levels. Danielsson found that girls with autism were relatively much more likely than boys to suffer from epilepsy (Danielsson *et al.* 2005). In a large American series of 302 children with autism, Tuchman *et al.* (1991) reported that epilepsy occurred in 14%. In this series, girls were affected more frequently than boys (24% vs 11%). (When cognitive and motor disabilities were excluded, the risk of epilepsy in children with autism was only 6%.) Elia *et al.* (1995) also found females to be more frequently affected by seizures than males in an Italian series of subjects with autism and mental retardation.

A review and meta-analysis of all published reports 1963–2006 of epilepsy in autism concluded that females are at relatively much higher risk of the combination of epilepsy and autism than are males, and that epilepsy is much more common (21%) in intellectually disabled children with autism than in those with normal levels of intelligence (8%) (Amiet *et al.* 2008). Nevertheless, there was a much higher rate of epilepsy in the more high functioning group as well (8% versus 0.5% in the general population), indicating a strong link between autism '*per se*' and epilepsy (our conclusion).

5.4 Diagnostic/differential diagnostic aspects including EEG

Standard EEGs are helpful when they reveal frankly epileptiform activity (Rapin, 1997). Based on a review of the medical literature up to that time, Tsai *et al.* (1985) reported that the majority of children with autism have shown some kind of EEG abnormality whether they had seizures or not. However, if the abnormal EEG readings are limited to epileptiform findings, this figure declines. Rossi *et al.* (1995) examined 106 patients with autism and found that 23.6% had paroxysmal EEG abnormalities compared to 18.9% with actual clinical seizures. Chez *et al.* (2006) reporting on the largest autism-EEG cohort to date ($N = 889$), found 61% had epileptiform activity during sleep, in spite of having no diagnosed clinical seizure disorder (see also MEG findings, Chapter 4 (Section 4.3.1) of this volume).

When one looks at the picture from the public health point of view of how much epilepsy and mental retardation exist in a general population, there is the additional question of how much autism contributes to this cohort. An answer has been given by a population-based study of 6- to 13-year-olds which identified 98 children with active epilepsy and mental retardation and reported that an autistic disorder was present in 27% and an autistic-like disorder in 11% of these children (Steffenburg *et al.* 1995).

5.5 Autistic regression and epilepsy

About a fifth to one-third of autistic toddlers appear to regress in language, sociability, play and often cognition (Rapin 1995; Fernell *et al.* 2010). Some of this is probably not due to 'real' regression, but produced by the fact that children who develop 'normally' for about eighteen months or so thereafter do not have the communication 'building blocks' to develop more complex forms of language and cognition, and hence stop using what little language they may have had. The study by Billstedt *et al.* (2005) suggests that only about one in ten of all children with autism actually show some real regression early in life (and that another minority deteriorate in adolescence). Nevertheless, in a subgroup of all children with autism, regression is a real and very important phenomenon. In such cases, fluctuation in language or behaviour often raises the suspicion of epilepsy. Epilepsy or a paroxysmal EEG occasionally may be associated with autistic regression. However, according to one author, epilepsy probably plays a relatively minor, although non-negligible, pathogenetic role in autistic regression (Rapin, 1995). Others (Baird *et al.* 2006) have not found any evidence of a link. Nevertheless a prolonged sleep EEG that includes study of stage III and stage IV sleep is recommended for children without seizures who have regressed or who have fluctuating deficits and for mute and poorly intelligible children who may have verbal auditory agnosia (Tuchman and Rapin, 1997). In the medical literature, there is a rare subgroup of children with chronic motor tics who had both autistic regression and seizures as described by Nass *et al.* (1998). Seizures consisted of absence or myoclonic patterns, usually resistant to antiepileptic drugs. The patients had a specific pattern of occipital spiking on EEG.

After language is developed and after 2 years of age, a few children may undergo a rapid regression in language, sociability, play and apparent cognition. This has been called Childhood Disintegrative Disorder (Heller syndrome) and is thought by some to be a separate disorder from classic autism. We, however, have seen this phenotype starting as classical Landau-Kleffner syndrome.

5.6 Types of seizures

Many patterns of seizures are seen in patients with autism – infantile spasms, atonic seizures, myoclonic seizures, atypical absence, complex partial and generalised tonic–clonic seizures. Most known EEG patterns are also found in this patient group including electrical status epilepticus in slow wave sleep (ESES). Infantile spasms and complex partial seizures are relatively more common than other seizure types.

In the first few months of life, infantile spasms is the seizure pattern most likely, by far, to be associated with later development of autistic symptoms. However, there is a case in the literature of a child with EEG and clinical symptoms that met the criteria of benign familial neonatal convulsions who later developed autism (Alfonso *et al.* 1997).

5.6.1 *Atonic seizures*

Atonic seizures refer to generalised seizures in which the dominant motor manifestation is loss of postural tone, associated with loss of consciousness, usually for several minutes. They are simply grand mal seizures with limpness – rather than stiffness and repetitive jerking. Such cases have been reported in children with autism in the Tuchman *et al.* (1991) series.

5.6.2 *Myoclonic epilepsies of early childhood (minor motor seizures)*

Myoclonic seizures refer to single or multiple brief, shock-like jerking movements of the head, trunk or extremities. The infant form of these epilepsies begins in infancy or pre-school years and is often seen in combination with tonic–clonic patterns. It may be associated with bursts of slow 1- to 2.5-per-second spike-and-wave complexes on EEG.

Myoclonic seizures are seen in patients with autism but it is unusual to find them as an isolated seizure type. Most often they are found in combination with other seizure patterns, particularly tonic–clonic, and are classified as the myoclonic epilepsies (Gillberg and Steffenburg 1987; Olsson *et al.* 1988). As the exception to the rule, there are several cases in the medical literature of solitary myoclonic seizures and autism (Boyer *et al.* 1981; Gillberg *et al.* 1984). The Gillberg *et al.* (1984) case is a description of a boy with classical autism, XYY syndrome, and myoclonic seizures who became seizure-free on valproic acid, and thereafter quickly improved regarding both his severe behavioural symptoms and his language disturbances.

5.6.3 *Absence epilepsy (petit mal)*

Absence seizures refer to staring spells, usually less than 20 seconds in duration, sometimes with slight flickering of the eyes. There are associated bilateral 2 to 4 Hz spike-and-slow wave complexes on EEG. EEGs are indicated for children in whom epilepsy is suspected, but it should be kept in mind that non-epileptic staring spells are much more common than absence seizures (Rapin, 1997).

There are a few studies which have found absence seizures in patients with autism (Ritvo *et al.* 1990; Tuchman *et al.* 1991). The absence seizures may be described as atypical. There is a case in the literature of an 8-year-old boy where absence seizures were reported to 'masquerade' as autism. He had almost continuous bilateral synchronous 3 Hz spike-and-slow wave on EEG and improved dramatically – both psychiatrically and neurologically – with ethosuximide monotherapy (Gillberg and Schaumann, 1983).

5.6.4 *Complex partial seizures (psychomotor epilepsy)*

If a child blanks out or stares, there are two possible seizure types to consider. One is absence seizures, as described above. The other is complex partial seizures which usually last between 30 seconds and two minutes and are accompanied by a variety of automatisms, such as lip smacking, hand wringing or plucking at clothes. Other signs of a partial complex seizure might be a temporary 'dreamy state' or impaired consciousness with an affective disturbance such as fear or anger. The EEG may show either unilateral or bilateral foci, usually frontal or temporal.

It is easy to see how such seizure activity might be hard to pick out in a child with autism. Corbett (1982) raised the question about how likely it was that such seizure activity might be under-reported in non-verbal children with autism. A population-based study of epilepsy in pre-pubertal children with autism or autistic-like conditions found that complex partial seizures were present in 71% of those that had an onset of seizures in early childhood (Olsson *et al.* 1988). In another study of young people with autism, aged 16 to 23 years, Gillberg and Steffenburg (1987) found the majority of those with epilepsy and a prepubertal onset had complex partial seizures. Danielsson *et al.* (2005) in their very long-term prospective follow-up study of children with autism found complex partial seizures (with or without generalisation) to be the most common type of epilepsy throughout the follow-up period.

5.6.5 *Generalised tonic–clonic seizures (grand mal)*

In seizure parlance, the word 'tonic' refers to a stiffening of the body with rigid extension of the trunk and extremities. The word 'clonic' refers to generalised seizures with repetitive bilateral clonic jerking of the extremities. In tonic–clonic (grand mal) seizures, there is typically alternate stiffening and jerking associated with loss of consciousness.

Generalised tonic–clonic seizures are the most frequent form of epilepsy in the general population. They are relatively common in children and adolescents with autism (Carod *et al.* 1995; Olsson *et al.* 1988; Tuchman *et al.* 1991). In autism, tonic–clonic seizures may be associated with other types of seizures, either as sequelae after infantile spasms or immediately following complex partial seizures (Gillberg and Steffenburg, 1987; Olsson *et al.* 1988).

5.7 Early onset epilepsy syndromes with developmental regression

We now review specific early onset epilepsy syndrome in which developmental regression occurs. This may be on the basis of normal early development or in some lesional cases in which early development may be slow. Some are strongly genetic and regression may theoretically be epileptically driven or genetic.

5.7.1 *Infantile spasms and hypsarrhythmia (West syndrome)*

Infantile spasms begin in early infancy with runs of spasms. The EEG changes have a characteristic picture of abundant spike and polyspikes along with high voltage slowing. The association of infantile spasms with this EEG picture of 'hypsarrhythmia' has become known as West syndrome, referring to the physician who first described the features in his own son. At the time of presentation eye contact and verbalisation are commonly lost.

Despite effective treatment of infantile spasms in many with corticosteroids and vigabatrin, the child is often left with cognitive impairment and autistic symptoms. The percentage of patients with infantile spasms who later show the symptoms of autism varies in different studies from 2% (Prats *et al.* 1991) to 16%

(Riikonen and Amnell, 1981). Looking at the problem from a different perspective, one could ask what percentage of patients with autism with all forms of epilepsy have infantile spasms? In the large series of 302 patients with autism studied by Tuchman *et al.* (1991), infantile spasms occurred in 12% of those patients with autism who also had epilepsy.

Patients with infantile spasms who later develop an autistic syndrome may have one of a number of different disease entities, which include tuberous sclerosis, neurofibromatosis 1, Down syndrome, phenylketonuria and minor hydrocephalus. Tuberous Sclerosis is one of the more common aetiologies underlying autism in epilepsy. In a study of 38 patients with tuberous sclerosis and epilepsy, 17 had infantile spasms (Ohtuska *et al.* 1998). A number of patients with neurofibromatosis 1 also have been reported with infantile spasms (Millichap, 1997). Saemundsen in an Icelandic study found that the odds of developing autism was about 5–6 times raised after infantile spasms, but that much of this risk was associated with a symptomatic origin of the seizures (Saemundsen *et al.* 2008).

One study suggests that both temporal lobes often appear to be involved in those patients with infantile spasms who will later develop autism (Chugani *et al.* 1996). This follow-up study of 14 babies with infantile spasms and a PET study which showed bitemporal hypometablism revealed that 10 had developed autism. We also have ERP evidence of delay and blunting of responses to novelty stimuli in the temporal lobe (Werner *et al.* 2005).

5.7.2 *Landau-Kleffner (acquired epileptic aphasia) syndrome and ESES (electric status epilepticus in slow sleep)*

Landau-Kleffner syndrome is an acquired epileptic aphasia or verbal auditory agnosia affecting children between 2 and 5 years of age who already have developed speech. There are seizures and/or an often bilateral paroxysmal EEG pattern. In the classical Landau-Kleffner syndrome, aphasia is acquired and other higher cortical functions usually do not deteriorate. In a variation of the syndrome called 'epilepsy with continuous spike-waves during slow wave sleep' (CSWS) or Electric Status Epilepticus in Slow Sleep (ESES), speech is disturbed in 50% of the cases and intellectual deterioration occurs with psychiatric symptoms, often reminiscent of autism, developing. According to Hirsch *et al.* (1990), they are probably variations of a single syndrome. Corticosteroids are usually tried in this patient group and may have at least a temporary – sometimes dramatic – beneficial effect. There is also an experimental surgical therapy called subpial intracortical transection (Cross and Neville, 2009; Morrell *et al.* 1995; Nass *et al.* 1998).

5.7.3 *Dravet syndrome (severe myoclonic epilepsy in infancy)*

Dravet syndrome is a catastrophic form of epilepsy which begins with seizures, often hemiclonic status epilepticus with fever, during the first year of life (Nolan *et al.* 2008). Development remains normal during the first year and until the onset of habitual seizures, usually in the second year. These seizures include myoclonic, atypical absences, partial and secondarily generalised. Psychomotor retardation, autistic features often satisfying full criteria for autism, hyperactivity and other neurological deficits occur in affected children, and are usually obvious in the second to fourth year of life. A considerable proportion of all affected individuals have missense or truncated mutation of the sodium channel gene SCN1A. Seizures are often triggered by fever and children with very early onset, long-lasting (> 10 mins) 'febrile seizures' should always be suspected of Dravet syndrome. Unfortunately, most treatments for seizures in Dravet syndrome have been relatively unsuccessful, although stiripentol combined with sodium valproate and sometimes a benzodiazepine appears to hold promise (Chiron *et al.* 2000). During the first year of normal development the interictal EEG is usually normal but becomes abnormal during the second phase of regression.

In addition to these specific epilepsy syndromes at high risk of autism and cognitive impairment there is a generally higher rate of autism in unselected series of children with active epilepsy. Specialist referral units for childhood epilepsy are accustomed to autism and ADHD being unrecognised for several years despite obvious problems at home and school. It is therefore clear that all children with intractable epilepsy should be screened for these problems including ASD so that they can be fully diagnosed and managed. The simplest broad screen is the Strengths and Difficulties questionnaire (Goodman, 1999). The Autism Spectrum Screening questionnaire can be used for more precise identification (Ehlers and Gillberg, 1993).

5.8 The phenotype of ASD with epilepsy

Until recently the issue of whether the ASD associated with epilepsy is the same as that without epilepsy had not been addressed. We already know that cognitive level was lower with epilepsy. A study of this subject is difficult for several reasons:

- The two quite separate pathways outlined above may not be included in the study design
- The criteria for the diagnosis of ASD will influence the phenotype as an outcome measure
- The co-existence of other behavioural characteristics (e.g. of attention, impulsivity, obsessive and manipulative behaviour) will have to be handled in the study design in a way which answers the question. This is difficult because of the arbitrary nature of the definitions of ASD used.

In a recent study comparing the features of autism between those with and without epilepsy there were difficulties in controlling for IQ (Turk *et al.* 2009). The factors that were more evident in those with epilepsy were a relatively greater proportion of girls, more motor difficulties but no difference in aloofness and passivity, but the writers acknowledge the difficulties of this type of study.

One method of dealing with this would be a description of the elements of behaviour in children with epilepsy at different cognitive levels without attempting to control data.

5.9 Investigation and management

In early onset epilepsies with regression an urgent EEG including sleep is essential with a view to treatment particularly of sub-clinical seizure activity with benzodiazepine and corticosteroids. It is important that response to such treatment is monitored using standardised measures of verbal and non-verbal abilities and autism features. Details of the medical management of epilepsy are outside the remit of this text. It is important, however, that the epilepsy and psychiatric management are integrated. Neurological regression requires neurological investigation which will include MRI scanning and biochemical investigation.

5.10 Place of EEG in the investigation of autism

Despite the evidence of higher than expected rates of epileptic activity in autism without seizures no studies have shown that routine EEGs, waking or sleep, help in diagnosis or management of the patient and it may be quite testing to obtain a good record. In the main this conclusion also applies to those who show typical autistic regression in the second year of life. If, however, the regression is atypical or occurs with seizures EEG monitoring is indicated as it is with children with autism and seizures. Treatment with antiepilepsy drugs in the latter situation aims to reduce or stop seizures and no change in autism features is expected. There are, however, situations where clear features of autism recede with intensive treatment:

- In Landau-Kleffner syndrome obvious features of autism may remit with medical or surgical treatment.
- Early onset lesional epilepsy particularly dysembryoplastic temporal lobe lesions showing autistic regression which may remit with early effective surgery (Gillberg *et al.* 1996; Neville *et al.* 1997).

5.11 Pathogenesis of autistic regression in epilepsy

There are several strands of evidence that support the view that the developing temporal lobe is not able to make appropriate language and social communication connections in the presence of high rates of epileptic discharges. This evidence includes:

- West syndrome caused by tuberous sclerosis shows a relationship between temporal lobe tubers and autism (Bolton and Griffiths, 1997).
- Abnormal temporal lobe generator ERPs to novelty (Thivierge *et al.* 1990).
- A high rate of autistic features in LKS which is predominantly a disturbance of function and structure in the superior temporal gyrus.
- Strong association between temporal lobe lesions, particularly right sided, and autism in patients coming for epilepsy surgery (Taylor *et al.* 1999).
- The FDG PET evidence of temporal lobe hypometabolism in patients with tuberous sclerosis and autism (Asano *et al.* 2001).
- Interestingly, as well as acute regression at about 4 months with infantile spasms and tuberous sclerosis, this regression with the appearance of autism has occurred with recurrence of seizures in the second year of life (Humphrey *et al.* 2006).

This evidence, however, only applies to autistic regression which is led by a severe early onset epilepsy syndrome. We have no current explanation for the high rates of epilepsy and epileptic EEG abnormality in developmental autism. Stating that in autism generally there appears to be a reduced threshold for epilepsy may be doing no more than repeating the above evidence.

5.12 References

Alfonso, I., Hahn, J.S., Papazian, O., *et al.* (1997). Bilateral tonic-clonic epileptic seizures in non-benign familial neonatal convulsions. *Pediatric Neurology*, **16**: 249–251.

Amiet, C., Gourfinkel-An, I., Bouzamondo, A., *et al.* (2008). Epilepsy in autism is associated with intellectual disability and gender: evidence from a meta-analysis. *Biological Psychiatry*, **64**: 577–582.

Asano, E., Chugani, D.C., Muzik, O., *et al.* (2001). Autism in tuberous sclerosis complex is related to both cortical and subcortical dysfunction. *Neurology*, **57**: 1269–1277.

Baird, G., Simonoff, E., Pickles, A., *et al.* (2006). Prevalence of disorders of the autism spectrum in a population cohort of children in South Thames: The Special Needs and Autism project (SNAP). *Lancet*, **368**: 210–215.

Billstedt, E., Gillberg, I.C., Gillberg, C. (2005). Autism after adolescence: population-based 13- to 22-year follow-up study of 120 individuals with autism diagnosed in childhood. *Journal of Autism and Developmental Disorders*, **35**: 351–360.

Bolton, P.F., Griffiths, P.D. (1997). Association of tuberous sclerosis of temporal lobes with autism and atypical autism. *Lancet*, **349**: 392–395.

Bolton, P.F., Park, R.J., Higgins, J.N., Griffiths, P.D., Pickles, A. (2002). Neuro-epileptic determinants of autism spectrum disorders in tuberous sclerosis complex. *Brain*, **125**: 1247–1255.

Boyer, J-P., Deschatrette, A., Delwarde, M. (1981). Autisme convulsif? *Pédiatrie*, **5**: 353–368.

Carod, F.J., Prats, J.M., Garaizar, C., Zuazo, E. (1995). Clinical-radiological evaluation of infantile autism and epileptic syndromes associated with autism. (in Spanish) *Review of Neurology*, **23**: 1203–1207.

Chez, M.G., Loeffel, M., Buchanan, C.P., Field-Chez, M. (1998). Pulse high-dose steroids as combination therapy with valproic acid in epileptic aphasia patients with pervasive developmental delay or autism. *Annals of Neurology*, **44**: 539.

Chiron, C., Marchand, M.C., Tran, A., *et al.* (2000). Stiripentol in severe myoclonic epilepsy in infancy: a randomised placebo controlled syndrome-dedicated trial. STICLO study group. *Lancet*, **356**: 1638–1642.

Chugani, H.T., Da Silva, E., Chugani, D.C. (1996). Prognostic implications of bitemporal hypometabolism on positron emission tomography. *Annals of Neurology*, **39**: 643–649.

Corbett, J. (1982). Epilepsy and the electroencephalogram in early childhood psychosis. In *Handbook of Psychiatry*, Vol. 3. London: Cambridge University Press, pp. 198–202.

Cross, J.H., Neville, B.G. (2009). The surgical treatment of Landau-Kleffner syndrome. *Epilepsia*, **50 (Suppl 7)**: 63–67.

Danielsson, S., Gillberg, I.C., Billstedt, E., Gillberg, C., Olsson, I. (2005). Epilepsy in young adults with autism; a prospective population-based follow-up study of 120 individuals diagnosed in childhood. *Epilepsia*, **46**: 918–923.

Ehlers, S., Gillberg, C. (1993). The epidemiology of Asperger Syndrome. A total population study. *Journal of Child Psychology and Psychiatry*, **34**: 1327–1350.

Elia, M., Musumeci, S.A., Ferri, R., Bergonzi, P. (1995). Clinical and neurophysiological aspects of epilepsy in subjects with autism and mental retardation. *American Journal of Mental Retardation*, **100**: 6–16.

Engel, J. Jr. (2001). International League against Epilepsy (ILAE). A proposed diagnostic scheme for people with epileptic seizures and with epilepsy. Report of the ILAE Task Force on Classification and Terminology. *Epilepsia*; **42**: 796–803.

Fernell, E., Hedvall, A., Norrelgren, F., *et al.* (2010). Developmental profiles in preschool children with autism spectrum disorders referred for intervention. *Research in Developmental Disabilities*, **31**: 790–799.

Gillberg, C., Schaumann, H. (1983). Epilepsy presenting as infantile autism? Two case studies. *Neuropediatrics*, **14**: 206–212.

Gillberg, C., Steffenburg, S. (1987). Outcome and prognostic factors in infantile autism and similar conditions: a population-based study of 46 cases followed through puberty. *Journal of Autism and Developmental Disorders*, **17**: 273–287.

Gillberg, C., Winnergård, I., Wahlström, J. (1984). The sex chromosomes – one key to autism? An XYY case of infantile autism. *Applied Research in Mental Retardation*, **5**: 353–360.

Gillberg, C., Persson, E., Grufman, M., Themnér, U. (1986). Psychiatric disorders in mildly and severely mentally retarded urban children and adolescents: epidemiological aspects. *British Journal of Psychiatry*, **149**: 68–74.

Gillberg, C., Uvebrant, P., Carlsson, G., Hedstrom, A., Silfvenius, H. (1996). Autism and epilepsy (and tuberous sclerosis?) in two pre-adolescent boys: neuropsychiatric aspects before and after epilepsy surgery. *Journal of Intellectual Disability Research*, **40**: 75–81.

Gillberg, C., Billstedt, E., Sundh, V., Gillberg. I.C. (2010). Mortality in autism: a prospective longitudinal community-based study. *Journal of Autism and Developmental Disorders*, **40**: 352–357.

Goodman, R. (1999). The extended version of the strengths and difficulties questionnaire as a guide to child psychiatric caseness and consequent burden. *Journal of Child Psychology and Psychiatry*, **40**: 791–799.

Herder, G.A. (1993). Infantile autism among children in the county of Nordland: Prevalence and etiology. (in Norwegian) *Tidsskrif for Norsk Laegeforening*, **113**: 2247–2249.

Hirsch, E., Marescaux, C., Maquet, P., *et al.* (1990). Landau-Kleffner syndrome: a clinical and EEG study. *Epilepsia*, **31**: 756–767.

Humphrey, A., Neville, B.G.R., Bolton, P.F. (2006). Autistic regression associated with seizure onset in an infant with tuberous sclerosis. *Developmental Medicine and Child Neurology*, **48**: 942–944.

Kanner, L. (1943). Autistic disturbances of affective contact. *Nervous Child*, **2**: 217–250.

Kanner, L. (1971). Follow-up study of eleven children originally reported in 1943. *Journal of Autism and Childhood Schizophrenia*, **1**: 119–145.

Morrell, F., Whisler, W.W., Smith, M.C., *et al.* (1995). Landau-Kleffner syndrome: Treatment with subpial intracortical transection. *Brain*, **118**: 1529–1546.

Nass, R., Gross, A., Devinsky, O. (1998). Autism and autistic epileptiform regression with occipital spikes. *Developmental Medicine and Child Neurology*, **40**: 453–458.

Neville, B.G., Harkness, W.F., Cross, J.H., *et al.* (1997). Surgical treatment of severe autistic regression in childhood epilepsy. *Pediatric Neurology*, **16**: 137–140.

Nolan, K., Camfield, C.S., Camfield, P.R. (2008). Coping with a child with Dravet syndrome: insights from families. *Journal of Child Neurology*, **23**: 690–694.

Ohtsuka, Y., Ohmori, I., Oka, E. (1998). Long-term follow-up of childhood epilepsy associated with tuberous sclerosis. *Epilepsia*, **39**: 1158–1163.

Olsson, I., Steffenburg, S., Gillberg, C. (1988). Epilepsy in autism and autistic-like conditions: a population-based study. *Archives of Neurology*, **45**: 666–668.

Prats, J.M., Garaizar, C., Rua, M.J., Garcia-Nieto, M.L., Madoz, P. (1991). Infantile spasms treated with high doses of sodium valproate: initial response and follow-up. *Developmental Medicine and Child Neurology*, **33**: 617–625.

Rapin, I. (1995). Autistic regression and disintegrative disorder: how important is the role of epilepsy? *Seminars in Pediatric Neurology*, **2**: 278–285.

Rapin, I. (1997). Autism. *New England Journal of Medicine*, **337**: 97–104.

Riikonen, R., Amnell, G. (1981). Psychiatric disorders in children with earlier infantile spasms. *Developmental Medicine and Child Neurology*, **23**: 747–760.

Ritvo, E.R., Freeman, B.J., Pingree, C., *et al.* (1990). The UCLA-University of Utah epidemiological survey of autism prevalence. *American Journal of Psychiatry*, **146**: 194–199.

Rossi, P.G., Parmeggiani, A., Bach, V., Santucci, M., Visconti, P. (1995). EEG features and epilepsy in patients with autism. *Brain and Development*, **17**: 169–174.

Saemundsen, E., Ludvigsson, P., Rafnsson, V. (2008). Risk of autism spectrum disorders after infantile spasms: a population-based study nested in a cohort with seizures in the first year of life. *Epilepsia*, **49**: 1865–1870.

Steffenburg, U., Hagberg, G., Viggedal, G., Kyllerman, M. (1995). Active epilepsy in mentally retarded children. I. Prevalence and additional neuro-impairments. *Acta Paediatrica*, **84**: 1147–1152.

Taylor, D.C., Neville, B.G., Cross, J.H. (1999). Autistic spectrum disorders in childhood epilepsy surgery candidates. *European Child and Adolescent Psychiatry*, **8**: 189–192.

Thivièrge, J., Bedard, C., Côté, R., Maziade, M. (1990). Brainstem auditory evoked response and subcortical abnormalities in autism. *American Journal of Psychiatry*, **147**: 1609–1613.

Tsai, L.Y., Tsai, M.C., August, G.J. (1985). Brief report: implication of EEG diagnoses in the subclassification of infantile autism. *Journal of Autism and Childhood Schizophrenia*, **15**: 339–344.

Tuchman, R.F., Rapin, I. (1997). Regression in pervasive developmental disorders: seizures and epileptiform electroencephalogram correlates. *Pediatrics*, **99**: 560–565.

Tuchman, R.F., Rapin, I., Shinnar, S. (1991). Autistic and dysphasic children. II: epilepsy. *Pediatrics*, **88**: 1219–1225.

Turk, J., Bax, M., Williams, C., Amin, P., Eriksson, M., Gillberg, C. (2009). Autism spectrum disorder in children with and without epilepsy: impact on social functioning and communication. *Acta Paediatrica*, **98**: 675–681.

Werner, K., Scott, R., Baldweg, T., Boyd, S., Neville, B.G.R. (2005). Auditory evoked potential abnormalities in infants with infantile spasms. *Developmental Medicine and Child Neurology*, **101** (Suppl): 47.

Wing, L. (1981). Sex ratios in early childhood autism and related conditions. *Psychiatry Research*, **5**: 129–137.

Wong, V. (1993). Epilepsy in children with autistic spectrum disorder. *Journal of Child Neurology*, **8**: 316–322.

6

Biochemistry of autism: changes in serotonin, reelin and oxytocin

ELIZABETA B. MUKAETOVA-LADINSKA, JODIE WESTWOOD AND ELAINE PERRY

Autism is a neurodevelopmental disorder characterised by impaired social skills, communication deficits and repetitive behaviours. Alterations in a number of neurotransmitter signalling systems and neuroregulatory proteins have been reported in individuals with autism spectrum disorders (ASD). The most compelling evidence seems to suggest an imbalance in excitatory and inhibitory impulses in the premature autistic brain, combined with defects in secondary neurotransmitter systems, resulting in autistic traits. Serotonin, known to be disrupted in ASD, facilitates the release of both reelin and oxytocin, with excessive levels of serotonin resulting in a decrease in reelin and oxytocin. Deficits in developmental growth factors, such as reelin, may regulate or be regulated by oxytocin, thus contributing to both neurodevelopmental arrest and altered social behaviour, characteristic for the autistic spectrum. In this review we therefore concentrate on the role of the serotonin neurotransmitter and the two neuroregulatory proteins (reelin and oxytocin), and evaluate the pharmacological interventions available at the moment, associated with the latter neurochemical changes in autism.

6.1 Introduction

Autism is regarded as a heterogeneous neurodevelopmental disorder, characterised by a spectrum of impaired social skills, communication deficits, repetitive behaviour and frequently associated with co-morbid disorders (e.g. obsessive compulsive disorder, epilepsy, Tourette syndrome, attention deficit hyperactivity disorder, tuberous sclerosis and Fragile X syndrome, among others; Gillberg and Billstedt, 2000). A significant number of individuals with autism also show

Researching the Autism Spectrum: Contemporary Perspectives, ed. I. Roth and P. Rezaie. Published by Cambridge University Press.

hyperactivity, anxiety and self-injurious behaviours. The degree of the characteristic symptoms can vary profoundly, from an extremely affected individual with significant learning difficulties, to a high functioning individual with Asperger syndrome, giving rise to the 'autism spectrum'. The onset of the symptoms can also vary: some children have developmental delay within the first 18 months of life, whereas 25–40% of children (Goldberg *et al.* 2003) will have a 'regressive' phenotype, characterised by near-normal development until 18–24 months, following which they regress. Autism incidence rates are currently predicted as 1:150 births (Centers for Disease Control and Prevention, CDCP USA, 2007), with an overall prevalence estimate of 1:100 children (see Chapter 1), and a three- to four-fold higher prevalence in males.

The diversity and degree of severity of the various symptoms associated with ASD contribute to difficulties in studying these conditions. Similarly, the use of different diagnostic criteria limits continuity between studies. The heterogeneity of the autism spectrum is further supported by the various alterations in neurochemicals (signalling molecules in the nervous system) and neurotransmitters (molecules that travel across a synapse between pre- and post-synaptic nerve terminals). Thus, deficits in serotonergic, cholinergic, glutamatergic, gamma-aminobutyric acid (GABA)-ergic and oxytocin systems (McNamara *et al.* 2008), as well as reelin and *N*-acetylaspartate, have been documented (Blaylock and Strunecka, 2009; Fatemi *et al.* 2005; Martin-Ruiz *et al.* 2004; McNamara *et al.* 2008; Oblak *et al.* 2009).

Serotonin, a neurotransmitter shown to be disrupted in ASD, facilitates the release of both reelin and oxytocin. Thus, excessive levels of serotonin result in decreased reelin levels (Janusonis *et al.* 2004) and oxytocin-containing neurons (McNamara *et al.* 2008). Furthermore, deficits in developmental growth factors, such as reelin, may regulate or be regulated by oxytocin (Carter, 2007; Liu *et al.* 2005), and contribute towards altered social behaviours associated with the autism spectrum. Changes in the expression of serotonin, reelin and oxytocin may underlie altered neurodevelopment in autism. In this review we will concentrate on the role of serotonin and these two neuroregulatory proteins (reelin and oxytocin), and evaluate the pharmacological interventions that are currently available, targeting these latter neurochemical changes in autism.

6.2 Serotonin neurochemistry in autism

Serotonin, or 5-hydroxytryptamine (5-HT), is a signalling molecule found throughout the body (transported by platelets; Anderson *et al.* 1987), and in the brain where it acts as a neurotransmitter. It is derived from the amino acid tryptophan, hydroxylated by tryptophan hydroxylase (TPH) to form 5-hydroxytryptophan (5-HTT), the rate limiting step in the production of serotonin. An aromatic amino acid decarboxylase then catalyses the conversion of 5-HTT to serotonin. Serotonin has many physiological functions and impacts on many human behaviours, including eating, sleeping, mood, hostility, temperament, body temperature and hormone release (reviewed by Keltikangas-Järvinen and Salo, 2009)).

6.2.1 *Serotonin dysfunction*

It has long been established that serotonin plays a role in autism. Acting as a developmental signal in the immature brain, prior to the time it assumes the role as a neurotransmitter, serotonin influences a range of brain developmental changes, including inhibition of serotonergic neurons (in an autocrine manner), promotion of neurite outgrowth, synaptogenesis, neurogenesis in target neurons, differentiation and organisation of the brain network (reviewed by McNamara *et al.* 2008). The impact of serotonin on atypical neurodevelopment in autism may be reflected, therefore, in brain overgrowth, poor cortical lamination, smaller neuronal cell size, as well as poor dendritic arborisation and synaptic expression (Amaral *et al.* 2008; Mukaetova-Ladinska *et al.* 2004).

Acute depletion of dietary tryptophan increases the symptoms of autism (McDougle *et al.* 1996a). Children exposed *in utero* to drugs that increase serotonin levels, such as cocaine, are reported to have a higher incidence of autism than is normally expected (Davis *et al.* 1992; Kramer *et al.* 1994). These findings have led to the development of a rat 'hyperserotonaemia' model of autism, in which high levels of serotonin in the blood precede loss of serotonin terminals within the brain, acting through a negative feedback process. Serotonergic functions are consequently disrupted, with widespread changes affecting the hypothalamus and amygdala (McNamara *et al.* 2008). This animal model has much in common with several social and behavioural changes inherent in autism, e.g. lack of maternal and sibling bonding, diminution of adult pro-social behaviours in the social interactions and stereotyped behaviour and with certain neuropathological changes observed at post-mortem within the brain of individuals with ASD (Adolphs *et al.* 2002; Howard *et al.* 2000). Interestingly, post-mortem analysis in an animal model also found loss of oxytocin-containing neurons within the paraventricular nucleus of the hypothalamus (McNamara *et al.* 2007). These results may correspond to the hypothalamic and amygdalar changes in the human ASD and suggest that the hyperserotonaemia model of autism may be a valid model which produces many of the social, behavioral and peptide changes inherent to autism. However, these findings need to be examined further in human neuropathological studies in ASD.

Dysfunction of the serotonin system may also arise from abnormal cholesterol metabolism, which could in turn lead to the range of social and behavioural problems associated with individuals with ASD (reviewed by Aneja and Tierney, 2008). Cholesterol is a constituent of the lipid rafts of the serotonin transporter (Allen *et al.* 2007), and disruption of lipid rafts by cholesterol-interfering agents can lead to as much as a 50% reduction in the rate of GABA, 5-HT and glutamate transporters (Saher *et al.* 2005). A role for cholesterol in abnormal serotonergic neuronal development associated with ASD is further supported by a mouse model of Smith-Lemli-Opitz syndrome (Waage-Baudet *et al.* 2003). Furthermore, bioinformatics and gene ontological analyses of available data in ASD implicate a number of genes involved in nervous system development, inflammation and cytoskeletal organisation, in addition to genes relevant to gastrointestinal or other physiological symptoms often associated with autism. Most importantly, these processes appear to be modulated by cholesterol/steroid metabolism, especially at the level of androgenic hormones (Hu *et al.* 2009), and may thus explain the greater susceptibility to ASD in male subjects.

6.2.2 *Positron emission tomography (PET) studies*

PET studies have been used to determine serotonin synthesis in the brain, using an α-[^{11}C] methyl-L-tryptophan ([^{11}C]AMT) tracer. In a study by Chugani *et al.* (1997), seven boys with autism were analysed using PET and compared to their unaffected siblings. In autism, areas with unusual serotonin synthesis levels included the frontal cortex (decreased synthesis), cerebellar dentate nucleus (increased synthesis) and the thalamus (decreased synthesis), all connected via the dentatothalamocortical pathway, thought to be involved in speech production and sensory integration. Typically developing children have 200% higher serotonin synthesis levels than adults up to the age of five, with the levels then gradually decreasing with age to normal adult levels (Chugani *et al.* 1999). Similar findings of decreased cortical serotonin 5-HT$_{2A}$ receptor binding in a number of cortical areas (associated with impaired social communication) were reported in adults with Asperger syndrome using SPECT (Murphy *et al.* 2006). However, in ASD, serotonin synthesis capacity gradually increases from 2 years of age up to 15 years, being 1.5 times greater than typical adult levels (Chugani *et al.* 1999). This suggests that high brain serotonin synthesis occurs during childhood, but this developmental mechanism could be significantly altered in children with ASD. Lower cortical 5-HT$_2$ receptor density is also present in parents of children with autism (Goldberg *et al.* 2008), suggesting an underlying association.

6.2.3 *Plasma blood serotonin levels in autism*

Hyperserotonaemia (elevated blood serotonin levels) has been shown to consistently occur in 25–33% of individuals with autism (Mulder *et al.* 2004; Takahashi *et al.* 1976; Table 6.1). The disequilibrium in the peripheral and central turnover of serotonin, accompanied by an increase in neurotoxic glucocorticoids (Croonenberghs *et al.* 2008), appears to play an important role in autism. Despite efforts to link hyperserotonaemia to a possible clinical sub-group of autism, results have varied. Interestingly, about 20% of individuals with ASD also have

Table 6.1 *Hyperserotonaemia studies with autistic patients*

Study	Participants	Limitations	Criteria for diagnosis of autism	Main findings
Takahashi, *et al.* (1976)	30 children with early infantile autism, 30 age matched control children, 45 children with various neurological disorders (age range unknown)	Sample sizes; lack of accuracy of diagnosis	Kanner's criteria	Platelet serotonin levels higher in children with autism. Elevated in some of the other groups with hyperactivity. Higher levels observed in under school age children with autism
McBride *et al.* (1998)	77 (aged 2–37 years) with autistic disorder, 22 with ID or otherwise cognitively impaired children. 65 controls	Lack of accuracy of diagnosis; sample sizes	DSM-III-R ADOS-G ABC	Platelet serotonin levels were higher in pre-pubertal children with autism, compared to controls. Hyperserotonaemia only evident in individuals with autistic features (not ID)
Mulder *et al.* (2004)	81 (aged 3–20 years) with autism, Asperger syndrome or PDD-NOS. 54 with ID, 60 controls	Medication; sample sizes; lack of accuracy of diagnosis	ADI-R ADOS DSM-IV-R ABC	Platelet serotonin levels higher in ASD group. Not found in majority of individuals with ID. No behavioural correlates
Hranilovic *et al.* (2007)	53 with ASDs (aged 16–45 years) of whom 48 were diagnosed with autism, 1 Asperger, 4 PDD-NOS. 45 controls (aged 20–55 years)	Most with ASD were medicated (those taking SSRIs were excluded); male to female ratio and mean age were lower in ASD group; lack of accuracy of diagnosis	DSM-IV Speech development was clinically evaluated	Platelet serotonin levels were significantly higher in the ASD group. Negative correlation between platelet serotonin levels and language development

PDD-NOS: pervasive developmental disorders not otherwise specified; ASD: autistic spectrum disorders; ID: intellectual disability; DSM-III-R: diagnostic and statistical manual of mental disorders-III-revised; ADOS: autism diagnostic observation schedule; ABC: aberrant behaviour checklist; ADI-R: autism diagnostic interview-revised.

hypocholesterolaemia, and this is not due to gastrointestinal disturbances or abnormal diets, but is a result of decreased cholesterol synthesis (Aneja and Tierney, 2008).

6.2.4 *Genetics and serotonin*

As blood hyperserotonaemia is evident in many people with autism, candidate genes among the serotonin pathways have been identified and studied. The most extensively studied gene is SLC6A4, which encodes the serotonin transporter (chromosomal location 17q12). Several polymorphisms have been identified in this gene, the most significant so far being 5-HTTLPR, a functional polymorphism in the 5' promoter region of the gene. The two forms of this polymorphism can be identified by the insertion or deletion of 44 base pairs, resulting in the short ('s') or the long ('l') allele (the 's' allele being the dominant of the two). Over-transmission of either the 's' or 'l' allele has varied among different studies (Table 6.2). Possible reasons for these differences include ethnic differences, since they are one of the most probable explanations for the variability of the serotonergic polymorphisms in ASD, as well as the genetic heterogeneity of autism (reviewed by Cho *et al.* 2007).

More recent studies have attempted to link the serotonin genotype and phenotype in ASD. In a study by Brune *et al.* (2006), the participants were analysed according to their genotype groups (s/s, s/l and l/l) and were then clinically studied and assessed using the autism diagnostic interview (ADI-R) and autism diagnostic observation schedule (ADOS) methods. Participants with the s/s or s/l phenotype scored significantly more severely than the l/l genotype in the B1 (failure to use non-verbal behaviours to regulate social interaction) subdomain of the ADI-R (Figure 6.1). The l/l genotype group was more impaired in the ADI-R D3 (stereotyped and repetitive motor mannerisms) subdomain. Parents of the participants in both genotypic groups confirmed that these behaviours (specific to their child's genotype) were what first caused them concern about their child's development. These results need to be repeated on a larger sample to be further validated.

Since platelets are considered to be a good model for neurons, a study by Cross *et al.* (2008) investigated the relationship between platelet serotonin levels and polymorphisms in various autism candidate genes. The participants were categorised into three groups. Group one was homozygous for haplotypes containing the T allele at both SLC6A4 single nucleotide polymorphism (SNP) 10 and SNP 11 (5-HTTLPR s/s and s/l). The second group consisted of individuals who were homozygous for the 5-HTTLPR long allele polymorphism, and group three had combinations of other haplotypes. Differences were observed between different haplotype groups at SLC6A4 for transporter K_m and V_{max}. Participants with the s/s and s/l genotypes (TT/TT) were shown to have higher transporter K_m and V_{max}

Table 6.2 *Serotonin transporter SLC6A4 studies*

Study	Participants	Criteria for diagnosis of autism	Main findings
Klauck *et al.* (1997)	Probands with autistic disorder and both parents, 65 trios	ADI-R ADOS	Preferential transmission of the long allele
Cook *et al.* (1997)	Probands with autistic disorder and both parents, 86 trios	Not disclosed	Preferential transmission of the short allele
Yirmiya *et al.* (2001)	34 trios	ADI-R, ADOS, DSM-III-R, DSM-IV	Preferential transmission of the long allele
Conroy *et al.* (2004)	84 trios	Not disclosed	Preferential transmission of the short allele
Guhathakurta *et al.* (2006)	61 trios, 18 duos	DSM-IV CARS	Preferential transmission of the short allele
Ramoz *et al.* (2006)	272 multiplex families and 80 simplex families, with 645 affected subjects	ADI-R	No association of the 5-HTTLPR locus with autism
Cho *et al.* (2007)	126 trios	DSM-IV K-CARS	Preferential transmission of the long allele

Duos: one parent with one affected child; trios: two parents with one affected child; multiplex families: families with multiple affected children; simplex families: families with only one affected child.

ADI-R: autism diagnostic interview; ADOS: autism diagnostic observation schedule; DSM-III-R: diagnostic and statistical manual of mental disorders-III-revised; DSM-IV: diagnostic and statistical manual of mental disorders-IV; (K-) CARS: (Korean) childhood autism rating scale.

than the other two haplotypes. This is in contrast to previous studies which found that the s/s and s/l genotype is associated with lower serotonin transporter V_{max} than other haplotypes (Anderson *et al.* 2002; Greenburg *et al.* 1999). The TT haplotype may be associated with functional variants elsewhere in the gene, or it may have an unknown function, for example altering gene expression or protein trafficking. Despite the correlation between the TT phenotype and the transporter kinetics, this group was not associated with a change in whole blood serotonin, which suggests that hyperserotonaemia in autism has a heterogeneous aetiology. This theory is further validated by other results from the study with regards to tryptophan hydroxylase 1 (TPH1), as different polymorphisms in this gene were found to have different levels of whole blood serotonin (Cross *et al.* 2008).

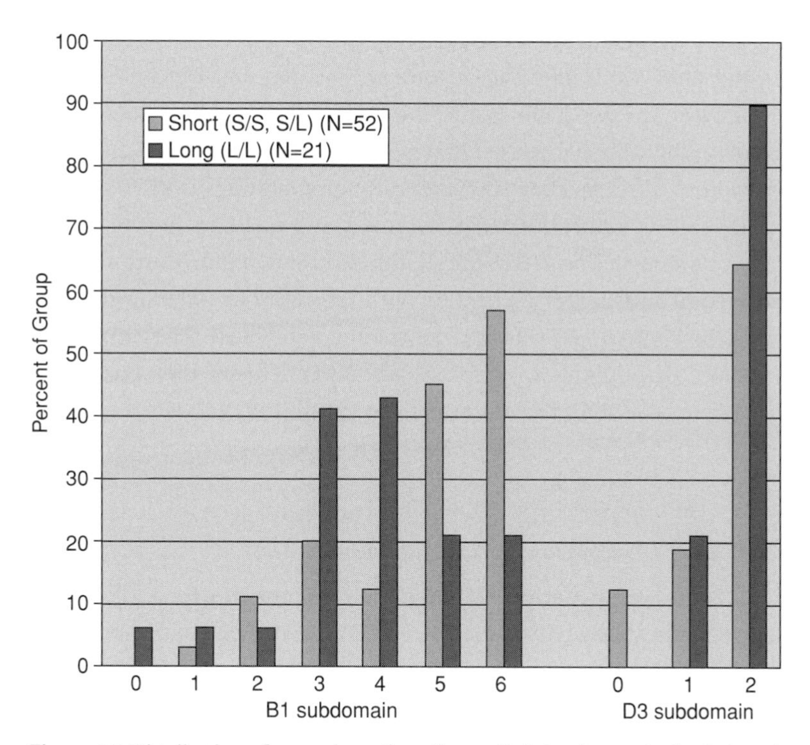

Figure 6.1 Distribution of scores in autism diagnostic interview-revised sub-domains by short and long allele 5-HTTLPR genotype group (adapted from Brune *et al.* 2006). B1 subdomain is the failure to use non-verbal communication to regulate social interaction (statistical analysis: significant difference between genotype groups $F = 7.12$, $df = 1, 73$, $P = 0.01$). D3 subdomain is stereotyped and repetitive mannerisms (statistical analysis: significant difference between genotype groups $F = 4.25$, $df = 1, 73$, $P = 0.04$).

Another candidate gene is ITGB3 (chromosomal location 17q21.32), which encodes the integrin β3 substrate (a subunit of the platelet heterodimeric fibrinogen receptor). ITGB3 is associated with high blood serotonin levels in ASD. While these variants in ITGB3 do not explain hyperserotonaemia, it is very possible that they contribute to it (Weiss *et al.* 2006a). Selective serotonin reuptake inhibitor (SSRI) medications are found to be effective in 50% of patients with autism (McDougle *et al.* 1996b), despite only 25–33% of affected individuals showing hyperserotonaemia (Table 6.1). It is therefore possible that variations in the ITGB3 gene could still be present in an individual with autism, and affect the broader serotonin system, despite normal platelet serotonin levels, thus providing further evidence for the heterogeneity underlying the phenomenon of hyperserotonaemia in ASD.

While it is established that β3 integrin has a function within platelets, it also has a role in synapse maturation within the hippocampus (Chavis and Westbrook,

2001). Both ITGB3 and SLC6A4 have been identified as male quantitative trait loci (QTL) and both are implicated in autism. This has spurred investigation of epistasis between the two genes (Coutinho *et al.* 2007; Weiss *et al.* 2006b). Specifically, Weiss *et al.* (2006a) hypothesised that genetic variation at ITGB3 may influence the expression of SLC6A4. They showed that expression levels of ITGB3 and SLC6A4 are correlated in several tissues in humans and mice (including the brain). Furthermore, a non-coding ITGB3 single nucleotide polymorphism (SNP) previously implicated in autism (via association with serotonin levels) may genetically interact with the SLC6A4 5-HTTPLR polymorphism to increase the risk of autism (Weiss *et al.* 2006b). Although these findings are not conclusive they do offer an insight into possible genetic factors for autism susceptibility, linked to serotonin.

6.2.5 *Serotonergic interventions in autism*

Selective serotonin reuptake inhibitors (SSRIs)

There are currently no effective medical remedies for autism, though there are some medications which may serve to alleviate certain symptoms associated with autism. Moreover, many if not most of these medications have potentially serious side effects, which must be taken into account in evaluating them.

Many individuals with autism, as well as their first- and second-degree relatives (Veenstra-VanderWeele *et al.* 2000) are treated with and respond well to selective serotonin reuptake inhibitors (SSRIs). SSRIs are found to be effective in around 50% of individuals with ASD (McDougle *et al.* 1996b). Their site of action is the serotonin transporter, and the drugs function by increasing the amount of serotonin available in the synaptic cleft. SSRIs can be therapeutic in ASD by reducing a range of symptoms, including anxiety, aggression and stereotypical/repetitive behaviours. However, the variable extent of improvement of mood and mood-associated behaviours even in the responders is also associated with a high incidence of a number of side effects (occurring in up to 50% of treated individuals with ASD) (reviewed by West *et al.* 2009a).

Fluoxetine and fluvoxamine have been highlighted as SSRIs which are particularly useful (Kolevzon *et al.* 2006). A double-blind, placebo controlled, crossover study of 44 children and adolescents with autism highlighted the usefulness of fluoxetine in reducing repetitive behaviours (Hollander *et al.* 2005), with some increase in hyperactivity, irritability, insomnia and lethargy described as adverse effects (Fatemi *et al.* 1998; Hollander *et al.* 2005). In a 10-week open labelled clinical study involving 18 children and adolescents with autism, fluvoxamine was shown to significantly improve obsessive-compulsive or anxiety-related symptoms in only 3 children, whereas 5 had only partial responses, with akathisia, behavioural activation and agitation reported as adverse effects (Martin *et al.* 2003). In contrast, a double-blind, placebo-controlled study of fluvoxamine in 30 adults with autistic disorder reported that half of the treated group were responders, showing significant reduction of repetitive thoughts, behaviour and aggression (McDougle *et al.* 2000). The findings of these two studies raise the possibility that fluvoxamine might have a better efficacy in older individuals with ASD.

Another SSRI, sertraline, was found to produce a similar rate of reduction in repetitive and aggressive behaviours to fluvoxamine in an open trial, with adult autistic individuals with Prader-Willi syndrome responding better than those with a clinical diagnosis of Asperger syndrome (Hellings *et al.* 1996). The efficacy of other SSRIs – paroxetine, citalopram and escitalopram – needs to be further investigated in larger studies.

Serotonin and noradrenaline reuptake inhibitors (SNRIs)

A recent case report on the use of another type of antidepressant, mirtazepine (a selective serotonin and noradrenaline reuptake inhibitor, SNRI), also points towards the usefulness of these types of antidepressants in adjusting sexual behaviour in ASD (Coskun and Mukaddes, 2008; Nguyen and Murphy, 2001). The benefits of SNRIs for improving inattention and hyperactivity in autism have been documented in a series of case reports (Carminati *et al.* 2006; Hollander *et al.* 2000).

Pharmacological manipulation of serotonin levels using SSRIs and SNRIs can affect distinct neuroregulatory proteins (e.g. increase plasma levels of oxytocin; Magalhães-Nunes *et al.* 2008) and neuronal signalling mechanisms, including glycogen synthetase kinase 3β(GSK3β) signalling. Inhibition of GSK3β appears to inhibit some behaviours, especially aggression (Beaulieu *et al.* 2008). This raises the possibility of developing further therapies that target GSK3β and its related signalling events to manage behavioural changes related to serotonin deficiency.

Tryptophan

Using tryptophan as a supplement has also been considered to enhance serotonin release and/or reuptake inhibition. Reduction in tryptophan has been documented to cause significant deterioration in people with autism (Cook and Leventhal, 1996). Although there is evidence for differences between individuals with autism and controls with respect to peripheral metabolism of 5-hydroxytryptophan after an oral challenge (Croonenberghs *et al.* 2005), the clinical efficacy of this intervention still needs to be assessed. Similarly, the cofactor tetrahydrobiopterin, which plays a role in the biosynthesis of catecholamines and serotonin, and enhances synaptic release of various neurotransmitters, showed a small, but statistically significant improvement in the ability of participants to interact socially, and in their IQs in a small double-blind, placebo-controlled, crossover study involving 12 children with autism (Danfors *et al.* 2005).

Risperidone

Risperidone is an atypical antipsychotic drug that blocks serotonergic 2A ($5HT_{2A}$) receptors and dopaminergic D2 receptors post-synaptically. Although predominantly used in schizophrenia, it has found its place in the treatment of certain symptoms in autism, thus providing further evidence for the role of 5-HT and dopamine in autism. Thus, short-term risperidone intervention is effective for ameliorating/improving a variety of behaviours associated with ASD, including aggression, hyperactivity, social skills and self-injurious behaviour (Capone *et al.* 2008; Nagaraj *et al.* 2006). About 66–83% of autistic children treated with risperidone will have substantial improvements in compulsive and stereotypic behaviour, affective reactions, sensory response and motor behaviours; with 68% of them maintaining a positive response during a 4-month drug maintenance phase (reviewed in West *et al.* 2009b). However, variable response to treatment between individuals and for distinct core symptoms of autism has also been noted (West *et al.* 2009b). An 18-month-long randomised, placebo-controlled, double-blind study also showed the benefits of risperidone intervention for children with autism (2–9 years of age), with improvement in social responsiveness and non-verbal communication, reduction of hyperactivity and aggression (Nagaraj *et al.* 2006). Improvement in social withdrawal was noted as early as 3 months after starting treatment (Capone *et al.* 2008).

Studies examining long term treatment (6 and 18 months) with risperidone report mild to substantial weight gain in patients (Martin *et al.* 2000; 2004; Nagaraj *et al.* 2006). Although risperidone appears to ameliorate some autistic symptoms, and it has been proven to be one of the rare interventions with which results can be replicated in intervention studies (reviewed in Parikh *et al.* 2008), the weight gain, alongside somnolence and hyperglycaemia (reviewed in Scott and Dhillon, 2007), may be too large an adverse effect to consider it as a long term intervention, and further studies are needed to establish the clinical relevance of this intervention for ASD.

6.3 Reelin

Reelin is a serine protease glycoprotein, essential for normal brain development (Quattrocchi *et al.* 2002). It has three receptors: $\alpha3\beta1$ integrin, very low density lipoprotein receptor (VLDLR) and apolipoprotein E receptor 2 (ApoER2). Disabled 1 (Dab-1) is a cytoplasmic adapter associated with reelin. In the prenatal brain, reelin is secreted by Cajal Retzius cells, interacting with other proteins to ensure correct laminar organisation in the neocortex, hippocampus and cerebellum (Ogawa *et al.* 1995). In adults, reelin is secreted from GABAergic interneurons throughout the brain (Pesold *et al.* 1998; Roberts *et al.* 2005), neurons which are believed to be disrupted in autism (Oblak *et al.* 2009).

Reelin is not only essential during development; it is also utilised for memory formation and higher cognitive function (D'Arcangelo, 2005; Krueger *et al.* 2006), which can be affected in autism. Serotonin, shown to be disrupted in ASD, facilitates the release of reelin. However, excessive levels of serotonin (as discussed above, see Table 6.1) may also decrease reelin levels, and could alter neurodevelopment (Janusonis *et al.* 2004).

6.3.1 *Reelin animal models*

Studies with reelin knockout (KO) mice (reeler mice) have shown the importance of reelin in neurodevelopment, with the KO mice displaying severe deficiencies in social behaviour and cognitive impairments, reminiscent of autism (Falconer 1951). Reelin KO mice have reduced numbers of cerebellar Purkinje cells – a finding that is common in post-mortem studies on autism. When reelin was ectopically expressed in developing reeler mice, some of the expected behavioural impairments (also noted in ASD) were avoided, especially the ataxic gait and deficiency in positional cue (Magdaleno *et al.* 2002), thus proving the importance of reelin in cognitive function in mice.

6.3.2 *Reelin and autism*

In a study examining blood reelin levels in 28 autistic twins, unprocessed reelin (410 KDa) was decreased by 70%. Levels were also decreased in their parents (mothers 72%, fathers 62%) and normal siblings (70%) compared to controls (Fatemi, 2002). Similar findings have been reported in related neurodevelopmental conditions, such as schizophrenia and mood disorders (Fatemi *et al.* 2001a). A later post-mortem study compared cerebellar cortices from five adults with ASD and eight age-matched controls, using SDS-gel electrophoresis and Western blotting. Reelin was found to be reduced by 43% in the ASD group (Fatemi *et al.* 2001b). These data suggest that the reelin blood decrease may reflect the reelin brain abnormalities. However, to date there are no comparative studies on blood and brain reelin expression.

In a more recent study, these authors examined various sections of the brain at post-mortem from 7 adult individuals with ASD (19–56 years of age at death) and 10 age-matched controls (20–36 years of age at death) (Fatemi *et al.* 2005). In the ASD group, levels of full-length reelin within the superior frontal cortices were 71% lower than controls. In the cerebellum in ASD, reelin levels were 39% lower, and in the parietal cortex levels of reelin were 72% lower than controls (Fatemi *et al.* 2005). mRNA levels were measured for reelin, VLDLR, Dab-1 and GSK3 (found downstream in the reelin signalling pathway, see Table 6.3 and Figure 6.2).

Table 6.3 *mRNA levels for Reelin, VLDLR, Dab-1, and GSK3β in autism. Abbreviations: M, male; F, female; GOI, gene of interest (adapted from Fatemi* et al. *2005)*

Brain area	mRNA	GOI relative to age matched control	*P* value
Superior frontal cortex (Brodmann Area 9) 6M controls and 7 ASD (6M, 1F)	VLDLR	+14.2	<0.01
	GSK3β	+1.9	NS
	Reelin	−4.7	<0.035
	Dab-1	−5.4	<0.01
Cerebellum 9 controls (8M, 1F) and 7 ASD (6M, 1F)	VLDLR	+2.8	<0.04
	GSK3β	+1	NS
	Reelin	−3.9	<0.01
	Dab-1	−3.4	<0.001

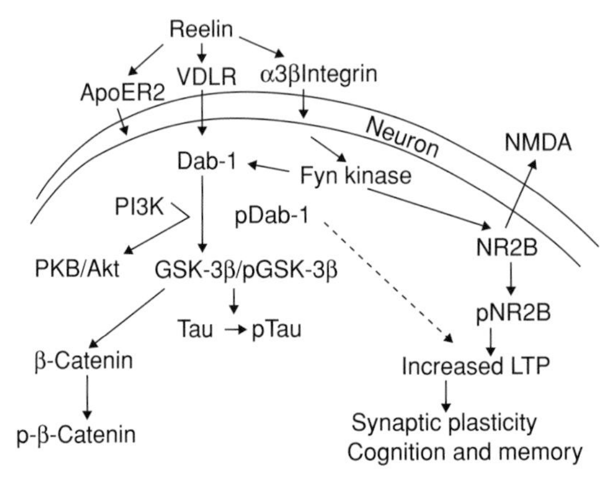

Figure 6.2 The Reelin signalling system (adapted from Fatemi *et al.* 2005).

Levels of reelin and Dab-1 mRNA were significantly decreased within the superior frontal cortex (Brodmann Area 9 in the dorsolateral part of the frontal lobe) and cerebellum in the ASD group compared to controls, whereas the levels of VLDLR were significantly increased.

These studies suggest that reelin signalling is impaired in autism (Figure 6.2). Thus, lower production of reelin (Fatemi *et al.* 2001b; Fatemi, 2002) and reduction in reelin mRNA levels (Fatemi *et al.* 2005) will result in lower activation of receptors. The increase in VLDLR mRNA in the ASD group may possibly reflect a response to lowered reelin levels – the body attempts to adapt by providing more receptors for the ligand to bind to. Dab-1 mRNA levels were also reduced – either due to the lack of positive feedback from reduced levels of reelin, or increased negative feedback from the upregulated VLDLR (Fatemi *et al.* 2005). However, these findings are somewhat difficult to interpret in the light of not being replicated since, and although the decrease in reelin mRNA seems to parallel the protein decrease, their relationship was not addressed directly in the latter study (Fatemi *et al.* 2005). It is of interest to note that the GSK3β mRNA levels were not significantly different between ASD and control group, and one of the explanations for this may be that levels of phosphorylated GSK3β are altered in autism similar to the same phenomenon reported in schizophrenia (Emamian *et al.* 2004).

6.3.3 *Reelin and genetic studies*

Abnormalities affecting reelin and its signalling pathway have been associated with autism. Taken together with the behavioural deficits (highlighted above) observed in reeler mice, these findings suggest a role for reelin in the aetiology of autism. Various studies have implicated the RELN gene (chromosomal location 7q22) as a susceptibility gene for autism (Serajee *et al.* 2006; Skaar *et al.* 2005; Zhang *et al.* 2002). However, other studies have shown no association between polymorphisms in the RELN gene and autism (Devlin *et al.* 2004; Dutta *et al.* 2008; Krebs *et al.* 2002; Li *et al.* 2004). It may be that RELN polymorphisms are only present in a subset of the autistic population.

6.4 Oxytocin neurochemistry in autism

Oxytocin (OT) is a nine amino acid neuropeptide and hormone, synthesised in the paraventricular nucleus and the supraoptic nucleus in the brain, and is the product of a series of cleavage events from a prohormone. The last step in the process is the cleavage of C-terminal extended peptides, OT-Gly, OT-Gly-Lys and OT-Gly-Lys-Arg (or OT-X) to oxytocin. Receptors for oxytocin are found throughout the limbic system, forebrain and autonomic centres in the brainstem. The function of oxytocin receptors is modulated by cholesterol (Gimpl *et al.* 2002). Low levels of cholesterol are thought to perturb oxytocin receptors and may contribute to problems in social functioning in autism (Aneja and Tierney, 2008).

6.4.1 *Oxytocin and animal studies*

Several animal studies have implicated oxytocin in social affiliative behaviours, such as mating, pair-bond formation, parental/maternal behaviour, social memory and recognition, separation distress and various other forms of attachments (reviewed by Tom and Assinder, 2010). Differences in behavioural profile in these animal models are due largely to different mouse strains being used, as well as different techniques to disrupt the OT gene or its receptor. Thus, oxytocin knockout (KO) mouse pups are less vocal when separated from the dam, and adult oxytocin KO mice are unable to recognise familiar peers even after several social encounters (Winslow and Insel, 2002). However, after oxytocin is administered this social deficit is reversed. A recent study extended these findings, using them to separate OT KO mouse strains, and showed that the lack of OT does not alter general prosocial behaviour in the mutant, neither does it confer an anxiety-related phenotype, but selectively impairs the ability to remember having previously met a novel mate (Crawley *et al.* 2007). Increased aggressive behaviour has also been reported in OT KO mice (Ragnauth *et al.* 2005).

6.4.2 *Oxytocin in humans*

There is a relationship between oxytocin and human social behaviour. A person's willingness to trust another individual (accepting social risks; Kosfeld *et al.* 2005) and the ability to interpret subtle social cues (Domes *et al.* 2007) have been shown to increase following oxytocin administration. In another study, participants administered oxytocin were found to be more generous when deciding how to split a sum of money than those on the placebo (Zak *et al.* 2007).

Altered oxytocin levels have been documented in certain neuropsychiatric conditions. People with obsessive-compulsive disorder (OCD), a condition with repetitive behaviours, have elevated levels of oxytocin in their cerebrospinal fluid (Leckman *et al.* 1994). Similarly, schizophrenic patients have decreased levels of plasma oxytocin, relating to the affected individual's ability to identify facial emotions – a process that is also impaired in individuals with ASD (Goldman *et al.* 2008). Although not specific to a particular disorder, these findings could relate to neurobiological mechanisms underlying clinical symptoms that are shared in various psychiatric conditions, including autism, OCD and schizophrenia

6.4.3 *Oxytocin and autism*

Plasma oxytocin levels were measured in 29 boys with autism (aged 6 to 11) and compared to 30 age matched controls (Modahl *et al.* 1998). All of the ASD participants were diagnosed using DSM-IV criteria. The boys all completed three cognitive tests, and additionally the parents of the autistic children were given two interview questionnaires (the Vineland Adaptive Behaviour Scales and a background questionnaire) and interviewed about their child's behaviour. Despite a considerable overlap of values, the ASD group showed on average lower plasma oxytocin levels than the controls. A number of children ($N = 10$) with autism had undetectable levels of oxytocin. The lower levels of oxytocin in ASD children were not associated with the medication the children were taking. In the control but not the ASD group, there was a positive correlation between levels of plasma oxytocin and age. In contrast to the controls who had positive correlation between plasma oxytocin levels and social skills (except in expressive language), children with autism showed negative association (Modahl *et al.* 1998). These results suggest that there may be deficits in oxytocin receptors or upstream regulators in children with ASD. The low expression of oxytocin is hypothesised to contribute to the delay in brain maturation in autism (Campbell *et al.* 1980). Similar observations were made in an independent study involving Saudi Arabian children with autism (Al-Ayadhi, 2005).

To further investigate plasma oxytocin levels in boys with autism, participants recruited in the previous study (Modahl *et al.* 1998) were examined to see whether isoforms of oxytocin were present at different levels in the ASD group when compared to controls (Green *et al.* 2001). OT antisera which react with either oxytocin or the C-terminal extended oxytocin (OT-X) isoforms were used. Similar to previous findings, the ASD group showed lower levels of oxytocin than the control group. However, OT-X levels were higher in the group with autism, with a more than two-fold higher OT-X to OT ratio. OT-X levels were also positively associated with age in the ASD group, but not the controls (Green *et al.* 2001). These results suggest that children with autism may have deficits in oxytocin processing.

An inability to completely process mature oxytocin may result in elevated amounts of OT-X. Studies examining the function of OT-X have shown that it is not an effective agonist at OT receptor sites (Mitchell *et al.* 1998), meaning that OT-X is not an adequate substitute for decreased levels of oxytocin in children with autism. In contrast to the studies conducted in children, a study in adults with ASD reported higher plasma levels of oxytocin (Jansen *et al.* 2006), suggesting that the maturation process may affect the level of oxytocin expression. However, the variations in oxytocin levels were large, and the participant groups were small (10 ASD and 14 controls). This study (Jansen *et al.* 2006) was also conducted on high functioning ASD adults, in contrast to previous studies conducted on children with variable cognitive functioning (Modahl *et al.* 1998). However, further studies are needed to elucidate the reasons for the differences between the young and adult autistic populations.

6.4.4 Oxytocin and genetic studies in autism

A study screening the Autism Genetic Resource Exchange (AGRE) samples and a Finnish autism sample identified the oxytocin receptor gene, OXTR, as a candidate susceptibility gene in autism (Ylisaukko-oja *et al.* 2005). The OXTR gene is located on 3p25.3, within the 3p25–27 loci identified in the study. Two single nucleotide polymorphisms (SNP) located within the OXTR gene in 195 Chinese Han autism trios (two parents with one affected child) were found to be significantly associated with autism (Wu *et al.* 2005), further implicating OXTR in the condition. In contrast to the Chinese Han population, Caucasian children and adolescents with autism have overtransmission of the G allele, rather than the reported overtransmission of the A allele (Jacob *et al.* 2007). This discrepancy may be due to a different pattern of linkage disequilibrium between the genetic marker and the susceptibility variant in the OXTR gene. An additional study has again shown a significant association between SNPs on the OXTR gene and autism susceptibility, also analysing any linkage between the SNPs and cognition (Lerer *et al.* 2007). The study reports that there is an association between IQ and Vineland Adaptive Behaviour Scales and OXTR, suggesting that the OXTR gene affects skills such as communication and daily living skills.

6.4.5 Oxytocin as a therapeutic agent

The deficit of oxytocin in oxytocin KO mice, in which impairments in social recognition and discrimination have been demonstrated, can be reversed by infusion of oxytocin within the amygdala (Ferguson *et al.* 2001). In a clinical study, Hollander *et al.* (2003) administered synthetic oxytocin (pitocin) or placebo to six adults with autism (diagnosed according to DSM-IV and ADI-R criteria) and nine adults with Asperger disorder (aged 19–55 years). Repetitive behaviours were significantly reduced over time, as well as the number of different types of repetitive behaviours, after pitocin had been administered. In a later study, these authors reported that intervention with oxytocin led to improvements in 'appropriate use of emotional intonations' in the speech within a group of individuals with ASD (Hollander *et al.* 2007). In this study, six adults with autism and nine adults with Asperger syndrome were enrolled, and they all showed improvement in comprehension of affective speech (e.g. happy, indifferent, angry and sad). A recent functional imaging study showed that intervention with oxytocin reduced activation within the amygdala, and also reduced 'coupling' of amygdala to brainstem regions that are implicated in autonomic and behavioural manifestations of fear (Kirsch *et al.* 2005).

The results of these studies reinforce the notion that the oxytocin system is affected in autism, and may contribute towards repetitive and emotional behaviours. Although these studies have been carried out on only a very small number of individuals, the potential therapeutic use of oxytocin for treating some of the symptoms of autism seems promising. However, this intervention may have some restrictions in a clinical setting – pitocin is administered intravenously, and monitoring social behaviour would require involvement of a number of people (family members, teachers, carers).

An interesting theory that has been proposed recently is that high levels of oxytocin which are released during childbirth in the mother (i.e. during labour), and the use of oxytocin in inducing labour, could also influence brain development in the infant. Thus, elevated oxytocin levels may be transferred to the infant via the maternal–fetal circulation during this critical period, and cross over from the blood into the infant brain (which lacks a fully developed blood–brain barrier at this stage) (reviewed by Rojas Wahl, 2004). The hypothesis is that raised levels of oxytocin can lead to desensitisation of oxytocin receptors within key areas of the infant brain. *In vitro* studies have shown that within 5–10 minutes following agonist stimulation, more than 60% of the oxytocin receptor is internalised, thus becoming unavailable for further oxytocin binding and corresponding signal transduction cascades (reviewed by Zingg and Laporte (2003)). The excess of oxytocin, in turn, downregulates oxytocin receptor mRNA (Jo and Fortune, 2002). According to a study in 1998, about 61% of children with autism were reported to have had a history of induced labour (Hollander *et al.* 1998), three-fold higher than the national average. However, an independent study found similar rates of pitocin-induced labour among ASD and matched control children (Gale *et al.* 2003). This hypothesis needs to be explored in further prospective studies to determine whether oxytocin-induced labour may indeed influence the incidence of autism.

6.5 Conclusions

In this review we have discussed alterations in serotonergic neurotransmitters and two neuroregulatory proteins, reelin and oxytocin, in ASD. The studies predominantly come from reports on people with autism from 5 years old and upward. The reasons for this are manifold; e.g. children younger than five (with or without ASD) often prove more difficult to study clinically because of their inattention and lower IQ (Mayes and Calhoun, 2003); post-mortem samples from infants are limited. However, discovering the causes of ASD may ultimately depend on data obtained from infants between 2 and 4 years (age range at which autism is usually diagnosed) and even younger, when symptoms first become apparent.

The heterogeneity of the autism spectrum, alongside the lack of well characterised clinico-pathological and biochemical studies, small sample sizes, and lack of coverage of the various developmental stages of the spectrum, all contribute to difficulties in understanding the neurobiology of autism. It is difficult to be conclusive in allocating distinct neurotransmitter alterations to a distinct clinical symptom. Although a number of neurotransmitter systems have been investigated and found to be altered in autism, the resultant pharmacological interventions on their own do not appear to regulate all the characteristic clinical symptoms of the syndrome. Due to the percentage of autistic patients found to be hyperserotonaemic (25–33%, see Table 6.1), and compelling evidence from genetic studies implicating the serotonin transporter gene, SLC6A4, in ASD (Table 6.2), the serotonergic system appears to be significantly involved in ASD. Although perhaps not a cause, disruptions to the serotonergic system may worsen the behavioural phenotype of an individual with autism. As serotonin facilitates the release of reelin, and excess serotonin may decrease reelin levels (Janusonis *et al.* 2004), an individual with ASD who is hyperserotonaemic may also have reelin deficits. Since these factors are among the most consistent biochemical changes reported in autism, it would be of interest to explore further their contribution towards the aetiology of ASD.

Oxytocin is involved in human social behaviour (Kosfeld *et al.* 2005; Zak *et al.* 2007). It is, therefore, not surprising that altered levels of oxytocin are reported in autism, and correlate with the altered social behaviour, one of the core symptoms. Various genetic studies also implicate the oxytocin receptor gene in autism (Jacob *et al.* 2007; Lerer *et al.* 2007), suggesting that deficits in the oxytocin system contribute towards the clinical phenotype. Intravenous administration of oxytocin has had some success as a pharmacological trial for certain symptoms associated with autism (Hollander *et al.* 2003; 2007). Improvements noted in repetitive behaviours and expressive speech may be beneficial, and the potential for oxytocin to improve social behaviour, a trait associated with autism that has not been targeted by drug therapy, looks promising from animal studies (Winslow and Insel, 2002), as well as human trials (Kosfeld *et al.* 2005).

Although oxytocin replacement therapy, as well as SSRI/SNRI, appears to be useful in regulating some of the clinical features of autism, larger clinical and neuropathological studies are now needed not only to replicate these findings, but also to put together the distinct neurotransmitter and neurochemical profiles in autism, and relate them to distinct (or group of distinct) clinical symptoms. This will help in understanding the neurobiochemical changes behind the clinical phenotype of autism, and will contribute to novel development of symptom-targeted medical interventions.

While the heterogeneity of 'autism' is accepted, we are still far from understanding the specific causes of the condition and subsequently developing appropriate pharmacological interventions that would be of benefit to individuals on the autism spectrum, especially those with significantly altered behaviour and cognition. Further evidence is needed from larger, multi-centre clinical studies that can be replicated, in order to accept such medical interventions within a clinical setting.

6.6 Acknowledgement

We would like to thank Mrs Christine Bohanan for secretarial support.

6.7 References

Adolphs, R., Baron-Cohen, S., Tranel, D. (2002). Impaired recognition of social emotions following amygdala damage. *Journal of Cognitive Neuroscience*, **14**: 1264–1274.

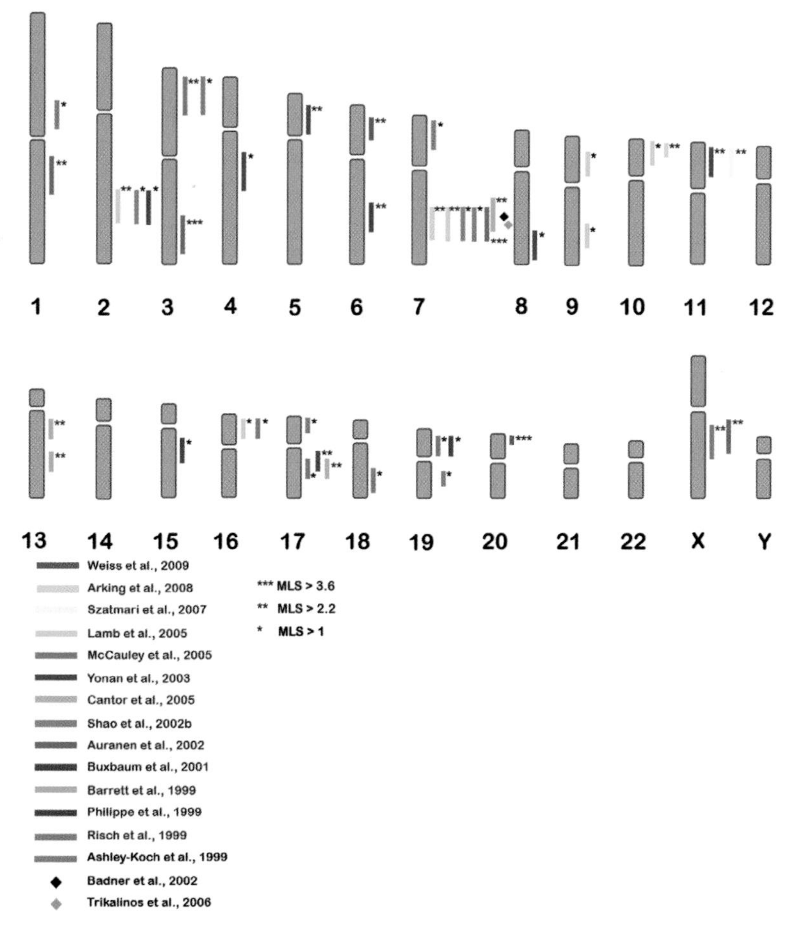

Figure 2.1 Ideogram representing linkage findings in eleven genome-wide screens for autism. Each scan is represented by differently coloured bars in the respective chromosomal regions and the two meta-analyses by diamond shaped symbols. The results indicated are followed by *** if MLS > 3.6, by ** if MLS > 2.2, and by * if MLS > 1.

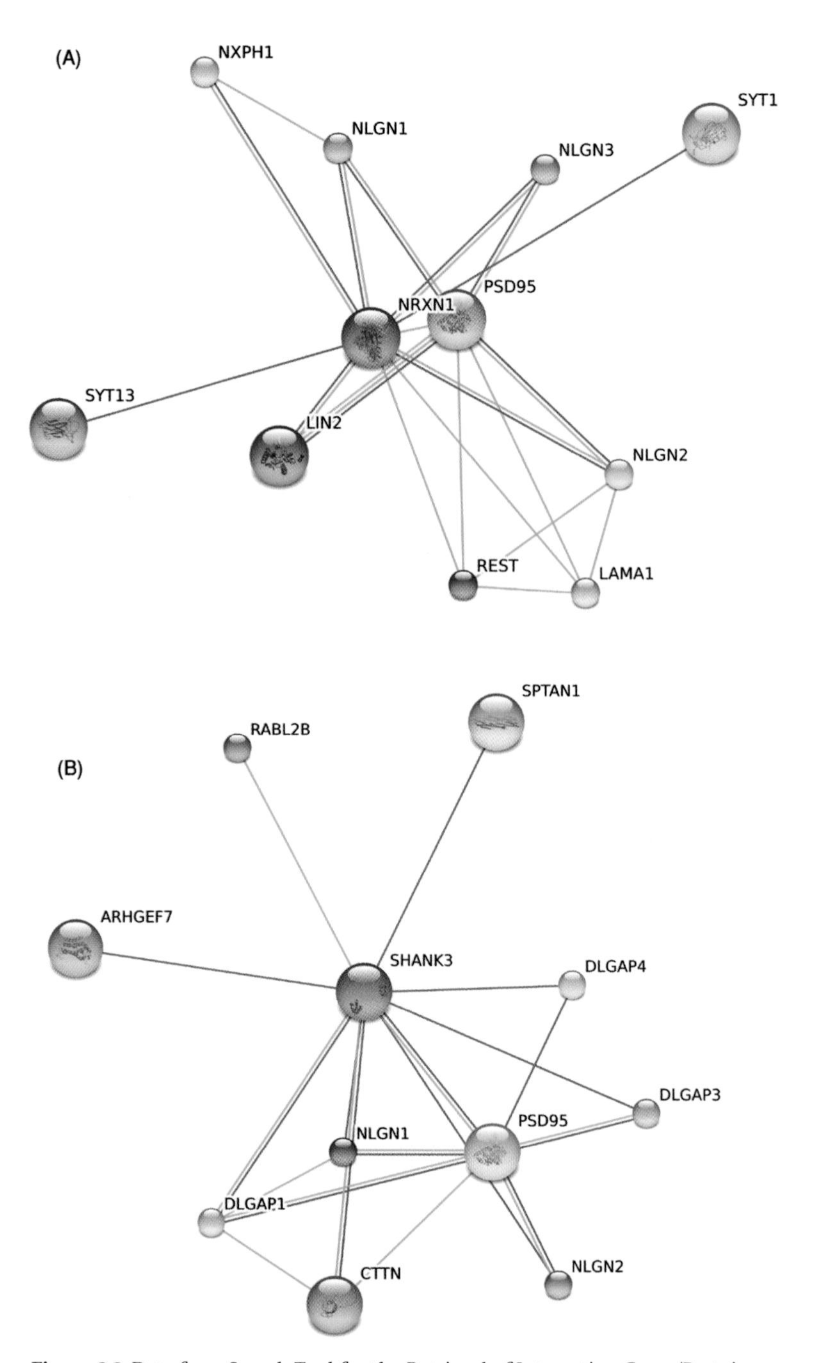

Figure 2.2 Data from Search Tool for the Retrieval of Interacting Genes/Proteins (http://string.embl.de/). Spheres represent specific genes/proteins. Lines represent evidence for associations from experimental data (pink), text mining (green) or homology studies (blue). (**A**) Network of proteins that interact with *NRXN1*. (**B**) Network of proteins interacting with *SHANK3* (von Mering *et al.* 2007).

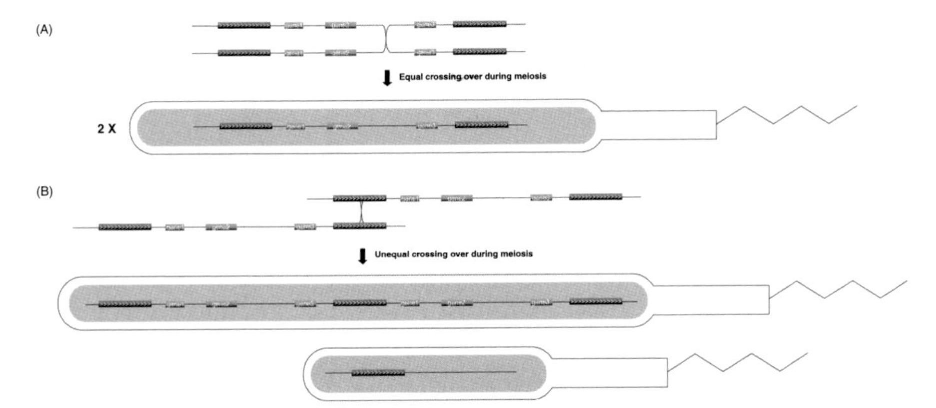

Figure 2.3 CNVs arise by unequal crossing over during meiosis. Schematic diagram showing 3 genes in green, flanked by segmental duplications in orange. (**A**) Equal crossing over leads to gametes with a single copy of the three genes.
(**B**) Unequal crossing over results in gametes with 0 or 2 copies of these genes.

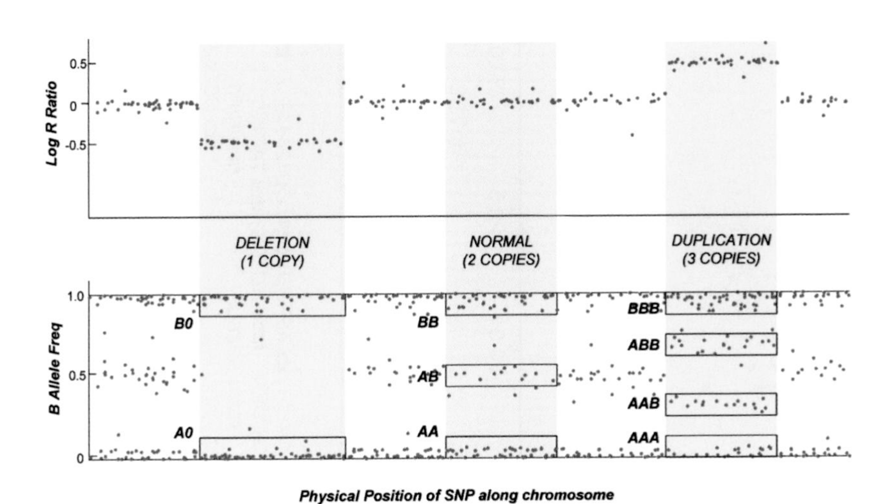

Figure 2.4 Hypothetical data along an autosome demonstrating how results from SNP arrays can be used to detect CNVs. A drop in the log R ratio, combined with a lack of heterozygous SNP calls is suggestive of a deletion. In contrast, segments which demonstrate increased log R ratios and B allele frequencies clustering around 1/3 and 2/3 suggest a duplication. Real experimental data are usually noisier than this schematic diagram, and moving window average analysis of log R ratio is often carried out to detect changes. 'Log R Ratio' is a measure of the combined fluorescent intensity signals from both sets of probes/alleles at each SNP, whereas 'B Allele Frequency' is the relative ratio of fluorescent signals between the two probes/alleles.

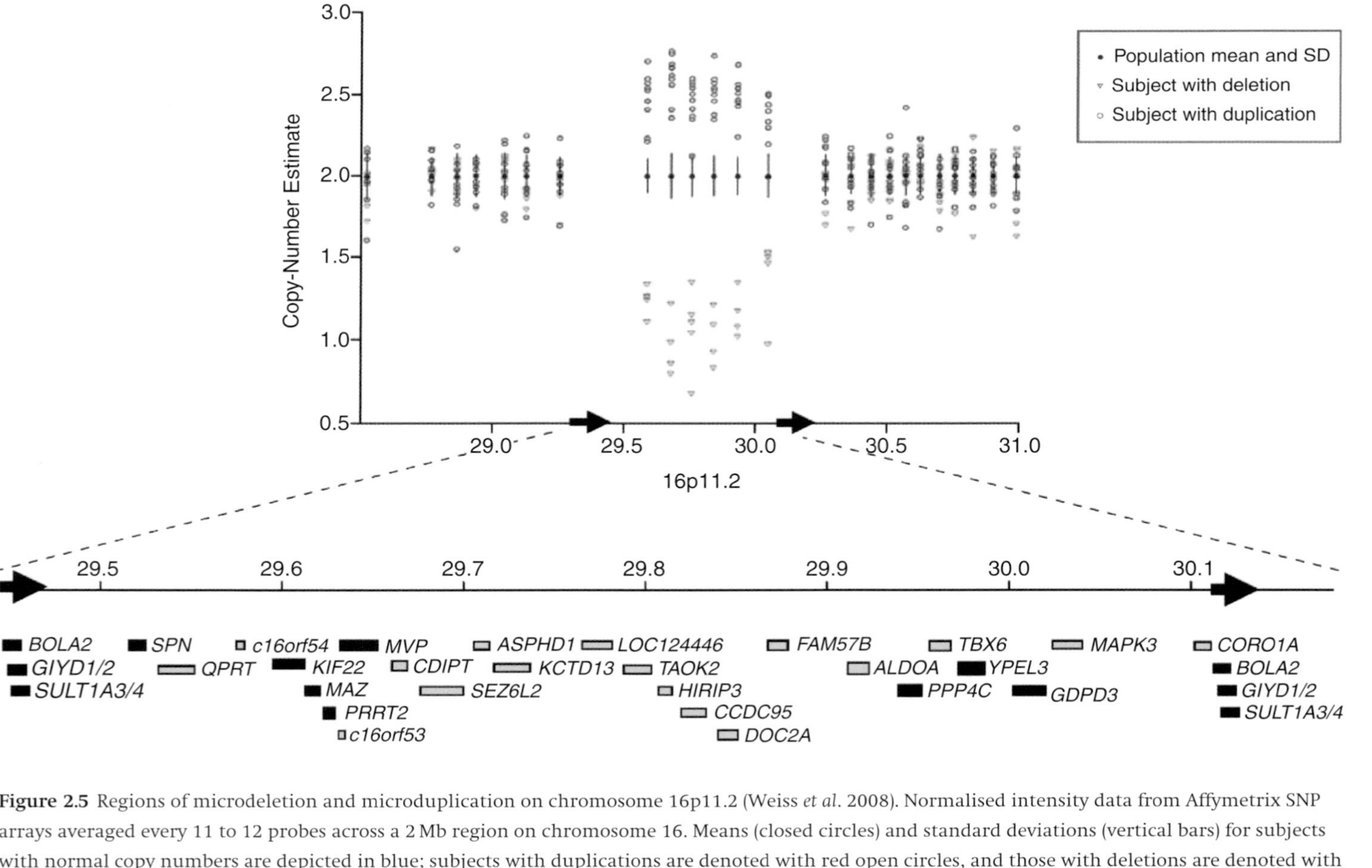

Figure 2.5 Regions of microdeletion and microduplication on chromosome 16p11.2 (Weiss *et al.* 2008). Normalised intensity data from Affymetrix SNP arrays averaged every 11 to 12 probes across a 2 Mb region on chromosome 16. Means (closed circles) and standard deviations (vertical bars) for subjects with normal copy numbers are depicted in blue; subjects with duplications are denoted with red open circles, and those with deletions are denoted with green triangles. Annotated genes in the region of interest are shown (not to scale), with grey denoting brain expression and black denoting unknown or little brain expression. Arrows represent the segmental duplications mediating the rearrangements, with three genes located within the segmental duplication. Reproduced with kind permission.

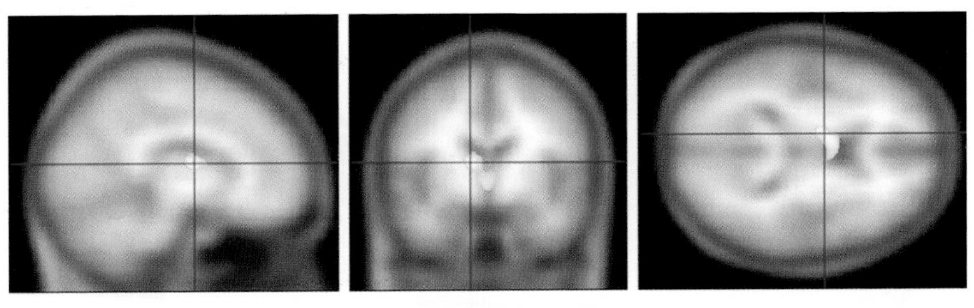

Figure 3.3 Reduced thalamic grey matter density as measured using voxel-based morphometry in intellectually disabled adolescents with autistic features as compared to controls scoring below the threshold for ASD. From left to right, the three images illustrate the same findings on sagittal, coronal and axial sections, respectively. The coronal image is displayed in neurological convention (i.e. left is left). (Adapted from Spencer, M.D., Moorhead, T.W.J., Lymer, G.K.S., *et al.* (2006). Structural correlates of intellectual impairment and autistic features in adolescents. Neuroimage, 33: 1136–1144, with permission of the copyright holder, Elsevier Limited.)

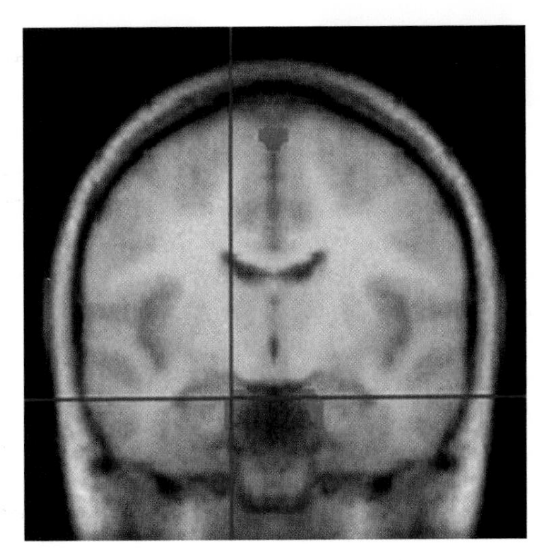

Figure 3.4 Significant positive correlation between score on Autism Behavioural Checklist and grey matter density in the junction area between the amygdala, hippocampus and entorhinal cortex of children with autism spectrum disorder. (Reprinted from Salmond, C., Ashburner, J., Connelly, A., Friston, K.J., Gadian, D.G., Vargha-Khadem, F. (2005). The role of the medial temporal lobe in autistic spectrum disorders. European Journal of Neuroscience, 22, 764–772, with permission of the copyright holder, John Wiley and Sons.)

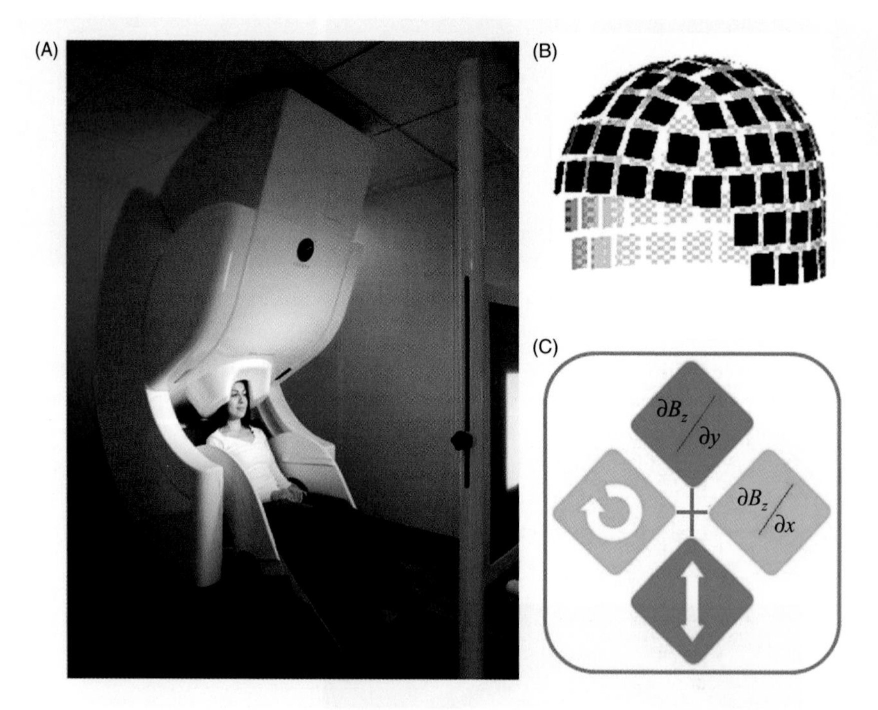

Figure 4.1 The MEG scanner at the Oxford Centre for Human Brain Activity. The scanner itself is shown in (**A**). The system features a helmet-shaped array of 102 detectors (black plates, totalling 306 sensors) covering the whole head (**B**). Each detector consists of one magnetometer (grey loop) which measures the magnetic field, and two first-order planar gradiometers (diamonds) which measure magnetic field gradients along orthogonal directions (**C**). The outputs of the latter are most sensitive to the tangential current flow in the region directly below the detectors. The root-mean-square signal summed over the two readings is a measure of current strength. Comparing the head to a globe, $\partial B_z/\partial y$ gradiometers measure the variation of the magnetic field (more precisely its z-component perpendicular to the head) along longitudinal directions, and $\partial B_z/\partial x$ gradiometers measure along latitudinal directions.

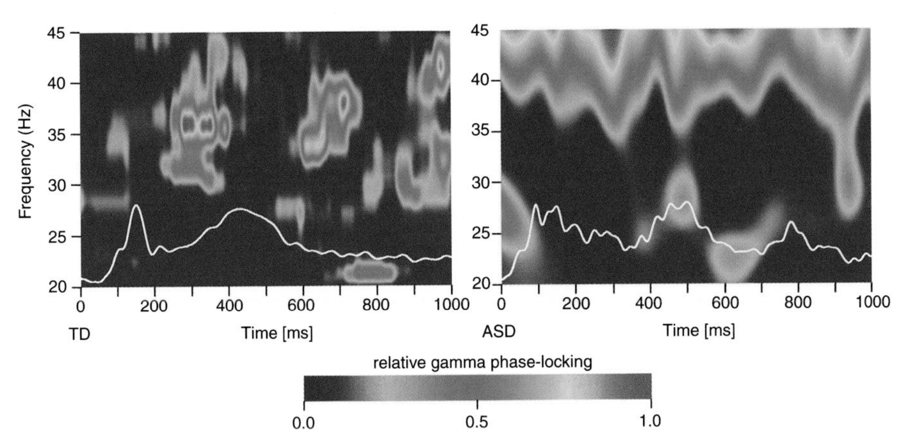

Figure 4.2 This figure shows time-frequency plane (t-f plane) representations of the phase-locked gamma-responses following incongruous words. The planes take into account the data from all typically developing individuals (left) and all individuals with ASD (right) studied in Braeutigam *et al.* (2008). For each plane, the corresponding root-mean-square signals (evoked power = total brain activation) have been superimposed for reference. Remarkably, in individuals with autism spectrum disorders, gamma phase-locking to incongruous words is observed within a very long interval independent of evoked power. (The effects here are significant, but the underlying statistical argument is beyond the scope of this chapter.)

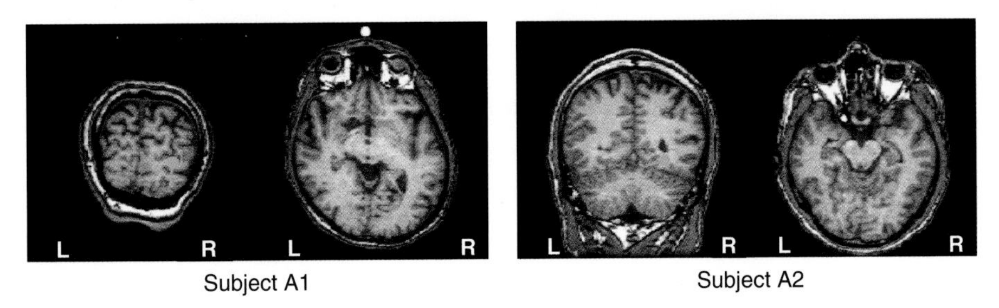

Figure 4.3 The images show the equivalent-current-dipole locations (orange dots) for responses to statically presented images of faces at about 150 ms after stimulus in two subjects with autism spectrum disorders. The dipoles have been superimposed on individual structural (MRI) scans. These figures (adapted from Bailey *et al.* 2005) illustrate that the generator of the N170 response might locate more towards the medial aspects of the (inferior) temporal lobe and more towards striate cortex than in typically developing subjects. There is little consistency in dipole orientation (orange line), which suggests a greater-than-normal heterogeneity in individuals with ASD.

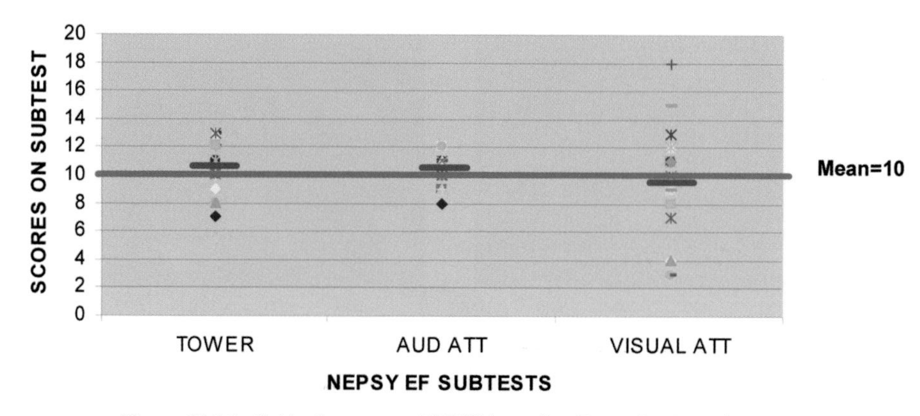

Figure 11.1 Individual scores on NEPSY Attention/Executive Function Domain sub-tests.

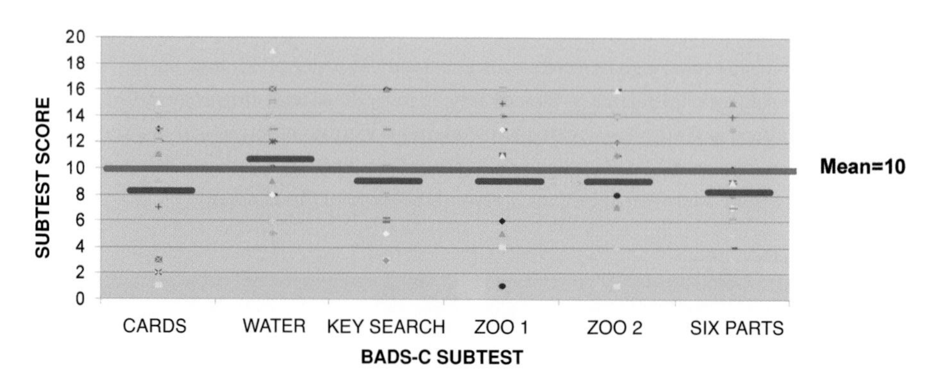

Figure 11.2 Individual Bads-C sub-test scores.

Al-Ayadhi, L.Y. (2005). Altered oxytocin and vasopressin levels in autistic children in central Saudi Arabia. *Neuroscience*, **10**: 47–50.

Allen, J.A., Halverson-Tamboli, R.A., Rasenick, M.M. (2007). Lipid raft microdomains and neurotransmitter signalling. *Nature Reviews Neuroscience*, **8**: 128–140.

Amaral, D.G., Schumann, C.M., Nordahl, C.W. (2008). Neuroanatomy of autism. *Trends in Neurosciences*, **31**: 137–145.

Anderson, G.M., Freedman, D.X., Cohen, D.J., *et al.* (1987). Whole blood serotonin in autistic and normal subjects. *Journal of Child Psychology and Psychiatry*, **28**: 885–900.

Anderson, G.M., Gutknecht, L., Cohen, D.J. *et al.* (2002). Serotonin transporter promotor variants in autism: functional effects and relationship to platelet hyperserotonemia. *Molecular Psychiatry*, **7**: 831–836.

Aneja A., Tierney, E. (2008). Autism: The role of cholesterol in treatment. *International Review of Psychiatry*, **20**: 165–170.

Beaulieu, J.-M., Zhang, X., Rodriguiz, R.M., *et al.* (2008). Role of GSK3β in behavioral abnormalities induced by serotonin deficiency. *Proceedings of the National Academy of Sciences USA*, **105**: 1333–1339.

Blaylock, R.L., Strunecka, A. (2009). Immune-glutamatergic dysfunction as a central mechanism of the autism spectrum disorders. *Current Medicinal Chemistry*, **16**: 157–170.

Brune, C.W., Kim, S.J., Salt, J., *et al.* (2006). 5-HTTLPR Genotype-specific phenotype in children and adolescents with autism. *American Journal of Psychiatry*, **163**: 2148–2156.

Campbell, M., Petti, T.A., Greene, W.H., *et al.* (1980). Some physical parameters of young autistic children. *Journal of the American Academy of Child Psychiatry*, **19**: 193–212.

Capone, G.T., Goyal, P., Grados, M., Smith, B., Kammann, H. (2008). Risperidone use in children with Down syndrome, severe intellectual disability and comorbid autistic spectrum disorders: a naturalistic study. *Journal of Developmental and Behavioral Pediatrics*, **29**: 106–116.

Carminati, G.G., Deriaz, N., Bertschy, G. (2006). Low-dose venlafaxine in three adolescents and young adults with autistic disorders improves self-injurious behavior and attention deficit/hyperactivity disorders (ADHD)-like symptoms. *Progress in Neuropsychopharmacology and Biological Psychiatry*, **30**: 312–315.

Carter, C.S. (2007). Sex difference in oxytocin and vasopressin: implications for autism spectrum disorders? *Behavioral Brain Research*, **176**: 170–186.

Chavis, P., Westbrook, C. (2001). Integrins mediate functional pre- and postsynaptic maturation at a hippocampal synapse. *Nature*, **411**: 317–321.

Cho, I.H., Yoo, H.J., Park, M., Lee, Y.S., Kim, S.A. (2007). Family-based association study of 5-HTTLPR and the 5-HT2A receptor gene polymorphisms with autism spectrum disorder in Korean trios. *Brain Research*, 1139: 34–41.

Chugani, D.C., Muzik, O., Rothermel, R., *et al.* (1997). Altered serotonin synthesis in the dentatothalamocortical pathway in autistic boys. *Annals of Neurology*, **42**: 666–669.

Chugani, D.C., Muzik, O., Behen, M., *et al.* (1999). Developmental changes in brain serotonin synthesis capacity in autistic and nonautistic children. *Annals of Neurology*, **45**: 287–295.

Conroy, J., Meally, E., Kearney, G., *et al.* (2004). Serotonin transporter gene and autism: a haplotype analysis in an Irish autistic population. *Molecular Psychiatry*, **9**: 587–593.

Cook, E.H., Leventhal, B.L. (1996). The serotonin system in autism. *Current Opinion in Pediatrics*, **8**: 348–354.

Cook Jr., E.H., Courchesne, R., Lord, C., *et al.* (1997). Evidence of linkage between the serotonin transporter and autistic disorder. *Molecular Psychiatry*, **2**: 247–250

Coskun, M., Mukaddes, N.M. (2008). Mirtazepine treatment in a subject with autistic disorder and fetishism. *Journal of Child and Adolescent Psychopharmacology*, **18**: 206–209.

Coutinho, A.M., Sousa, I., Martins, M., *et al.* (2007). Evidence for epistasis between SLC6A4 and ITGB3 in autism etiology and in the determination of platelet serotonin levels. *Human Genetics*, **121**: 243–256.

Crawley, J.H., Chen, T., Puri, A., *et al.* (2007). Social approach behaviours in oxytocin knockout mice: comparison of two independent lines tested in different laboratory environments. *Neuropeptides*, **41**: 145–163.

Croonenberghs, J., Verkerk, R., Scharpe, S., Deboutte, D., Maes, M. (2005). Serotonergic disturbances in autistic disorder: L-5-hydroxytryptophan administration to autistic youngsters increases the blood concentrations of serotonin in patients but not in controls. *Life Sciences*, **76**: 2171–2183.

Croonenberghs, J., Spass, K., Wauters, A., *et al.* (2008). Faulty serotonin-DHEA interactions in autism: results of the 5-hydroxytryptophan challenge test. *Neuroendocrinology Letters*, **29**: 385–390.

Cross, S., Kim, S.J., Weiss, L.A., *et al.* (2008). Molecular genetics of the platelet serotonin system in first-degree relatives of patients with autism. *Neuropsychopharmacology*, **33**: 353–360.

Danfors, T., von Knorring, A.L., Hartvig, P., *et al.* (2005). Tetrahydrobiopterin in the treatment of children with autistic disorder: a double-blind placebo-controlled crossover study. *Journal of Clinical Psychopharmacology*, **25**: 485–489.

D'Arcangelo, G. (2005). Apoer2: A Reelin receptor to remember. *Neuron*, **47**: 471–473.

Davis, E., Fennoy, I., Laraque, D., *et al.* (1992). Autism and developmental abnormalities in children with perinatal cocaine exposure. *Journal of the National Medical Association*, **84**: 315–319.

Devlin, B., Bennett, P., Dawson, G., *et al.* (2004). Alleles of a Reelin CGG repeat do not convey liability to autism in a sample from the CPEA Network. *American Journal of Medical Genetics Part B: Neuropsychiatric Genetics*, **126B**: 46–50.

Domes, G., Heinrichs, M., Michel, A., Berger, C., Herpertz, S.C. (2007). Oxytocin improves 'mind-reading' in humans. *Biological Psychiatry*, **61**: 731–733.

Dutta, S., Sinha, S., Ghosh, S., *et al.* (2008). Genetic analysis of reelin gene (RELN) SNPs: No association with autism spectrum disorder in the Indian population. *Neuroscience Letters*, **441**: 56–60.

Emamian E.S., Hall, D, Birnbaum, M.F., *et al.* (2004). Convergent evidence for impaired AKT1-GSK3 beta signaling in schizophrenia. *Nature Genetics*, **36**: 131–137.

Falconer, D.S. (1951). Two new mutants, Trembler and 'Reeler' with neurological actions in the house mouse. *Journal of Genetics*, **50**: 182–201.

Fatemi, S.H. (2002). The role of Reelin in pathology of autism. *Molecular Psychiatry*, **7**: 919–920.

Fatemi, S.H., Realmuto, G.M., Khan, L., Thuras, P. (1998). Fluoxetine in treatment of adolescent patients with autism: a longitudinal open trial. *Journal of Autism and Developmental Disorders*, **28**: 303–307.

Fatemi, S.H., Kroll, J.L., Stary, J.M. (2001a). Altered levels of Reelin and its isoforms in schizophrenia and mood disorders. *Neuroreport*, **12**: 3209–3215.

Fatemi, S.H., Stary, J.M., Halt, A.R., Realmuto, G.R. (2001b). Dysregulation of Reelin and Bcl-2 proteins in autistic cerebellum. *Journal of Autism and Developmental Disorders*, **31**: 529–535.

Fatemi, S.H., Snow, A.V., Stary, J.M., *et al.* (2005). Reelin signaling is impaired in autism. *Biological Psychiatry*, **57**: 777–787.

Ferguson, J.N., Aldag, J.M., Insel, T.R., Young, L.J. (2001). Oxytocin in the medial amygdala is essential for social recognition in the mouse. *Journal of Neuroscience*, **21**: 8278–8285

Gale, S., Ozonoff, S., Lainhart, J. (2003). Brief report: pitocin induction in autistic and nonautistic individuals. *Journal of Autism and Developmental Disorders*, **33**: 205–208.

Gillberg, C., Billstedt, E. (2000). Autism and Asperger syndrome: coexistence with other clinical disorders. *Acta Psychiatrica Scandinavica*, **102**: 321–330.

Gimpl, G., Wiegand, V., Burger, K., Fahrenolz, F. (2002). Cholesterol and steroid hormones: modulators of oxytocin receptor function. *Progress in Brain Research*, **139**: 43–55.

Goldberg, J., Anderson, G.H., Zwaigenbaum, L., *et al.* (2008). Cortical serotonin type-2 receptor density in parents of children with autism spectrum disorders. *Journal of Autism and Developmental Disorders*, **39**: 97–104.

Goldberg, W., Osann, K., Filipek, P., *et al.* (2003). Language and other regression: Assessment and timing. *Journal of Autism and Developmental Disorders*, **33**: 607–616.

Goldman, M., Marlow-O'Conner, M., Torres, I., Carter, C.S. (2008). Diminished plasma oxytocin in schizophrenic patients with neuroendocrine dysfunction and emotional deficits. *Schizophrenia Research*, **98**: 247–255.

Green, L. A., Fein, D., Modahl, C., *et al.* (2001). Oxytocin and autistic disorder: alterations in peptide forms. *Biological Psychiatry*, **50**: 609–613.

Greenburg, B., Tolliver, T., Huang, S., *et al.* (1999). Genetic variation in the serotonin transporter promotor region affects serotonin uptake in human blood platelets. *American Journal of Medical Genetics*, **88**: 83–87.

Guhathakurta, S., Ghosh, S., Sinha, S., *et al.* (2006). Serotonin transporter promoter variants: Analysis in Indian autistic and control population. *Brain Research*, **1092**: 28–35.

Hellings, J.A., Kelley, L.A., Gabrielli, W.F., Kilgore, E., Shah, P. (1996). Sertraline response in adults with mental retardation and autistic disorder. *Journal of Clinical Psychiatry*, **57**: 333–336.

Hollander, E., Cartwright, C., Wong, C., *et al.* (1998). A dimensional approach to the autism spectrum. *CNS Spectrums*, **3**: 22–39.

Hollander, E., Kaplan, A., Cartwright, C., Reichman, D. (2000). Venlafaxine in children, adolescents, and young adults with autism spectrum disorders: an open retrospective clinical report. *Journal of Child Neurology*, **15**: 132–135.

Hollander, E., Novotny, S., Hanratty, M., *et al.* (2003). Oxytocin infusion reduces repetitive behaviours in adults with autistic and Asperger's disorders. *Neuropsychopharmacology*, **28**: 193–198.

Hollander, E., Phillips, A., Chaplin, W., *et al.* (2005). A placebo controlled crossover trial of liquid fluoxetine on repetitive behaviors in childhood and adolescent autism. *Neuropsychopharmacology*, **30**: 582–589.

Hollander, E., Bartz, J., Chaplin, W., *et al.* (2007). Oxytocin increases retention of social cognition in autism. *Biological Psychiatry*, **61**: 498–503.

Howard, M.A., Cowel, P.E., Boucher, J., *et al.* (2000). Convergent neuroanatomical and behavioural evidence of an amygdala hypothesis of autism. *Neuroreport*, **11**: 2931–2935.

Hranilovic, D., Bujas-Petkovic, Z., Vragovic, R., *et al.* (2007). Hyperserotonemia in adults with autistic disorder. *Journal of Autism and Developmental Disorders*, **37**: 1934–1940

Hu, V.W., Nguyen, A., Kim, K.S., *et al.* (2009). Gene expression profiling of lymphoblasts from autistic and nonaffected sib pairs: altered pathways in neuronal development and steroid biosynthesis. *PLoS One*, **4**: e5775.

Jacob, S., Brune, C.W., Carter, C.S., *et al.* (2007). Association of the oxytocin receptor gene (OXTR) in Caucasian children and adolescents with autism. *Neuroscience Letters*, **417**: 6–9.

Jansen, L.M.C., Gispen-de Wied, C.C., Wiegant, V.M., *et al.* (2006). Autonomic and neuroendocrine responses to a psychosocial stressor in adults with autistic spectrum disorder. *Journal of Autism and Developmental Disorders*, **36**: 891–899.

Janusonis, S., Gluncic, V., Rakic, P. (2004). Early serotonergic projections to Cajal-Retzius cells: relevance for cortical development. *Journal of Neuroscience*, **24**: 1652–1659.

Jo, M., Fortune, J.E. (2002) Changes in oxytocin receptor in bovine preovulatory follicles between the gonadotropin surge and ovulation. *Molecular and Cellular Endocrinology*, **200**: 31–43.

Keltikangas-Järvinen, L., Salo, J. (2009). Dopamine and serotonin systems modify environmental effects on human behavior: a review. *Scandinavian Journal of Psychology*, **50**: 574–582.

Kirsch, P., Esslinger, C., Chen, Q., *et al.* (2005). Oxytocin modulates neural circuitry for social cognition and fear in humans. *Journal of Neuroscience*, **25**: 11489–11493.

Klauck, S.M., Poustka, F., Benner, A., Lesch, K.P., Poustka, A. (1997). Serotonin transporter (5-HTT) gene variants associated with autism? *Human Molecular Genetics*, **6**: 2233–2238

Kolevzon, A., Mathewson, K.A., Hollander, E. (2006). Selective serotonin reuptake inhibitors in autism: a review of efficacy and tolerability. *Journal of Clinical Psychiatry*, **67**: 407–414.

Kosfeld, M., Heinrichs, M., Zak, P.J., Fischbacher, U., Fehr, E. (2005). Oxytocin increases trust in humans. *Nature*, **435**: 673–676.

Kramer, K., Azmitia, E.C., Whitaker-Azmitia, P.M. (1994). In vitro release of [3H]5-hydroxytryptamine from fetal and maternal brain by drugs of abuse. *Developmental Brain Research*, **78**: 142–146.

Krebs, M.O., Betancur, C., Leroy, S., *et al.* (2002). Absence of association between a polymorphic GGC repeat in the 5' untranslated region of the reelin gene and autism. *Molecular Psychiatry*, **7**: 801–804.

Krueger, D.D., Howell, J.L., Hebert, B.F., *et al.* (2006). Assessment of cognitive function in the heterozygous reeler mouse. *Psychopharmacology*, **189**: 95–104.

Leckman, J.F., Goodman, W.K., North, W.G., *et al.* (1994). Elevated cerebrospinal fluid levels of oxytocin in obsessive-compulsive disorder. Comparison with Tourette's syndrome and healthy controls. *Archives of General Psychiatry*, **51**: 782–792.

Lerer, E., Levi, S., Salomon, S., *et al.* (2007). Association between the oxytocin receptor (OXTR) gene and autism: relationship to Vineland Adaptive Behaviour Scales and cognition. *Molecular Psychiatry*, **13**: 980–988.

Li, J., Nguyen, L., Gleason, C., *et al.* (2004). Lack of evidence for an association between WNT2 and RELN polymorphisms and autism. *American Journal of Medical Genetics Part B: Neuropsychiatric Genetics*, **126B**: 51–57.

Liu, W., Pappas, G.D., Carter, C.S. (2005). Oxytocin receptors in brain cortical regions are reduced in haploinsufficient (+/–) reeler mice. *Neurological Research*, **27**: 339–345.

Magalhães-Nunes, A.P., Badauê-Passos, D. Jr., **Rizo Ventura, R.**, *et al.* (2008). Sertraline, a selective serotonin reuptake inhibitor, affects thirst, salt appetite and plasma levels of oxytocin and vasopressin in rats. *Experimental Physiology*, **92**: 913–922.

Magdaleno, S., Keshvara, L., Curran, T. (2002). Rescue of ataxia and preplate splitting by ectopic expression of Reelin in reeler mice. *Neuron*, **33**: 573–586.

Martin, A., Landau, J., Leebens, P., *et al.* (2000). Risperidone-associated weight gain in children and adolescents: a retrospective chart review. *Journal of Child and Adolescent Psychopharmacology*, **10**: 259–268.

Martin, A., Koenig, K., Anderson, G.M., Scahill, L. (2003). Low-dose fluvoxamine treatment of children and adolescents with pervasive developmental disorders: a prospective, open-label study. *Journal of Autism and Developmental Disorders*, **33**: 77–85.

Martin-Ruiz, C.M., Lee, M., Perry, R.H., *et al.* (2004). Molecular analysis of nicotinic receptor expression in autism. *Molecular Brain Research*, **123**: 81–90.

Mayes S.D., Calhoun S.L. (2003) Ability profiles in children with autism: Influence of age and IQ. *Autism* **7**: 65–80.

McBride, P.A., Anderson, G.M., Hertzig, M.E., *et al.* (1998). Effects of diagnosis, race and puberty on platelet serotonin levels in autism and mental retardation. *Journal of the American Academy of Child and Adolescent Psychiatry*, **37**: 767–776.

McDougle, C.J., Naylor, S.T., Cohen, D.J., *et al.* (1996a). Effects of tryptophan depletion in drug-free adults with autistic disorder. *Archives of General Psychiatry*, **53**: 993–1000.

McDougle, C.J., Naylor, S.T., Cohen, D.J., *et al.* (1996b). A double-blind, placebo-controlled study of fluvoxamine in adults with autistic disorder. *Archives of General Psychiatry*, **53**: 1001–1008.

McDougle, C.J., Scahill, L., McCracken, J.T., *et al.* (2000). Research Units on Pediatric Psychopharmacology (RUPP) Autism Network. Background and rationale for an initial controlled study of risperidone. *Child and Adolescent Psychiatric Clinics of North America*, **9**: 201–224.

McNamara, I.M., Borella, A.W., Bialowas, L.A., Whitaker-Azmitia, P.M. (2008). Further studies in the developmental hyperserotonemia model (DHS) in autism: Social, behavioral and peptide changes. *Brain Research*, **16**: 203–214.

Mitchell, B.F., Fang, X., Wong, S. (1998). Role of carboxy-extended forms of oxytocin in the rat uterus in the process of parturition. *Biology of Reproduction*, **59**: 1321–1327.

Modahl, C., Green, L., Fein, D., *et al.* (1998). Plasma oxytocin levels in autistic children. *Biological Psychiatry*, **43**: 270–277.

Mukaetova-Ladinska, E.B., Arnold, H., Jaros, E., Perry, R., Perry, E. (2004). Laminar cytoarchitectonic changes and depletion of MAP2 expression in dorsolateral prefrontal cortex in adult autistic individuals. *Neuropathology and Applied Neurobiology*, **30**: 615–623.

Mulder, E.J., Anderson, G.M., Kema, I.P., *et al.* (2004). Platelet serotonin levels in pervasive developmental disorders and mental retardation: diagnostic group differences within group distribution and behavioural correlates. *Journal of the American Academy of Child and Adolescent Psychiatry*, **43**: 491–499.

Murphy, D.G.M., Daly, E., Schmitz, N., *et al.* (2006). Cortical serotonin 5-HT2A receptor binding and social communication in adults with Asperger's syndrome: an in vivo SPECT study. *American Journal of Psychiatry*, **163**: 934–936.

Nagaraj, R., Singhi, P., Malhi, P. (2006). Risperidone in children with autism: randomized, placebo-controlled, double-blind study. *Journal of Child Neurology*, **21**: 450–455.

Nguyen, M., Murphy, T. (2001). Mirtazepine for excessive masturbation in an adolescent with autism. *Journal of the American Academy of Child and Adolescent Psychiatry*, **40**: 868–869.

Oblak, A., Gibbs, T.T., Blatt, G.J. (2009). Decreased GABAA receptors and benzodiazepine binding sites in the anterior cingulate cortex in autism. *Autism Research*, **2**: 205–219.

Ogawa, M., Miyata, T., Nakajima, K., *et al.* (1995). The reeler gene-associated antigen on Cajal-Retzius neurons is a crucial molecule for laminar organization of cortical neurons. *Neuron*, **14**: 899–912.

Parikh, M.S., Kolevzon, A., Hollander, E. (2008). Psychopharmacology of aggression in children and adolescents with autism: a critical review of efficacy and tolerability. *Journal of Child and Adolescent Psychopharmacology*, **18**: 157–178.

Pesold, C., Impagnatiello, F., Pisu, M.G., *et al.* (1998). Reelin is preferentially expressed in neurons synthesizing gamma-aminobutyric acid in cortex and hippocampus of adult rats. *Proceedings of the National Academy of Sciences USA*, **95**: 3221–3226.

Quattrocchi, C.C., Wannenes, F., Persico, A.M., *et al.* (2002). Reelin is a serine protease of the extracellular matrix. *Journal of Biological Chemistry*, **277**: 303–309; erratum **277**: 11616.

Ragnauth, A.K., Devidze, N., Moy, V., *et al.* (2005). Female oxytocin gene-knockout mice, in a semi-natural environment, display exaggerated agressive behaviour. *Genes Brain and Behavior*, **4**: 229–239.

Ramoz, N., Reichert, J.G., Corwin, T.E., *et al.* (2006). Lack of evidence for association of the serotonin transporter gene SLC6A4 with autism. *Biological Psychiatry*, **60**: 186–191.

Roberts, R.C., Xu, L.Y., Roche, J.K., Kirkpatrick, B. (2005). Ultrastructural localization of reelin in the cortex in post-mortem human brain. *Journal of Comparative Neurology*, **482**: 294–308.

Rojas Wahl, R.U. (2004). Could oxytocin administration during labour contribute to autism and related behavioral disorders? – A look at the literature. *Medical Hypothesis*, **63**: 456–460.

Saher, G., Brugger, B., Lapper-Siefke, C., *et al.* (2005). High cholesterol level is essential for myelin membrane growth. *Nature Neuroscience*, **8**: 468–475.

Scott, L.J., Dhillon, S. (2007). Risperidone: a review of its use in the treatment of irritability associated with autistic disorder in children and adolescents. *Pediatric Drugs*, **9**: 343–354.

Serajee, F.J., Zhong, H., Mahbubul Huq, A.H.M. (2006). Association of Reelin gene polymorphisms with autism. *Genomics*, **87**: 75–83.

Skaar, D.A., Shao, Y., Haines, J.L., *et al.* (2005). Analysis of the RELN gene as a genetic risk factor for autism. *Molecular Psychiatry*, **10**: 563–571.

Takahashi, S., Kanai, H., Miyamoto, Y. (1976). Reassessment of elevated serotonin levels in blood platelets in early infantile autism. *Journal of Autism and Childhood Schizophrenia*, **6**: 317–326.

Tom, N., Assinder, S.J. (2010). Oxytocin in health and disease. *International Journal of Biochemistry and Cell Biology*, **42**: 202–205.

Veenstra-VanderWeele, J., Anderson, G.M., Cook, E.H. Jr. (2000). Pharmacokinetics and the serotonin system: initial studies and future directions. *European Journal of Pharmacology*, **410**: 165–181.

Waage-Baudet, H., Lauder, J.M., Dehart, D.B., *et al.* (2003). Abnormal serotonergic development in a mouse model for Smith-Lemli-Opitz syndrome: Implications for autism. *International Journal of Developmental Neuroscience*, **21**: 451–459.

Weiss, L.A., Kosova, G., Delahanty, R.J., *et al.* (2006a). Variation in ITGB3 is associated with whole blood serotonin level and autism susceptibility. *European Journal of Human Genetics*, **14**: 923–931.

Weiss, L.A., Ober, C., Cook Jr, E.H. (2006b). ITGB3 shows genetic and expression interaction with SLC6A4. *Human Genetics*, **120**: 93–100.

West, L., Brunssen, S.H., Waldrop, J. (2009a). Review of the evidence for treatment with children of autism with selective reuptake serotonin inhibitors. *Journal for Specialists in Pediatric Nursing*, **14**: 183–191.

West, L., Waldrop, J., Brunssen, S.H. (2009b). Pharmacologic treatment for the core deficits and associated symptoms of autism in children. *Journal of Pediatric Health Care*, **23**: 75–89.

Winslow, J.T., Insel, T.R. (2002). The social deficits of the oxytocin knockout mouse. *Neuropeptides*, **36**: 221–229.

Wu, S., Jia, M., Ruan, Y., *et al.* (2005). Positive association of the oxytocin receptor gene (OXTR) with autism in the Chinese Han population. *Biological Psychiatry*, **58**: 74–77.

Yirmiya, N., Pilowsky, T., Nemanov, L., *et al.* (2001). Evidence for an association with the serotonin transporter promoter region polymorphism and autism. *American Journal of Medical Genetics*, **105**: 381–386

Ylisaukko-oja, T., Alarcón, M., Cantor, R.M., *et al.* (2005). Search for autism loci by combined analysis of Autism Genetic Resource Exchange and Finnish families. *Annals of Neurology*, **59**: 145–155.

Zak, P.J., Stanton, A.A., Ahmadi, S. (2007). Oxytocin increases generosity in humans. *PLoS ONE*, **2**: e1128.

Zhang, H., Liu, X., Zhang, C., *et al.* (2002). Reelin gene alleles and susceptibility to autism spectrum disorders. *Molecular Psychiatry*, **7**: 1012–1017.

Zingg, H.H., Laporte, S.A. (2003) The oxytocin receptor. *Trends in Endocrinology and Metabolism*, **14**: 222–227

PART III COGNITION, DEVELOPMENT AND EDUCATION

7

Psychological models of autism: an overview

ELIZABETH PELLICANO

Autism is currently defined in terms of a core set of behaviours, including difficulties in social reciprocity and communication, and limitations in behavioural flexibility. In the past three decades, considerable efforts have been directed towards understanding the neurocognitive atypicalities that underlie these core behaviours. This chapter provides an overview of the major theoretical accounts of autism, especially the theory of mind hypothesis, the executive dysfunction hypothesis, and weak central coherence theory, each of which has aimed to explain autism in terms of a single underlying cognitive atypicality. Some of the reasons why researchers have become dissatisfied with these so-called 'single-deficit' accounts as explanatory models of autism will be analysed, before turning to more recent 'multiple-deficits' models to begin the task of outlining the additional challenges faced by such models. The chapter concludes by stressing the need to situate explanatory accounts of autism – single or multiple-deficit models – within a developmental context.

7.1 Introduction

Since the seminal experimental work of psychologists such as Hermelin and O'Connor (1970) and Frith (1970, 1972), considerable research efforts have been directed towards elucidating the psychological mechanisms underpinning the behavioural manifestations of autism spectrum disorder (hereafter 'autism')[1],

[1] The term 'autism spectrum disorder' includes Autistic Disorder, Asperger's Syndrome, Pervasive Developmental Disorder – Not Otherwise Specified and Atypical Autism, and has been adopted by clinicians and researchers to reflect the variability of these disorders in terms of intellectual functioning, language ability and degree of symptomatology.

Researching the Autism Spectrum: Contemporary Perspectives, ed. I. Roth and P. Rezaie. Published by Cambridge University Press.

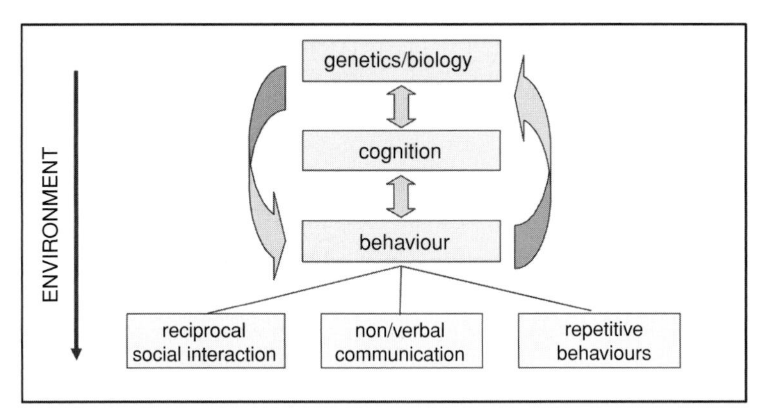

Figure 7.1 Causal model showing three levels of explanation: genetics/biology, cognition and behaviour (adapted from Frith *et al.* (1991)) encompassing a single primary cognitive deficit. In addition to interactions with the environment, there is likely to be a complex interplay between these explanatory levels, as the arrows indicate. For example, atypicalities in early cognitive development could have profound secondary effects on later brain and psychological development. Likewise, the premise of early behavioural intervention is that it should capitalise on the plasticity of the developing brain to alter underlying (atypical) brain processes.

including the often profound difficulties in social reciprocity and communication, and stereotyped, repetitive interests and activities. Historically, in the interests of parsimony, researchers focused their efforts on isolating a *single primary cognitive deficit* that could provide a unifying explanation for the constellation of symptoms that are unlikely to co-occur by chance (Morton and Frith, 1995) (see also Rutter, 1968; 1983). In the absence of specific genes or biological markers for autism, cognitive accounts of autism sought to further our understanding of autism by pinpointing the 'intervening variable' between biology and behaviour (Frith *et al.* 1991; Morton and Frith, 1995; 2001; Figure 7.1). Identification of a core cognitive marker could not only inform research at the genetic level by the discovery of 'endophenotypes' or vulnerability markers (Gottesman and Gould, 2003), but also provide insight into the brain bases of autism (Hill and Frith, 2003), and form the basis for intervention programmes.

The past few decades have witnessed researchers fervently pursuing the notion of a primary cognitive marker for autism, generating as they have done so numerous hypotheses concerning the nature of the cognitive deficit in autism, some of which have included atypical 'central' processes such as sequencing, concept formation and abstraction (Hermelin and O'Connor, 1970), core problems in language (Rutter, 1968), sensory and perceptual atypicalities (Ornitz and Ritvo, 1968), disruption of 'complex' information processing (Minshew *et al.* 1992;

Minshew *et al.* 1997), poor social responsiveness (Klin and Volkmar, 1993; Mundy and Sigman, 1989) and impairments in interpersonal relatedness (Hobson, 1989; 1993) (see also Hobson, 2002). Three additional theories have been particularly influential in the field largely due to their potential to explain autism in terms of a single underlying cognitive atypicality. These include: (1) the theory of mind hypothesis, which claimed that autism is caused primarily by a specific inability to impute mental states to oneself and to others (Baron-Cohen *et al.* 1985) (see Baron-Cohen *et al.* (2000) and Tager-Flusberg (2007), for reviews); (2) the executive dysfunction hypothesis, which proposed that the symptoms of autism are a result of a dysexecutive syndrome – a primary problem in the executive control of action (Hughes and Russell, 1993; Ozonoff *et al.* 1991), (see Hill (2004) and Russo *et al.* (2007) for reviews); and (3) 'weak' central coherence theory, which posited that individuals with autism have a tendency to focus on individual elements rather than wholes combined with an inability to integrate information into context (Frith, 1989; Frith and Happé, 1994) (see Happé and Booth (2008) and Happé and Frith (2006), for reviews).

These so-called 'single-deficit' theories have generated a huge amount of research, and, as a result, have brought autism research to the attention of mainstream developmental and cognitive neuroscience. Nevertheless, the notion of a single cause at the cognitive level of analysis has been challenged repeatedly by empirical investigations, which have cast considerable doubt on the validity of several of the theories' central claims. Consequently, there has been a recent shift from single-deficit accounts towards those espousing 'multiple deficits'. Proponents of these latter accounts argue that they could in principle provide a more adequate explanation of the diverse set of symptoms defining autism.

The goal of this chapter is to present an overview of each of the major single-deficit theories in turn, detailing the empirical reasons why researchers have become dissatisfied with these accounts as potential causal explanations of autism. In so doing, the often sophisticated conceptual accounts on which the theories depend will be introduced initially, before reviewing the extensive empirical literature that puts those theories to the test in such a way as to allow the reader direct access to the relevant results. The chapter also considers more recent multiple-deficits models, and begins the task of outlining the additional challenges faced by such models.

The chapter thus provides the reader with a comprehensive (although not, of course, exhaustive) survey and analysis of the most influential cognitive accounts of autism. Before it begins, however, it is necessary to outline the criteria specified by researchers, which have been used not only to guide and constrain single-deficit models of autism, but also to assess the veracity of these models' claims.

7.2 Criteria for explanatory accounts of autism

Michael Rutter (1983) first advocated the notion of a primary deficit for which he outlined several indicators, including universal manifestation, early appearance, prognostic significance, and the capacity to explain performance on a variety of tasks. Researchers have since refined the notion of a primary cognitive deficit as one which is 'universal, specific, and necessary and sufficient to cause the symptoms of the disorder ... in other words, the proximal cognitive cause of the behavioural symptoms of the disorder' (Pennington and Ozonoff, 1996, page 57). Similar to Rutter (1983), several authors have emphasised that the primary cognitive marker should also show causal priority; that is, it should have the capacity to explain the earliest-emerging features of autism (Boucher, 1996; Happé, 1994b; Tager-Flusberg, 2001).

The putative cognitive deficit should therefore:

1. Be universal, or near universal, among individuals with autism
2. Be unique to individuals with autism (i.e. not present in individuals with other developmental conditions)
3. Show causal precedence
4. Show explanatory power (i.e. the incidence and severity of the deficit should be directly related to the behavioural symptoms in each of the three domains)

These four criteria have been echoed in subsequent empirical and theoretical work (e.g. Bailey *et al.* 1996; Ozonoff and McEvoy, 1994; Turner, 1997), and will be used to evaluate each of the major theoretical accounts in the following sections. This set of criteria is by no means exhaustive. Additional criteria have been cited by several researchers, including presence of the putative deficit in the broader autism phenotype (individuals with a genetic liability for autism, who display autistic behaviours, albeit of a lesser degree than in autism itself) (Bailey *et al.*, 1996; Bailey and Parr, 2003; Hughes, 2001), and persistence or stability over time (Ozonoff and McEvoy, 1994; Rutter, 1983).

7.3 The Theory of Mind Hypothesis

The first major cognitive theory of autism focused on deficits in *theory of mind* (ToM) or 'mentalizing': the ability to attribute mental states to oneself and to others, which allows one successfully to predict and interpret others' behaviour (Dennett, 1978). A central focus of such work has been on children's understanding of beliefs, which often involves mistaken representations of reality, and is therefore held to signal the emergence of a representational understanding of mind (Wimmer and Perner, 1983). In a landmark study conducted more than two decades ago, Baron-Cohen *et al.* (1985) showed that 80% of their sample of children with autism displayed difficulties on the now classic false-belief task, despite the fact that the verbal mental age of these children was well beyond the 4- to 5-year-old level, when success on this task typically occurs. This evidence led to the proposal that the core features of autism could be explained by a single primary cognitive deficit in the ability to understand other minds (Baron-Cohen, 1993; 1995; Baron-Cohen *et al.* 1985; Frith *et al.* 1991; Leslie, 1987; 1991). Leslie (1987, 1991) and Leslie and Thaiss (1992) argued strongly that individuals with autism specifically lack the modular Theory of Mind Mechanism (ToMM), which in the typically developing child enables the formation of propositional attitudes (e.g. of the form, 'X believes that (. . .)'), and provides insight into others' behaviour.

In support of this position, a multitude of studies has since demonstrated that many persons with autism fail tasks that require a representational understanding of other minds (see Baron-Cohen *et al.* 2000, and Tager-Flusberg, 2001, 2007, for reviews), including those tapping the understanding of deception (Baron-Cohen, 1992; Russell *et al.* 1991; Sodian and Frith, 1992), knowledge (Baron-Cohen and Goodhart, 1994; Leslie and Frith, 1988), complex emotions, such as surprise (Baron-Cohen *et al.* 1993), intention (Phillips *et al.* 1998), in addition to recognition, comprehension and expression of mental state terms (Baron-Cohen *et al.* 1994; Tager-Flusberg, 1992; Ziatas *et al.* 1998).

The theory of mind hypothesis seemed to capture what Kanner (1943) first described as 'autistic aloneness'. Certainly, the inability to realise fully what it means to have a mind and to think, know, believe and feel differently from others should affect one's capacity to relate to others socially, and also should influence one's ability to communicate effectively (see Happé, 1993). Indeed, links were made between successful theory of mind task performance and pragmatic skills (Eisenmajer and Prior, 1991), in addition to 'real-life' social difficulties, including the ability to make or keep secrets, offer important information, and recognise surprise and embarrassment (Frith *et al.* 1994; Hughes *et al.* 1997; Tager-Flusberg, 2000). Furthermore, Leslie (1987, 1991) argued that a core 'metarepresentational' impairment in autism could also account for the lack of imaginative or pretend play in autism. The prospect that a core cognitive impairment in theory of mind could provide a causal explanation for autism caused a flurry of research. Yet it was soon met with various criticisms, which are outlined below.

7.3.1 *Universality*

Initial research showed that not all individuals with autism fail false belief tasks. In Baron-Cohen *et al.*'s (1985) original study, 20% of children with autism passed the critical false belief question[2]. In subsequent studies, this percentage varied from 15% (e.g. Reed and Peterson, 1990) to 55% (e.g. Prior *et al.* 1990), with 90% of participants with autism passing in one study (Dahlgren and Trillingsgaard, 1996). The presence of a theory of mind difficulties in some, but not all, individuals with the condition cast doubt over whether these difficulties played a causal role in the development of autism.

Proponents of the theory of mind hypothesis responded to this initial criticism by showing that although some individuals with autism could pass first-order false-belief tasks, they nevertheless failed more difficult second-order false-belief attributions (i.e. of the form 'Mary thinks that John thinks the icecream van is in the park'; Perner and Wimmer, 1985) despite being significantly older than the age at which such tasks are typically passed (6–7 years) (Baron-Cohen, 1989a; Perner *et al.* 1987; but see Bowler, 1992). These findings led Baron-Cohen (1989a) to suggest that the development of theory of mind is specifically delayed in autism rather than completely absent. Support for this view came from reports of a link between theory of mind success and autistic children's language skills (e.g. Charman and Baron-Cohen, 1992; Leekam and Perner, 1991) (see also Fisher *et al.* 2005 and Tager-Flusberg and Joseph, 2005). Indeed, in her review, Happé (1995) showed that the level of verbal ability necessary to pass standard false-belief tasks was considerably higher in children with autism (mental age (MA) of at least 12 years) than in typically developing children (MA of 4 years).

Some authors argued, however, that success by older individuals with autism on false-belief tasks did not provide unequivocal evidence that these individuals had in fact developed a theory of mind. Instead, these 'passers' could be using alternative compensatory routes to task success (Eisenmajer and Prior, 1991; Frith *et al.* 1991; Happé, 1995; Holroyd and Baron-Cohen, 1993; Ozonoff *et al.* 1991). Subsequent studies have provided indirect support for this idea. Behavioural studies have shown that older individuals with autism who pass standard false-belief tasks nevertheless show poor performance on more naturalistic tests of theory of mind, including understanding of irony (Happé, 1994a), and the attribution of mental states of moving geometric figures (Castelli *et al.* 2002; Klin, 2000). Neuroimaging studies have further shown that, while typical adults activate regions of the so-called social brain network (e.g. medial pre-frontal cortex and temporoparietal junction; Frith and Frith, 2003; Saxe *et al.* 2004) when solving theory of mind tasks, cognitively able adults with autism who pass such tasks show significantly less activation in these regions (e.g. Castelli *et al.* 2002) and may instead recruit

[2] Given the use of only two test trials in this study, it is plausible that the four children with autism who passed both trials may have done so due to random responding rather than a true understanding of other minds.

neural regions associated with general problem-solving skills (e.g. Happé *et al.* 1996), suggesting they might be using non-mentalistic strategies to help them reason about other peoples' behaviour.

Although more direct support for this proposal is still needed, a recent elegant study provides the most conclusive evidence to date that individuals with autism may genuinely show atypicalities in mentalising. Senju *et al.* (2009) used eye-tracking methodology to reveal the on-line processing of adults with Asperger syndrome as they watched an actor and puppet enact the classic false belief scenario. In an earlier study, the same authors had shown that, after having observed the puppet move a ball from one box to another unbeknown to the actor, typical 2-year-olds immediately looked to the empty box that the actor believes still holds the ball (Southgate *et al.* 2007). In their new study, adults with Asperger syndrome – who previously had passed standard versions of the false belief task – failed to anticipate accurately the box in which the actor will look for the ball, instead looking almost equally at the two boxes. Although older and more able individuals with autism may be able to solve standard false belief tasks, these findings strongly indicate that there may be less *spontaneous* mentalising in autism, the sort of processes automatically used by typical infants, children and toddlers to navigate everyday social interactions successfully. Future research using eye-tracking and functional imaging will help determine precisely what processes give rise to an implicit, intuitive theory of mind, and whether such additional processes might be atypical in autism.

7.3.2 *Uniqueness*

Researchers also showed that problems with theory of mind were not specific to autism. Researchers reported that a significant proportion of children with moderate learning difficulties without a diagnosis of autism also showed difficulties on false belief tasks (Benson *et al.* 1993; Yirmiya *et al.* 1996; Zelazo *et al.* 1996), and that problems with false belief understanding were present in children with other developmental disorders, such as oral deafness (Peterson and Siegal, 1995; 1999; Russell *et al.* 1998), congenital blindness (Brown *et al.* 1997; Green *et al.* 2004; Minter *et al.* 1998), and children with specific language impairment (Miller, 2001; but see Colle *et al.* 2007; Perner *et al.* 1989). This evidence called into question whether a specific deficit in theory of mind was necessary and sufficient to cause the behavioural symptoms of autism *per se*.

Proponents of the hypothesis have defended their position by claiming that it may be the severity of the impairment rather than the impairment itself that is unique to autism (e.g. Green *et al.* 2004; Yirmiya *et al.* 1998), or that the failure of the non-autistic clinical groups on false belief tasks might be due to reasons other than a genuine representational deficit (Baron-Cohen, 2000; Tager-Flusberg, 2001). For example, theory of mind difficulties might be the result of reduced conversational opportunities in the case of late or non-signing deaf children (Peterson and Siegal, 1999; 2000), or an inability to use visual cues, such as eye gaze or pointing gestures to 'read' other minds in the case of children with congenital blindness (Minter *et al.* 1998; Tager-Flusberg, 2001).

7.3.3 *Causal precedence*

One additional challenge for the theory of mind hypothesis was to account for how an impairment in theory of mind – as indexed by failure on false belief tasks usually passed by typically developing 4-year-olds – could explain the earliest symptoms of autism including atypicalities in social responsiveness and reciprocity, gaze behaviour, joint attention, and imitation often detected during infancy (e.g. Dawson and Adams, 1984; Klin *et al.* 1992; Mundy and Sigman, 1989; Volkmar *et al.* 1987). Leslie (1987) argued that pretence may be the earliest manifestation of theory of mind, emerging at around 18 months, and later authors suggested that earlier behaviours such as pointing to share interest in something (protodeclarative pointing) and joint attention may be precursors to a theory of mind (Baron-Cohen, 1989b; 1991) (see also see Leslie and Happé (1989)). Nevertheless, studies pointed towards early autistic symptoms that were non-representational in nature, including a failure to 'show anticipation of being picked up by a caregiver' or 'reach for familiar person' (Klin *et al.* 1992), which were interpreted instead as evidence in favour of a more primary affective, emotional or intersubjective impairment in autism (e.g. Hobson, 1993; Klin and Volkmar, 1993; Mundy *et al.* 1993).

Subsequent theoretical accounts have broadened the definition of theory of mind to respond to this challenge. Baron-Cohen (1994; 1995) proposed a more extensive 'mindreading' system, which included not only a module for understanding mental states, such as think, believe, know, but also other early-emerging 'precursor' modules, which include innate mechanisms for eye-gaze detection and shared attention. He proposed that one of these modules – the Shared Attention Mechanism – is specifically damaged in autism, which, as a result, fails to trigger the subsequent development of the Theory of Mind Module. Other theorists have proposed alternative models. Tager-Flusberg (2001) has interpreted the earliest symptoms of autism within a componential account of theory of mind, which encompasses a socio-cognitive system that allows for mental-state reasoning, and also a socio-perceptual system that includes eye-gaze perception, face recognition and emotion recognition, and imitation. Both systems are held to be impaired in autism, and dissociations among systems may be present in other neurodevelopmental conditions (e.g. William's syndrome; Tager-Flusberg and Sullivan, 2000). Others have postulated further that the social impairments in autism extend beyond the processing of mental state stimuli to include the on-line processing of social stimuli, including faces, voices and gestures (e.g. Klin *et al.* 2003). These broader theory of mind accounts represent attempts to provide a causal explanation of the *development* of autism. Nevertheless, it is important to note here that by broadening the definition of theory of mind to extend beyond false-belief understanding, these accounts introduce a degree of circularity in which the first signs of autism (poor gaze monitoring, failure to orient towards social stimuli) are, by definition, components of poor theory of mind (see Hughes and Leekam (2004) for discussion).

7.3.4 *Explanatory power*

Although the theory of mind hypothesis provides an intuitively appealing explanation of the core socio-communicative symptoms of autism, there has been limited direct evidence showing that the degree of theory of mind difficulties are linked to the nature and severity of the symptoms they purport to explain. Tager-Flusberg (2007) has attributed the series of negative findings (e.g. Pellicano *et al.* 2006; Travis *et al.* 2001) to the small numbers of individuals with autism included in these studies. Indeed, in the most comprehensive assessment thus far of the explanatory power of theory of mind difficulties, Tager-Flusberg (2003) reported significant longitudinal associations between performance on multiple theory of mind tasks and several behavioural outcome measures in 69 children with autism aged between 4 and 14 years. Early theory of mind performance emerged as a significant predictor of social and communicative functioning one year later, including real-life social functioning (as assessed by the Vineland Adaptive Behaviour Scales; Sparrow *et al.* 1984), conversational discourse (during a parent–child interaction) and degree of socio-communicative symptoms (as indexed by scores on the Autism Diagnostic Observation Schedules – Generic (ADOS-G); Lord *et al.* 2000) independent of age and verbal ability. Her findings suggest that the degree of impairments in theory of mind could explain in part the wide variation in socio-communicative symptoms in autism.

Despite such positive analysis, the theory of mind hypothesis has failed to address adequately the distinctive non-social symptoms in autism, particularly the repetitive behaviours and stereotyped interests also characteristic of the condition. Baron-Cohen (1989b) argued that the restricted repertoire of behaviours and interests are merely secondary consequences of a core mindreading deficit – the defence mechanisms that emerge to cope with the unpredictability of the social world. Yet rigid and repetitive behaviours are seen in individuals across the autism spectrum and across all levels of functioning. Furthermore, contrary to Baron-Cohen's (1989b) thesis, several early studies reported that individuals with autism show *fewer* repetitive behaviours and motor stereotypies in interpersonal situations than in situations in which the social demands are limited (e.g. Clark and Rutter, 1981). Moreover, several researchers have failed to find any relationship between scores on false belief tasks and symptoms in the repetitive behaviours domain (Joseph and Tager-Flusberg, 2004; Pellicano *et al.* 2006; Turner, 1997), questioning whether these atypicalities in mindreading are capable of accounting for the development of *all* autistic behaviours.

Overall, the theory of mind hypothesis has struggled to satisfy the criteria for an explanatory model of autism. Indeed, critics (e.g. Bloom and German, 2000) have stressed that the success of the hypothesis has centred largely on the validity of the false belief task as an index of theory of mind. They highlighted that failure on such tasks can of course occur for many reasons, and that in the case of autism, could be explained not by a fundamental theory of mind deficit but by deficits in more domain-general processing in executive function (see Section 7.4) or language ability (Bruner and Feldman, 1993; Tager-Flusberg, 2000). Although it was shown initially that children with autism succeed on tasks which have equivalent structure and demands to false belief (or other theory of mind) tasks but do not have mentalistic content (e.g. tests involving false photographs, drawings and models; Charman and Baron-Cohen, 1992; 1995; Leekam and Perner, 1991; Leslie and Thaiss, 1992), more recent analysis of these tasks has questioned whether the structure is in fact identical to standard false belief tasks; see Perner and Leekam (2008), and Sabbagh *et al.* (2006). One study using a false signs task, in which a sign falsely represents the location of an object, found that the difficulties that children with autism display on false belief task extend to the analogous false signs task, casting doubt on whether the children's difficulties on false belief tasks are due to a genuine difficulty in representing other minds (Bowler *et al.* 2005).

Although the theory's proponents have made some plausible arguments in defence of a single primary cognitive difficulty with theory of mind, which stretches beyond problems in false belief understanding, most authors would agree that autism in its entirety is not accounted for by theory of mind alone.

7.4 The Executive Dysfunction Hypothesis

Executive functions are a range of higher order functions, explicitly linked to the prefrontal cortex, which help guide flexible, goal-oriented behaviour, especially in novel circumstances (e.g. Lezak, 1995; Luria, 1966; Pennington and Ozonoff, 1996). Most theoretical models of executive function (e.g. Diamond, 2006; Miyake *et al.* 2000; Pennington, 1997; Shallice and Burgess, 1991) agree that the construct is componential in nature and includes inhibiting or resisting a natural response, working memory or the ability to hold information 'on-line' (in the mind) and mentally work with it, and the ability to flexibly shift one's attentional focus.

In what could be interpreted as one of the first demonstrations of a possible executive function impairment in autism, Frith (1972) showed that individuals with autism produced more rule-bound, repetitive and less unique patterns in a task of spontaneous colour and tone sequence production than comparison individuals. It was not until 1978, however, that Damasio and Maurer published an influential paper noting the striking resemblance between individuals with autism and patients with frontal lobe damage, including inflexible, perseverative behaviours, and concreteness in thought and language (Damasio and Maurer, 1978). Subsequent investigations using neuropsychological tasks such as the Wisconsin Card Sort Test (WCST), a test of cognitive flexibility, and the Tower of Hanoi (ToH) task, a test of higher order planning ability, showed that individuals with autism did in fact display remarkably poor performance on such tasks (Prior and Hoffmann, 1990; Rumsey and Hamburger, 1988). Ozonoff *et al.* (1991) confirmed these findings in an important study comparing performance on theory of mind and executive function tasks in cognitively able or 'high-functioning' children and adolescents with autism and Asperger syndrome. Individuals with autism performed poorly relative to comparison individuals on the WCST and ToH tasks, and Ozonoff *et al.* (1991) showed that executive function variables rather than theory of mind variables were best able to distinguish between individuals with autism and comparison individuals. This evidence led to the hypothesis that executive deficits might represent a single primary cognitive deficit in autism (Hughes and Russell, 1993; Ozonoff *et al.* 1991; Russell, 1997), and that the inflexible, 'stuck in set' problem solving strategies might explain autistic individuals' failure on theory of mind tasks. Furthermore, Ozonoff *et al.* (1991) pointed towards damage to the prefrontal cortex as the possible neuroanatomical underpinnings of executive (and theory of mind) problems in autism.

The executive dysfunction hypothesis has since generated numerous studies largely because of its promise as a candidate for a core cognitive marker in autism; see Hill (2004), O'Hearn *et al.* (2008), and Russo *et al.* (2007) for reviews. Indeed, in their review of studies on executive function in autism, Pennington and Ozonoff (1996) reported that 13 out of the 14 existing studies found evidence of disrupted performance on at least one executive task in autism. They also examined the magnitude of the group differences, and estimated the average effect size on executive tasks to be 0.98, and as high as 2.07 on the ToH task. Despite such promise, the hypothesis has faced a series of challenges, and these are outlined below.

7.4.1 *Universality*

Testing the criterion of universality has been more difficult in the case of executive dysfunction compared with theory of mind, largely because performance on executive tasks, unlike theory of mind tasks, is normally not reducible to 'pass' or 'fail'. Rather, typical executive variables include, for example, percent correct, time taken, number of perseverative responses, or number of rule violations. As a result, some researchers have used an arbitrary criterion of 'impairment' to determine the pervasiveness of executive deficits in autism. Ozonoff *et al.* (1991) calculated the proportion of individuals with autism who performed below the mean composite score of the comparison group for tasks of executive function. Remarkably, they found that impairments in executive function were almost universal in the autism group (96%). These authors, however, used quite a lenient criterion to determine the pervasiveness of executive difficulties. Indeed, if performance on the tasks was genuinely normally distributed, then one should expect to find half of the comparison group also showing 'impairments' in executive skills. When more conservative criteria are used, the proportions of individuals with autism demonstrating difficulties are not so striking. Liss *et al.* (2001) found that 57% of their group of high functioning autistic adolescents scored within 1 standard deviation of the mean number of perseverative errors of the comparison group on the WCST, and Pellicano (2007) reported that between 33% and 50% of her sample of cognitively able children with autism scored more than 1 standard deviation below the mean of the typically developing group on a range of executive function tasks. Other investigators have demonstrated that not all individuals with autism fail executive tasks (Hill and Bird, 2006; Hughes *et al.* 1994; Ozonoff and Jensen, 1999; Teunisse *et al.* 2001) (see also Guerts *et al.* 2009 for discussion), and have shown further that when task success does occur, it is usually in those individuals who are older (Ozonoff and Jensen, 1999) and/or have higher verbal ability (Liss *et al.* 2001; Ozonoff and McEvoy, 1994; Pellicano, 2007; but see Joseph *et al.* 2005).

7.4.2 *Uniqueness*

One other major challenge for the executive dysfunction hypothesis has been research showing that executive problems are not unique to autism but are present also in a variety of other developmental conditions, including, amongst others, conduct disorder, Attention Deficit Hyperactivity Disorder, early-treated phenylketonuria, and Tourette syndrome; see Hill (2004), and Pennington and Ozonoff (1996) for reviews. This so-called 'discriminant validity problem' (Pennington and Ozonoff, 1996) has called into question whether executive problems are necessary and sufficient to cause autistic symptomatology, and points towards the possibility that executive problems might be secondary in autism and possibly some of the other conditions – that is, that executive difficulties are a general consequence of having a developmental condition.

Proponents of the executive dysfunction hypothesis of autism have proposed instead that the development of distinct psychopathology could be explained by different severity and age of onset of executive impairment, and in particular, specific profiles of impairment on the various components of executive function (Ozonoff, 1997; Ozonoff *et al.* 1994; Pennington and Ozonoff, 1996). Since executive functions cover a range of different component processes, identifying the exact nature of the executive atypicality in autism has been the focus of more recent research. Ozonoff (1995) advocated the use of an information processing approach, which more precisely targets particular executive functions. For example, Hughes *et al.* (1994) administered the Intradimensional-Extradimensional shift task, a computerised test of cognitive flexibility, to children with and without autism. This task begins with a discrimination learning task, which becomes progressively more challenging such that shifts in discrimination are required either within-set (intradimensional; i.e. to a new set of stimuli) or between-set (extradimensional; i.e. to a new set of stimuli *and* a new set of dimensions). Hughes *et al.* (1994) found significant group differences only on the extradimensional shift stage of the task, which involves shifting cognitive set to *new* categories or rules and which places the most demands on executive resources, indicating a specific difficulty with cognitive switching in autism.

More recent studies making crucial cross-condition comparisons have delineated a profile of difficulties specific to autism in cognitive flexibility and planning (Guerts *et al.* 2004; Happé *et al.* 2006a; Ozonoff and Jensen, 1999), but not generativity (Bishop and Norbury, 2005a). It is less clear whether problems in inhibition are included in this profile since some studies have found problems in inhibitory control (e.g. Christ *et al.* 2007; Hughes, 1996; Rinehart *et al.* 2002; Williams *et al.* 2002), while others have not (e.g. Russell *et al.* 1999). Also, it remains controversial whether working memory problems form part of this profile. While some studies have reported difficulties in verbal (Bennetto *et al.* 1996) and non-verbal (Dawson *et al.* 1998; McEvoy *et al.* 1993) working memory tasks in persons with autism, other studies have failed to demonstrate autism-specific working memory problems in autism (Griffith *et al.* 1999; Guerts *et al.* 2004; Ozonoff and Strayer, 2001; Russell *et al.* 1996). Some theorists (e.g. Russell, 1997) have argued that these atypicalities emerge only if the task involves *both* inhibitory and working memory requirements.

The challenges faced by the executive dysfunction hypothesis with respect to the criterion of uniqueness raise an important methodological issue. Although executive function has a theoretical definition, it has nevertheless been difficult to operationalise for several reasons – see Hughes and Graham (2002) for discussion. First, unlike theory of mind, there is no 'gold standard' executive task (Burgess, 1997). Second, executive tasks are not process pure. Instead, 'non-executive' task factors are also likely to play a role in task performance, and these are notoriously difficult to disentangle from 'executive' factors. Third, since executive function tasks need to be sufficiently novel and demanding to engage controlled rather than automatic processing, their test–retest reliability is necessarily limited (Rabbitt, 1997). Indeed, since subsequent performance on the same tasks might be less challenging, it might not recruit the same executive processes as those involved in initial performance (e.g. Bishop *et al.* 2001). The lack of an operational definition for executive function (and for its component functions) therefore has made it difficult to pinpoint the precise profile of executive atypicalities which distinguish autism from other developmental conditions.

7.4.3 *Causal precedence*

If indeed executive functioning difficulties do play a causal role in autistic symptomatology, then it should be the case that deficits in these areas should be readily apparent in very young children with autism. McEvoy *et al.* (1993) administered a spatial reversal task to pre-schoolers with autism (mean age = 5 years 1 month). In this task, the child observes as the experimenter hides a reward in one of two identical containers placed to the left and right of the child's midline, concealed behind a screen. After the screen is removed, the child searches for the reward. Once the child retrieves the reward successfully for several consecutive trials (and forms an arbitrary stimulus–response mapping), the side of hiding is reversed, and it is on these so-called 'reversal' trials that he/she must shift to a new stimulus–response set. Pre-schoolers with autism in the study by McEvoy *et al.* (1993) made significantly more perseverative errors on this spatial reversal task. Dawson *et al.* (1998) assessed young children with autism (mean age = 5 years 5 months) on a version of the A-not-B task (see Diamond, 2002). In this task, the child observes as the experimenter hides a desired object in one of two places (e.g. location A). Following a delay (e.g. 5 seconds), the child is encouraged to find the object. After several successful searches, the child is shown the object again but this time the side of hiding is reversed (e.g. to location B). Young children with autism committed significantly more errors on 'reversal' trials compared to children with Down syndrome or typically developing children (Dawson *et al.* 1998).

Subsequent studies have failed, however, to find autism-specific executive difficulties at a young age. Griffith *et al.* (1999) tested young children with autism (mean age = 4 years 4 months) and children with developmental delay on a range of developmentally appropriate executive function tasks, including tasks measuring inhibition, set-shifting, spatial and object working memory, and action monitoring. Surprisingly, they found no group differences in performance on any executive function measure. Furthermore, a longitudinal follow-up of the same samples of children showed that autistic children's performance on the spatial reversal task did improve over the one-year period, and still no group differences were found at age 5 years. More recent studies have supported this conclusion (Dawson *et al.* 2002; Rutherford and Rogers, 2003; Stahl and Pry, 2002).

The apparently intact executive abilities of young children with autism suggest that executive difficulties cannot account for the earliest symptoms of autism, and instead suggest that executive problems may be acquired later, and could be a secondary consequence of other more primary cognitive atypicalities. If this were the case, then children with autism would show impaired performance on executive tasks compared with a group of typically developing children (rather than children with developmental delay; Griffith *et al.* 1999), and the magnitude of these group differences would increase with age. A recent study by Yerys *et al.* (2007) suggests, however, that this is not the case. They assessed the executive skills of the youngest autism sample to date (mean age = 2 years 11 months), and failed to find autism-specific difficulties on executive tasks when compared to either a group of children with developmental delay matched both in terms of mental and chronological age, or a group of chronological age-matched typically developing children. Yerys *et al.* (2007) suggested that executive problems are therefore an unlikely candidate for a primary cognitive deficit in autism and instead might emerge as a consequence of having autism (though see Ozonoff *et al.* (2004) for evidence of age-related increase in set-shifting problems in cognitively able adults with autism).

It remains possible that executive difficulties may have been missed in young children with autism because the tasks themselves are not sufficiently sensitive to detect what could be quite subtle difficulties in these young children with autism. Biró and Russell (2001) have noted that the tasks generally used with such young children do not invoke the use of arbitrary rules, which they assert is precisely the primary difficulty in autism. Also, executive problems might have been missed because researchers have not employed a thorough range of executive tasks. The past few years have seen the development of a range of reliable and valid tests to assess 'fledgling' executive skills in typically developing toddlers (Carlson *et al.* 2004a; Hughes and Ensor, 2005). It remains to be seen whether young children with autism will show problems on these tasks. Most of the studies reporting unimpaired executive function in young children have used tasks that have been linked directly to the dorsolateral prefrontal cortex (e.g. A-not-B task). One exception to this is work by Dawson *et al.* (1998; 2002) (see also Munson *et al.* 2008), which employed tasks that are known to activate the ventromedial prefrontal cortex, a region which has been linked to the processing of emotionally salient (rather than emotionally neutral) stimuli. Nevertheless, as it stands, this failure to demonstrate supporting evidence for an autism-specific problem in executive dysfunction at quite a young age challenges the idea that autistic symptomatology is a result of atypicalities in executive function.

7.4.4 *Explanatory power*

The executive dysfunction hypothesis has considerable face validity: it seems to easily explain the inherent rigidity and invariance of autistic behaviours, as a result of a reduced ability to generate novel, goal-directed behaviour. Indeed, evidence to support this claim has been reported for links between repetitive behaviours and measures of executive function. Turner (1997) showed that lower-level repetitive behaviours (e.g. motor stereotypies) were associated with perseverative responses on a set-shifting task, while higher-level repetitive behaviours (e.g. circumscribed interests) were related to the inability to switch cognitive set on the same task, and a reduced ability to generate new ideas. Similarly, López *et al.* (2005) found significant associations between restrictive and repetitive symptoms and indices of cognitive flexibility, inhibitory control and working memory, and, more recently, South *et al.* (2007) found a significant relationship between performance on the WCST and a measure of repetitive behaviour (see also Boyd *et al.* 2009; but see Pellicano *et al.* 2006; Joseph *et al.* 2005).

There have been less favourable findings, however, from studies investigating the strong version of the executive dysfunction hypothesis, that executive dysfunction has the power to explain also the persisting social handicaps in autism (Bennetto *et al.* 1996; Pennington *et al.* 1997; Rumsey, 1985; Russell, 1997; see section 7.6 below). There is some limited evidence for a link between performance on executive measures and measures of social functioning. McEvoy *et al.* (1993) found that performance on executive function tasks and joint attention behaviours were related in pre-school children with autism, and Griffith *et al.* (1999) demonstrated a significant association between early executive skills (performance on a spatial reversal task) and socio-communicative behaviour (bids for joint attention) in young children with autism, but not in children with developmental delay, both concurrently and longitudinally. Using more ecologically valid tests of executive function, Hill and Bird (2006) found that individual differences in performance on executive measures were significantly related to certain features of autistic symptomatology (specifically, pragmatic communication) in adults with Asperger syndrome. Joseph and Tager-Flusberg (2004) reported evidence of significant associations between a planning measure and communicative symptoms in children with autism, although this correlation failed to remain significant once variation in children's verbal ability was adjusted for (using partial correlations). Several other studies, however, have failed to find evidence of a link between executive function variables and specific features of autistic symptomatology (Bishop and Norbury, 2005b; Liss *et al.* 2001; Pellicano *et al.* 2006) when variance attributable to verbal and/or non-verbal ability was accounted for.

It is noteworthy that executive skills have been linked to a distinct aspect of outcome, adaptive functioning, typically measured by the Vineland Adaptive Behaviour Scales (Sparrow *et al.* 1984) in both cross-sectional and longitudinal work. Ozonoff *et al.* (2004) found a significant negative correlation between scores on a computerised version of the Tower of London task (the Stockings of Cambridge) and adaptive behaviour scores in a large group of adults with autism, in which poor executive skills were associated with fewer real-life adaptive skills (also see Gilotty *et al.* 2002). Happé *et al.* (2006a) reported significant links between certain executive measures and some aspects of concurrent adaptive functioning in adolescent boys with autism. In a 3-year follow-up study, Berger *et al.* (2003) found that, after controlling for verbal IQ, cognitive flexibility significantly predicted the social competence scores of high functioning young adults with autism in residential care. Similarly, in a long-term outcome study of cognitively able adults with autism, Szatmari *et al.* (1989) showed that a measure of cognitive flexibility, the WCST, upon initial testing was a strong predictor of adaptive functioning at follow-up between 11 and 27 years later. Although it remains unclear whether executive skills are a specific correlate of autistic symptomatology, these latter studies suggest that they may be one of a set of skills necessary for achieving later independence.

In sum, there have been numerous challenges to the executive dysfunction hypothesis in terms of its claims on universality, uniqueness, causal precedence and explanatory value, all of which are damaging to the notion that executive dysfunction plays a primary causal role in the development of autism. Critics of the executive dysfunction account have raised one other potential problem: if executive function difficulties are causally related to autistic symptomatology, then patients with acquired frontal lobe damage, who show executive function deficits, should meet diagnostic criteria for autism (see Bishop, 1993). A more appropriate comparison would be between children with autism and children who have sustained early damage to the prefrontal cortex, and therefore grown up with problems in executive function. Interestingly, these children do in fact show impairments in social interaction, spontaneous speech and pragmatic communication, and the production of novel, goal-directed behaviours but they do not actually go on to develop autism, more often displaying a condition resembling psychopathy or conduct disorder (Anderson *et al.* 1999; Eslinger *et al.* 1992; 1997). These findings point to the possibility that executive problems might be necessary but not sufficient to cause the full range of autistic symptomatology (see Section 7.6 for further discussion).

7.5 Central Coherence Theory

Frith (1989) identified one problem fundamental to these and other theories of autism which construed the condition in terms of deficits: they failed to explain the preserved or superior areas of skill present in individuals with autism. Initial clinical observations by Kanner (1943) and Asperger (1944) emphasised that, despite their impairments, many of their children with autism displayed special talents or 'islets of ability'. Indeed, the incidence of savant skills, that is, exceptional skills in the context of disability, in areas such as music, drawing, and mathematics, is much higher in individuals with autism than in those with intellectual difficulties (Heaton and Wallace, 2003; Hermelin, 2001; Rimland and Hill, 1984). Kanner (1943) highlighted other more common features, including excellent rote memory and a preoccupation with parts of objects, the latter of which has remained part of the current diagnostic criteria for autism (American Psychiatric Association, 1994; 2000). He also commented on children's remarkable ability to detect rapidly very minor modifications to their environment, and this peculiar attention to detail was considered to be one manifestation of what he termed 'insistence on sameness'.

Early empirical work also elucidated an unusual profile of performance on experimental tasks, where children with autism tended to do well on tasks where the stimuli were unarranged or devoid of meaning relative to tasks which entailed patterned or meaningful stimuli (Frith and Hermelin, 1969; Hermelin and O'Connor, 1967). Children were just as good, for example, at recalling jumbled sentences as coherent ones (Hermelin and O'Connor, 1967), and were as proficient at completing jigsaw puzzles upside-down as they were picture-side up (Frith and Hermelin, 1969). In an influential study, Shah and Frith (1983) tested children's performance on the Embedded Figures Test (EFT) (Witkin *et al.* 1971), where one must find hidden figures (e.g. a triangle) within larger meaningful drawings (e.g. a clock) as quickly as possible. Remarkably, autistic children's performance exceeded that of children with moderate learning difficulties (MLD), who were matched for non-verbal mental age.

The findings from these initial clinical and experimental reports led to Frith's (1989) formulation of central coherence theory. She described how typical individuals display 'central coherence': the natural propensity to process stimuli as Gestalts, which predominates over a local or piecemeal style of processing. In contrast, individuals with autism exhibit 'weak' central coherence – an inherent preference for processing local elements over the global whole. Frith (1989) and Frith and Happé (1994) argued that this local processing bias could effectively explain autistic children's enhanced performance on tasks such as the EFT since it enables them to focus immediately on the individual elements of stimuli. In contrast, typically developing individuals take longer to find the embedded figure because they become captured by the global meaning and need perceptually to resist the Gestalt. Frith and Happé (1994) explained further how weak central coherence in autism could account for another often-cited 'islet of ability' – superior performance on the Block Design task (Happé, 1994c; Tymchuk *et al.* 1977). Shah and Frith (1993) showed that pre-segmenting the to-be-copied designs, such that the individual blocks were immediately apparent, benefited the performance of control participants but did not confer any advantage to participants with autism. Enhanced performance on the standard task by individuals with autism seemed to be attributable to a natural facility for perceiving the design in terms of its constituent parts (see also Caron *et al.* 2006).

Central coherence theory (Frith, 1989; Frith and Happé, 1994) has engendered a significant amount of research during the past two decades. It makes two clear predictions. First, since (weak) central coherence is considered to be a domain-general information processing style, this particular cognitive style in autism is expected to pervade *all* areas of an individual's functioning, not just in the visuospatial domain. Second, the theory predicts that the relationship between local and global processing is reciprocal in nature. Accordingly, individuals with autism, who display weak central coherence, should demonstrate preserved or even enhanced performance on tasks where a local processing style is beneficial, but perform poorly on those tasks that necessitate the integration of information

Several lines of evidence show support for this cognitive style in individuals with the condition for a variety of different stimuli across several levels of functioning, including visuospatial, perceptual (visual and auditory), and to a lesser extent, verbal-semantic levels (see Frith and Happé (1994), Happé (1999), Happé and Booth (2008), and Happé and Frith (2006) for reviews). Yet this evidence has been tempered by a series of inconsistent findings, largely driven by repeated demonstrations of intact global or contextual processing in autism (e.g. Caron *et al.* 2006; López and Leekam, 2003; Mottron *et al.* 1999; 2003; Norbury, 2004; 2005; Ozonoff *et al.* 1991; Plaisted *et al.* 1998; 1999; Ropar and Mitchell, 1999; 2001). Indeed, several elegant studies using a variety of task paradigms have shown that individuals with autism can in fact process information at the global level *when they are instructed to do so* (López *et al.* 2004; Plaisted *et al.* 1999; Snowling and Frith, 1986).

Happé and Frith's (2006) review of existing empirical work led to a reappraisal of the notion of weak central coherence in autism. They asserted that 'the original suggestion of a core deficit in central processing, manifest in failure to extract global form and meaning, has changed from a primary problem to a more secondary outcome – with greater emphasis on possible superiority in local or detail-focused processing' (Happé and Frith, 2006; page 6, but see Behrmann *et al.* 2006, and Happé and Booth, 2008). Importantly, Happé and Frith (2006) stressed that this default can be overridden in the event of explicit situational demands to permit processing at the global level. Several researchers have responded to the shortfalls of this particular aspect of central coherence theory with alternative explanations of their own (Baron-Cohen, 2002; Baron-Cohen *et al.* 2005; Mottron and Burack, 2001; Mottron *et al.* 2006; Plaisted, 2000; 2001).

7.5.1 Universality

The theory predicts that a weak drive for coherence should be present in *all* individuals across the autism spectrum, regardless of age or ability (Happé, 1999). In support of this claim, weak central coherence has been demonstrated in autistic individuals with MLD (e.g. Hermelin and O'Connor, 1967; van Lang *et al.* 2006) and cognitively able individuals with autism (Happé, 1994c; 1997), and from early childhood (e.g. Morgan *et al.* 2003) to adulthood (e.g. Jolliffe and Baron-Cohen, 1997).

Numerous studies, however, have failed to find evidence in favour of weak central coherence in individuals with autism therefore questioning whether weak central coherence is in fact a universal feature of the condition (Bowler *et al.* 2000; Brian and Bryson, 1996; Burnette *et al.* 2005; López and Leekam, 2003; Norbury, 2004; 2005; Ozonoff *et al.* 1991; 1994; Ropar and Mitchell, 1999; 2001). An evaluation of these studies is beyond the scope of this overview but suffice to say that the studies vary considerably in terms of the populations sampled and the ages and abilities of the persons with autism, making it difficult to draw firm conclusions regarding the pervasiveness of the weak coherence bias. One alternative way to approach this issue is to examine the proportion of individuals who exhibit weak central coherence in those studies where supporting evidence has been reported. Happé demonstrated that almost all her sample of cognitively able children with autism exhibited a weak coherence bias as indexed by peak performance on the Block Design task (Happé, 1994c) or by poor use of context on the homograph task (Happé, 1997). Consistent with Happé, Pellicano *et al.* (2006) found that exceptional performance on three visuospatial coherence tasks (EFT, Block Design and Figure-Ground tasks) characterised between 78% and 92% of their group of young children with an ASD (aged 4 to 7 years).

Other findings, however, have indicated that weak coherence might be present in only a subset of individuals with autism. Teunisse *et al.* (2001) reported that 18 out of 35 of their sample of adolescents with autism exhibited this cognitive style.

Similarly, in a study on canonical counting, Jarrold and Russell (1997) showed that just under half of their sample of children with autism ($N = 22$) failed to adopt a local strategy (in their study, counting dot by dot). More recently, Caron *et al.* (2006) reported that almost half (42%) of their sample of adults with autism ($N = 92$) displayed a relative peak in performance on the Block Design task compared with 2% of their sample of typically developing individuals ($N = 112$). Although superior local processing might be more prevalent in autism than in typically developing populations, this latter finding indicates that this superiority might not be universal in more able adolescents and adults with autism.

7.5.2 *Uniqueness*

The few studies that have examined the specificity of weak central coherence in autism have yielded mixed results. In a study designed to test directly the criterion of uniqueness, Booth *et al.* (2003) administered a drawing task to children with autism, children with ADHD, and typical children. Only the children with autism were found to display a detail-focused drawing style, suggesting that this style might be unique to autism. Several other findings, however, have been less definitive. A local processing strategy has also been reported on perceptual coherence tasks by children with MLD (Jarrold and Russell, 1997; van Lang *et al.* 2006). Weak central coherence at the verbal-semantic level has been demonstrated in children with specific language impairment. Using either figures of speech or homographs, Norbury (2004; 2005) found that, akin to a subgroup of children with autism who exhibited concomitant language impairments, children with isolated (specific) language impairments also failed to use surrounding contextual cues to abstract higher-level meaning.

Researchers have also pointed towards a local processing style in children with Williams syndrome (Bihrle *et al.* 1989; though see Pani *et al.* 1999), casting further doubt on whether weak central coherence is specific to autism. Interestingly, unlike individuals with autism who demonstrate preserved or superior performance on the Block Design task due to a facility for segmentation (Shah and Frith, 1993), persons with Williams syndrome perform significantly worse on this task, relative to typically developing comparison individuals (Farran *et al.* 2001). These authors suggest that, for individuals with Williams syndrome the local bias most clearly hinders performance during the construction phase of the task, while for children with autism, the local bias seems to manifest itself at the initial segmentation or perceptual phase of the task, thus resulting in superior performance. It is surprising, however, that inferior and superior performance on the same task have been interpreted as reflecting a local processing bias; research designed to tease apart the different stages of processing for the Block Design task (e.g. Caron *et al.* 2006) across several developmental disorders is clearly desirable.

7.5.3 Explanatory power

In its strongest form (Frith, 1989), weak central coherence is held to play a primary causal role in the development of autistic symptoms. Frith described how an impaired ability to draw together complex information in the social environment in order to derive coherent and meaningful interpretations of social situations would result in 'an incoherent world of fragmented experience' (Frith, 1989; page 98). Similarly, she argued that an inability to extract meaning during a conversational exchange would impede an understanding of the 'deeper intentional aspects of communication' (Frith, 1989; page 124). She explained further that without the overriding drive for deriving coherence, automatic (maladaptive) behaviours could not be inhibited, thus resulting in rigidly structured and repetitive behaviour.

Very few studies have investigated whether indices of weak central coherence are related to autistic symptoms. One positive finding was reported by Briskman *et al.* (2001) in their investigation of weak central coherence in individuals with the broader autism phenotype. They demonstrated links between performance on coherence measures (e.g. un/segmented Block Design and EFT) and scores on a self-report questionnaire relating specifically to attention to detail in parents of children with autism (but not parents of children with dyslexia). Nevertheless there is limited evidence for a direct link between this cognitive style and behavioural symptoms (social or non-social) in individuals who meet diagnostic criteria for autism. Berger *et al.* (2003) investigated whether weak central coherence or executive dysfunction was best able to predict the functional outcomes of young adults with autism over a 3-year period. They found no support for a relationship between coherence measures and indices of social competence; instead, reduced set-shifting ability was significantly related to individuals' prognosis. Also, Pellicano *et al.* (2006) failed to find a significant link between performance on central coherence and a measure of autistic symptomatology (scores on the Autism Diagnostic Interview–Revised; Lord *et al.*, 1994) in their samples of children with autism (see also Burnette *et al.* (2005) and South *et al.* (2007)). These negative findings might be attributable to the rather crude measures of symptomatology used in these studies, and any such associations might be best elucidated by a more fine-grained assessment of behaviours of interest (e.g. insistence on sameness).

Although Frith (1989) originally considered weak central coherence to explain the non-social and the social symptoms of autism, subsequent findings led Frith and Happé (Frith and Happé, 1994; Happé and Frith, 2006) to no longer make strong claims about primacy. Initial findings revealed little association between weak central coherence and theory of mind in individuals with autism (Happé,

1994c; 1997). In one study, Happé (1994c) showed that superior performance on the Block Design task was characteristic of almost all individuals with autism in her sample, independent of theory of mind ability. Similarly, in a second study, the entire group of adults with autism displayed weak coherence on the homograph task, regardless of whether they were successful 'mindreaders' (Happé, 1997). In light of this evidence, Frith and Happé (1994) abandoned their earlier position, arguing that weak central coherence on its own was unable to provide a complete account of autism. In more recent work, they consider weak central coherence to be one of several primary cognitive atypicalities in autism, including problems in theory of mind and executive control (Happé and Frith, 2006) in which each atypicality is held to play a causal role in the development of some (but not all) symptoms.

7.5.4 *Causal precedence*

Very little attention has been paid to the development of a local processing bias either theoretically or empirically. The youngest age at which a local processing bias has been detected using common central coherence tasks comes from a study by Morgan *et al.* (2003). They reported superior performance on the Pre-school version of the EFT and Pattern Construction task (similar in nature to the Block Design task) in pre-schoolers with autism (mean age = 4 years 6 months) relative to typically developing children of similar age and non-verbal ability.

Although Happé and Frith (2006) do not elaborate on what might be the earliest manifestations of weak central coherence in autism, one rival account, Mottron *et al.*'s (2006) Enhanced Perceptual Functioning model, says something about the developmental course of a local processing bias. Mottron *et al.* (2006) proposed that autistic individuals' peaks in perceptual abilities derive from the overdevelopment of basic low-level perceptual processes, including local processing. Rather than being present from birth, enhanced local processing emerges early during the course of development and in response to diminished higher order processing operations. In a longitudinal study on children's cognitive skills, Pellicano (2010a) found that children with autism were no quicker to find the hidden figure on the CEFT than they were 3 years earlier, and that they made no improvements on the Pattern Construction task over time. This lack of improvement was in striking contrast to the significant gains made by typically developing children on both visuospatial coherence tasks, which implies, rather paradoxically, that typical children develop a more pronounced local processing bias over time. Other factors, however, are more likely to be driving this developmental change. For example, typical children's maturing executive skills might enable children to better resist interference from the overall Gestalt and therefore rapidly locate either the hidden figure (in the case of the CEFT) or the blocks necessary to reconstruct the design (in the case of the Pattern Construction task). For children with autism, local processing skills might be early-emerging and initially accelerated (cf. Mottron *et al.* 2006), and their concomitant problems in executive control might not limit performance on such tasks.

The notion of 'weak' central coherence in autism has been very influential. Not only has the theory generated a great deal of interest in local and global processing in autism, it also has forced researchers to reappraise their understanding of the condition as one with a specific pattern of weaknesses and strengths. In light of the significant challenges faced by the theory, the proponents no longer make strong claims about primacy. Rather than proposing that weak central coherence plays a unique causal role in the development of autism, the revised version of the theory espouses multiple cognitive atypicalities, including coexisting atypicalities in central coherence, theory of mind and executive function each of which might have their own distinctive causal pathways (see Section 7.6 for discussion) (Happé and Frith, 2006).

One putatively similar account that deserves mention here is Baron-Cohen's notion of Systemising (Baron-Cohen, 2002; Baron-Cohen *et al.* 2005). Proposing that autism is a result of an 'extreme male brain', Baron-Cohen postulates that autism is characterised by dual atypicalities: an underdeveloped ability to empathise and, most relevant to this discussion, a hyper-developed 'systemising' brain. The latter term systemising is defined as the predominantly male drive to analyse and control non-social systems. He argued that superior systemising can account for the non-social strengths, including savant abilities and attention to detail, and weaknesses, circumscribed interests and repetitive behaviours, that are characteristic of autism. Baron-Cohen's systemising–empathising theory distinguished itself from central coherence theory (Frith, 1989; Frith and Happé, 1994) by predicting superior local processing combined with *intact* (rather than impaired) integration in autism, the latter of which is essential to understanding both simple and complex rule-based systems. At present, the evidence for superior systemising is derived largely from self-ratings of preference and abilities (Baron-Cohen *et al.* 2002), though several authors have begun to establish links between behavioural task performance and scores on questionnaires tapping systemising and empathising (e.g. Brosnan *et al.* 2010; Lawson *et al.* 2004; see also Baron-Cohen *et al.* 2009). The theory has since been grounded in neurobiology (Baron-Cohen and Belmonte, 2005) – reduced functional connectivity to brain regions responsible for higher order social cognition combined with over-functioning of lower-level, perceptual processing. Although similar neural accounts have been proposed for weak central coherence in autism (see Happé and Frith, 2006), little has yet been said as to whether the account satisfies the criteria of universality, uniqueness and explanatory power.

7.6 Beyond single-deficit models of autism

It should be clear from the discussion above that all three cognitive accounts have struggled to meet the various criteria for primacy (particularly the criterion of explanatory power), which ultimately casts doubt on whether an atypicality in one of these domains alone is sufficient to cause such a complex behavioural phenotype. It remains possible of course that there might be other, as yet undiscovered candidates that could prove successful in explaining the full range of autistic symptoms. The shortcomings of these three cognitive accounts, together with emerging evidence that autism might not be a unitary construct, have led to a plea from some authors to 'give up on a single explanation of autism' (Happé *et al.* 2006b; page 1218) in favour of an explanation encompassing coexisting atypicalities in *multiple* cognitive domains.

The notion of 'multiple deficits' in autism is certainly not new. Wing and Wing (1971) first suggested that autism could arise due to multiple psychological deficits that were a result of multiple 'insults' at the neurological level. Subsequently, Goodman (1989) proposed that genetic and environmental insults could act upon distinct neural systems, which in turn could cause simultaneous 'abnormalities' at the cognitive level, each affecting a specific aspect of cognition. He suggested that it is 'synergistic interactions' between these cognitive 'abnormalities' that gives rise to the constellation of symptoms we call 'autism' (see also Bishop, 1989; Pennington *et al.* 1997).

Despite these early views, a multiple-deficits view has failed to capture the sustained attention of empirical researchers. This unwillingness to move beyond a single-deficit account is attributable largely to the fact that researchers and clinicians have traditionally assumed that the defining behavioural features of autism – both the socio-communicative symptoms *and* the non-social symptoms (repetitive behaviours and restricted activities) – occur together more often than what would be expected by chance, thus implicating a single underlying aetiology. Yet there is increasing agreement among researchers that this assumption may be unwarranted (see Boucher, 2006 and Mandy and Skuse, 2008 for discussion).

Two pieces of evidence argue against the traditional view. First, work on the broader phenotype of autism (Bailey *et al.* 1998) suggests that the relatives of people with autism do not tend to show a profile of symptoms that is qualitatively similar to (albeit milder than) autism in all three behavioural domains; instead, research suggests that the 'triad of impairments' may in fact be dissociable. While some relatives of people with autism display co-occurring behavioural symptoms (in the 'triad of impairments'), which are milder but qualitatively similar to those found in autism proper, the majority of these individuals show behaviours in isolated symptom domains (e.g. social difficulties or repetitive activities alone) (e.g. Bolton *et al.* 1994; Piven *et al.* 1997). This evidence suggests that the 'triad of impairments' might be fractionable, and inherited separately.

Second, research examining autistic traits in the general population further suggests that the behavioural features of autism might only be weakly related (Mandy and Skuse, 2008). Findings from a population-based study investigating autism-related social, communicative and repetitive traits in over 3000 7- to 9-year-old typically developing twin-pairs found that, rather than clustering together, the cross-trait genetic correlations were surprisingly modest-to-low (ranging from 0.4 down to 0.2) both across the general population and in children lying at the extreme end of the distributions, suggesting that largely independent genes may be operating on each aspect of the triad of impairments in autism (Ronald *et al.* 2006; see also Ronald *et al.* 2005). Although the defining behavioural features of autism were found to occur together more often than would be expected by chance alone, these authors also showed that a considerable number of children displayed behavioural difficulties in isolation (e.g. social difficulties only, communication problems alone).

Both sets of findings provocatively suggest that the components of the triad might have distinct underlying causes. Indeed, together with the failure to discover a single core cognitive marker for autism, their work led Happé *et al.* (2006b) to argue that researchers 'should abandon the attempt to find a single cognitive explanation, in favour of good accounts for each distinct aspect of the triad' (page 1219). They offered one candidate account of their own: independent cognitive atypicalities in three core domains – theory of mind, executive function and central coherence – are jointly necessary to produce autism, with each atypicality underpinning distinct aspects of the behavioural phenotype. For example, weak central coherence might best account for the perceptual and visuospatial anomalies associated with the condition; executive dysfunction might relate directly to the nature and severity of the repetitive behaviours, stereotypies and circumscribed interests, while a theory of mind deficit might best capture the difficulties in social reciprocity and communication (Figure 7.2). Since these atypicalities are held to be largely independent of each other both at the phenotypic and genetic levels, autistic symptomatology is therefore viewed as the result of multiple and distinct cognitive atypicalities.

Recent evidence partially supports this candidate multiple-deficits account. Pellicano *et al.* (2006) found that young children with an autism spectrum disorder ($N = 40$) did in fact demonstrate the cognitive profile proposed by Happé and colleagues, including difficulties in aspects of theory of mind (false-belief understanding) and executive function (planning, cognitive flexibility) accompanied by weak central coherence (i.e. enhanced local information processing), relative to age- and ability-matched typically developing children. This support at the group

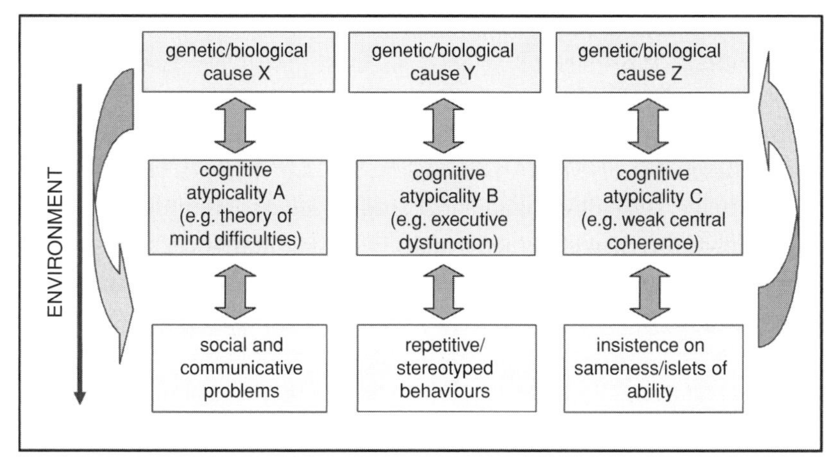

Figure 7.2 Causal model showing three levels of explanation: genetics/biology, cognition and behaviour (adapted from Frith *et al.* 1991) encompassing multiple deficits (cf. Happé *et al.* 2006b; Happé and Ronald, 2008).

level was somewhat tempered, however, by a failure to demonstrate the presence of this specific cognitive profile in each child with autism. These initial attempts to test the validity of this candidate account raised an important question: are multiple-deficits accounts confronted by the same set of criteria used to assess the veracity of single-deficit accounts? It is worth considering briefly these criteria in turn.

Should this profile of cognitive atypicalities be present in all, or nearly all, individuals with autism? Issues of task measurement and problems equating task difficulty can of course cloud whether a particular atypicality, or in this case a profile of atypicalities, is universal in individuals with the condition. There are also significant challenges inherent in defining atypicality (see Section 7.4.1), especially when examining individuals with developmental conditions, whose cognitive skills are unlikely to be 'all or none'. Rather than 'atypicality' being conceptualised categorically, Happé and colleagues (Happé *et al.* 2006b; Happé and Ronald, 2008) have conceived of the three cognitive domains as dimensions located (orthogonally) within a multivariate space. If one accepts a multidimensional version of this candidate multiple-deficits view, then the lack of universality of this particular cognitive profile may actually turn out to explain some of the heterogeneity in the condition. Indeed, the extent to which a person with autism shows a particular cognitive atypicality therefore should vary according to the place he/she occupies on that dimension, which in turn, should relate directly to the degree and nature of the behavioural symptoms it purports to explain.

It is easy to see how the criterion of uniqueness should apply to a multiple-deficits view. Since it is the co-occurrence of all three cognitive atypicalities that yields 'autism', one should expect that no other developmental condition should share all three atypicalities. It is plausible nevertheless that some conditions might show atypicalities in one or even two of the domains. For example, children with pragmatic language difficulties, who show similar socio-communicative symptoms to children with autism, show abnormalities in two putative cognitive dimensions – impairments in some aspects of executive function (generativity: Bishop and Norbury, 2005a) and difficulties understanding other minds (e.g. Shields *et al.* 1996).

It is also clear that the cognitive accounts held to explain each distinct aspect of the phenotype should show explanatory power. In a multidimensional model, one should expect that a cognitive atypicality should be shown by anyone displaying the relevant behavioural symptom, and that the degree of impairment within each dimension should be associated with the extent of symptomatology. Consideration of this issue in the sections above indicated, however, that there is limited evidence for a link between cognitive atypicality and behaviour for each of the three cognitive domains. A failure to establish links between performance on cognitive tasks and everyday behavioural symptoms in autism may be due to the difficulties inherent in acquiring a valid representation of the child's current symptomatology (see Bishop and Norbury (2002) and Pellicano *et al.* (2006) for discussion). Or it may reflect the possibility that there is no simple or direct relationship between current cognitive functioning and behavioural symptoms (Karmiloff-Smith *et al.* 2002). Further still – and most damaging for Happé *et al.*'s candidate multiple deficits account – it could indicate that these particular cognitive atypicalities, that is, difficulties in theory of mind, executive function and central coherence, are not sufficient to cause the triad of impairments. Establishing links between performance on cognitive tasks and everyday behavioural symptoms in autism is clearly a key challenge for future research.

In addition to satisfying these criteria, there are several additional challenges faced by a multiple deficit view. Current thinking assumes that these atypicalities in autism are largely independent of each other, and that different genes might contribute to each aspect of cognition (Happé *et al.* 2006b). These authors hint at the possibility that there might be interactions between cognitive functions but do not discuss the extent or nature of potential interactions between domains. This view is sharply contrasted with the developmental approach championed by several authors (e.g. Bishop, 1997; Karmiloff-Smith, 1998), which emphasises the dynamic nature of developing systems, where interactions between domains are likely to be the norm and where a selective difficulty at an early point during development is likely to have substantial knock-on effects on the subsequent development of other cognitive functions (see also Oliver *et al.*, 2000). On this view, the different cognitive atypicalities might be seen to occupy different positions in a causal chain.

In direct contrast to Happé *et al.*'s (2006) suggestion, significant associations have in fact been demonstrated between cognitive domains in both autism and in typical development (e.g. Carlson and Moses, 2001; Hughes, 1998a; 1998b; Jarrold *et al.* 2000; Ozonoff *et al.*, 1991; Pellicano, 2007; 2010b). Indeed, research on the typical development of theory of mind and executive function has consistently demonstrated a robust relationship between individual differences in tasks tapping theory of mind and tasks tapping several components of executive function, including mental flexibility, inhibitory control and working memory (but not planning ability), independent of age and IQ, in pre-schoolers (e.g. Carlson and Moses, 2001; Carlson *et al.* 2004b; Frye *et al.* 1995; Hughes, 1998a; 1998b), and more recently, in toddlers (Carlson *et al.* 2004a; Hughes and Ensor, 2007). These findings have prompted fervent theoretical discussion surrounding the functional link between these cognitive domains. For example, some theorists (e.g. Perner, 1998; Perner and Lang, 1999; see also Carruthers, 1996) argue that theory of mind is a prerequisite for the later development of executive control, while others (Moses, 2001; Russell, 1997) argue that the causal direction is reversed, such that executive function is a necessary precondition for understanding others' mental states. Findings from several longitudinal studies (e.g. Carlson *et al.* 2004a; 2004b; Flynn *et al.* 2004; Hughes, 1998b; Hughes and Ensor, 2007) demonstrate a functional relationship in one direction only, such that performance on executive function measures predicts developmental changes in performance on false-belief measures *but not vice versa*, therefore providing compelling evidence that early executive function plays a critical role in the emergence of theory of mind in typical development (cf. Moses, 2001; Russell, 1997).

There are fewer studies on the association between theory of mind and executive function in autism, although the very co-occurrence of such difficulties is suggestive of a link between domains. Significant theory of mind-executive function correlations have been documented, independent of age, verbal ability and non-verbal ability (e.g. Joseph and Tager-Flusberg, 2004; Ozonoff *et al.* 1991; Pellicano, 2007), and one cross-sectional study provided clues to developmental primacy, indicating that executive abilities might be especially important for theory of mind in children with autism (Pellicano, 2007).

Links between other cognitive domains are less clear. While some researchers have found evidence for the independence of theory of mind difficulties and weak central coherence in individuals with autism (Happé, 1997; Pellicano *et al.* 2006), others have not (Baron-Cohen and Hammer, 1997; Jarrold *et al.* 2000). Also, there is some evidence for a significant link between central coherence and executive function in children with autism (Pellicano *et al.* 2006; though see Booth *et al.* 2003), with some authors suggesting that one domain-general account could potentially be subsumed by the other (cf. Pennington *et al.* 1997).

Given the evidence for a significant link between some (though not all) of these domains, it might therefore be more plausible to expect that the dimensions within this candidate multiple-deficits model might not be orthogonal. Crucially, devising a theory that can take account of the interrelationships between aspects of cognition can only be accomplished within a developmental framework. At present, there are very few longitudinal studies examining the development of specific cognitive functions rendering it uncertain as to how this specific profile of cognitive atypicalities might manifest themselves during development. Remarkably, out of the multitude of studies published on autism every year, only five longitudinal investigations have traced developmental changes in theory of mind (Holroyd and Baron-Cohen, 1993; Ozonoff and McEvoy, 1994; Pellicano, 2010a; Serra *et al.* 2002; Steele *et al.* 2003), a mere three studies have charted changes in executive function (Griffith *et al.* 1999; Ozonoff and McEvoy, 1994; Pellicano, 2010a), and only one study has examined longitudinally changes in local processing in autism (Pellicano, 2010a). Consequently, there is very little knowledge about the development of these functions in individuals with autism. Does the full set of atypicalities co-exist at birth or do the different cognitive atypicalities emerge at different points during development? Moreover, *how* are these atypicalities related throughout development? This latter point raises the issue of developmental causal links between the three cognitive domains: do the three co-occurring cognitive atypicalities develop independently from one another or does one atypicality take precedence over another during development? It is possible that difficulties in one area (executive function, for example) might *cause* problems in another area (theory of mind, for example) during development, in which case we may come full circle to the notion of a 'single primary deficit'. Preliminary evidence suggests that this might be the case. In a 3-year follow-up study, Pellicano (2010b) found that individual differences in children's early skills in executive function and central coherence (Time 1) were longitudinally predictive of later theory of mind skills (Time 2), independent of age, language, non-verbal intelligence and early theory of mind skills. Predictive relations in the opposite direction, however, were not significant, and there were no developmental links between executive function and central coherence. Rather than viewing problems in these three domains as co-occurring, independent and predominantly static atypicalities in autism, these findings suggest that early domain-general skills might play a critical role in shaping the developmental trajectory of other functions (in this case, theory of mind). Since variation in both intellectual functioning and language ability plays a significant role in the development of the condition, attention should be directed towards elucidating the precise nature of this role, and how it relates to the cognitive capabilities in local processing and co-existing difficulties in theory of mind and executive function.

Traditionally, research was targeted towards specifying the single primary cognitive 'abnormality' to explain the development of autism. The field has since rejected this view in favour of a multiple-deficits account, which may be a more plausible explanation of autism given the extant heterogeneity evident at genetic, neurobiological and behavioural levels. It should be clear from this discussion that a multiple-deficits view of autism is confronted by a set of questions similar to those asked of a single-deficit account, as well as additional challenges, which require the analysis of concurrent *and* predictive relationships between cognitive functions. Teasing apart the complex (cognitive) mechanisms underlying the diverse set of autistic symptoms must be addressed longitudinally if we are to appreciate fully how these multiple atypicalities emerge during the development of the condition.

7.7 References

American Psychiatric Association. (1994). *Diagnostic and Statistical Manual of Mental Disorders*, 4th edn. Washington DC: American Psychiatric Association.

American Psychiatric Association. (2000). *Diagnostic and Statistical Manual of Mental Disorders, 4th Edn. Text Revision (DSMIV TR)*. Washington DC: American Psychiatric Association.

Anderson, S.W., Bechara, A., Damasio, H., Tranel, D., Damasio, A.R. (1999). Impairment of social and moral behavior related to early damage in human prefrontal cortex. *Nature Neuroscience*, **2**: 1032–1037.

Asperger, H. (1944). Die 'autistichen psychopathen' im kindersalter. *Archive fur psychiatrie und Nervenkrankheiten*, **117**: 76–136. (Reprinted in *Autism and Asperger Syndrome*, by U. Frith, 1991, Cambridge UK: Cambridge University Press).

Bailey, A., Parr, J. (2003). Implications of the broader phenotype for concepts of autism. In *Autism: Neural Basis and Treatment Possibilities*. Novartis Foundation Symposium 251. Chichester: John Wiley and Sons Ltd, pp. 26–47.

Bailey, A., Phillips, W., Rutter, M. (1996). Autism: Towards an integration of clinical, genetic, neuropsychological, and neurobiological perspectives. *Journal of Child Psychology and Psychiatry*, **37**: 89–126.

Bailey, A., Palferman, S., Heavey, L., Le Couteur, A. (1998). Autism: The phenotype in relatives. *Journal of Autism and Developmental Disorders*, **28**: 369–392.

Baron-Cohen, S. (1989a). The autistic child's theory of mind: A case of specific developmental delay. *Journal of Child Psychology and Psychiatry*, **30**: 285–297.

Baron-Cohen, S. (1989b). Perceptual role taking and protodeclarative pointing in autism. *British Journal of Developmental Psychology*, **7**: 113–127.

Baron-Cohen, S. (1991). Precursors to a theory of mind: Understanding attention in others. In *Natural Theories of Mind: Evolution, Development and Simulation of Everyday Mindreading*. Oxford: Blackwell, pp. 233–251.

Baron-Cohen, S. (1992). Debate and argument: On modularity and development in autism: A reply to Burack. *Journal of Child Psychology and Psychiatry*, **33**: 623–629.

Baron-Cohen, S. (1993). From attention-goal psychology to belief-desire psychology: The development of a theory of mind, and its dysfunction. In *Understanding Other Minds: Perspectives from Autism*. Oxford: Oxford University Press, pp. 59–82.

Baron-Cohen, S. (1994). How to build a baby that can read minds: Cognitive mechanisms in mindreading. *Cahiers de Psychologie Cognitive*, **13**: 513–552.

Baron-Cohen, S. (1995). *Mindblindness: An Essay on Autism and Theory of Mind*. Cambridge, MA: MIT Press.

Baron-Cohen, S. (2000). Theory of mind and autism: A fifteen year review. In *Understanding other Minds: Perspectives from Developmental Cognitive Neuroscience*, 2nd edn. London: Oxford University Press, pp. 3–20.

Baron-Cohen, S. (2002). The extreme male brain theory of autism. *Trends in Cognitive Sciences*, **6**: 248–254.

Baron-Cohen, S., Belmonte, M. (2005). Autism: A window onto the development of the social and the analytic brain. *Annual Review of Neuroscience*, **28**: 109–126.

Baron-Cohen, S., Goodhart, F. (1994). The 'seeing-leads-to-knowing' deficit in autism: The Pratt and Bryant probe. *British Journal of Developmental Psychology*, **12**: 397–401.

Baron-Cohen, S., Hammer, J. (1997). Is autism an extreme form of the 'male brain'? *Advances in Infancy Research*, **11**: 193–217.

Baron-Cohen, S., Leslie, A.M., Frith, U. (1985). Does the autistic child have a 'theory of mind'? *Cognition*, **21**: 37–46.

Baron-Cohen, S., Spitz, A., Cross, P. (1993). Can children with autism recognize surprise? *Cognition and Emotion*, **7**: 507–516.

Baron-Cohen, S., Ring, H., Moriarty, J., Schmitz, B., Costa, D., Ell, P. (1994). Recognition of mental state terms: Clinical findings in children with autism and a functional neuroimaging study of normal adults. *British Journal of Psychiatry*, **165**: 640–649.

Baron-Cohen, S., Tager-Flusberg, H., Cohen. D.J. (2000). *Understanding other Minds: Perspectives from Developmental Cognitive Neuroscience*. Oxford, UK: Oxford University Press.

Baron-Cohen, S., Wheelwright, S., Griffin, R., Lawson, J., Hill, J. (2002). The exact mind: Empathizing and systemizing in autism spectrum conditions. In *Handbook of Cognitive Development*. Malden, MA : Blackwell Publishers, pp. 491–508.

Baron-Cohen, S., Knickmeyer, R.C., Belmonte, M.K. (2005). Sex differences in the brain: Implications for explaining autism. *Science*, **310**: 819–823.

Baron-Cohen, S., Ashwin, E., Ashwin, C., Tavassoli, T., Chakrabarti, B. (2009). Talent in autism: hyper-systemising, hyper-attention to detail and sensory hypersensitivity. *Philosophical Transactions of the Royal Society: Biological Sciences*, **364**: 1377–1383.

Behrmann, M., Thomas, C., Humphreys, K. (2006). Seeing it differently: Visual processing in autism. *Trends in Cognitive Sciences*, **10**: 258–264.

Bennetto, L., Pennington, B.F., Rogers, S.J. (1996). Intact and impaired memory functions in autism. *Child Development*, **67**: 1816–1835.

Benson, G., Abbeduto, L., Short, K., Bibler-Nuccio, J., Maas, F. (1993). Development of a theory of mind in individuals with mental retardation. *American Journal of Mental Retardation*, **98**: 427–433.

Berger, H.J., Aerts, F.H., van Spaendonck, K.P., Cools, A.R., Teunisse, J.-P. (2003). Central coherence and cognitive shifting in relation to social improvement in high-functioning young adults with autism. *Journal of Clinical and Experimental Neuropsychology*, **25**: 502–511.

Bihrle, A.M., Bellugi, U., Delis, D., Marks, S. (1989). Seeing either the forest or the trees: Dissociation in visuospatial processing. *Brain and Cognition*, **11**: 37–49.

Biró, S., Russell, J. (2001). The execution of arbitrary procedures by children with autism. *Development and Psychopathology*, **13**: 97–110.

Bishop, D.V.M. (1989). Autism, Asperger‘s Syndrome and semantic-pragmatic disorder: where are the boundaries? *British Journal of Disorders of Communication*, **24**: 107–121.

Bishop, D.V.M. (1993). Annotation: Autism, executive functions and theory of mind: A neuropsychological perspective. *Journal of Child Psychology and Psychiatry*, **34**: 279–293.

Bishop, D.V.M. (1997). Cognitive neuropsychology and developmental disorders: Uncomfortable bedfellows. *Quarterly Journal of Experimental Psychology A*, **50A**: 899–923.

Bishop, D.V.M., Norbury, C.F. (2002). Exploring the borderlands of autistic disorder and specific language impairment: A study using standardised diagnostic instruments. *Journal of Child Psychology and Psychiatry*, **43**: 917–929.

Bishop, D.V.M., Norbury, C.F. (2005a). Executive functions in children with communication impairments, in relation to autistic symptomatology: I: Generativity. *Autism*, **9**: 7–27.

Bishop, D.V.M., Norbury, C.F. (2005b). Executive functions in children with communication impairments, in relation to autistic symptomatology: II: Response inhibition. *Autism*, **9**: 29–43.

Bishop, D.V.M., Aamodt-Leeper, G., Creswell, C., McGurk, R., Skuse, D.H. (2001). Individual differences in cognitive planning on the Tower of Hanoi task: Neuropsychological maturity or measurement error? *Journal of Child Psychology and Psychiatry*, **42**: 551–556.

Bloom, P., German, T. (2000). Two reasons to abandon the false belief task as a test of theory of mind. *Cognition*, **77**: B25–B31.

Bolton, P., Macdonald, H., Pickles, A., *et al.* (1994). A case-control family history study of autism. *Journal of Child Psychology and Psychiatry*, **35**: 877–900.

Booth, R., Charlton, R., Hughes, C., Happé, F. (2003). Disentangling weak coherence and executive dysfunction: planning drawing in autism and attention deficit/hyperactivity disorder. *Philosophical Transactions of the Royal Society of London Part B*, **358**: 387–392.

Boucher, J. (1996). What could possibly explain autism? In *Theories of Theories of Mind*. Cambridge: Cambridge University Press, pp. 223–241.

Boucher, J. (2006). Letter to the Editor: Is the search for a unitary explanation of autistic spectrum disorders justified? *Journal of Autism and Developmental Disorders*, **36**: 289.

Bowler, D.M. (1992). 'Theory of mind' in Asperger's syndrome. *Journal of Child Psychology and Psychiatry*, **33**: 877–893.

Bowler, D.M., Gardiner, J.M., Grice, S., Saavalainen, P. (2000). Memory illusions: false recall and recognition in adults with Asperger's syndrome. *Journal of Abnormal Psychology*, **109**: 663–672.

Bowler, D.M., Briskman, J., Gurvidi, N., Fornells-Ambrojo, M. (2005). Understanding the mind or predicting signal-dependent action? Performance of children with and without autism on analogues of the false-belief task. *Journal of Cognition and Development*, **6**: 259–283.

Boyd, B.A., McBee, M., Holtzclaw, T., Baranek, G.T., Bodfish, J.W. (2009). Relationships among repetitive behaviours, sensory features, and executive functions in high-functioning autism. *Research in Autism Spectrum Disorders*, **3**: 959–966.

Brian, J.A. Bryson, S.E. (1996). Disembedding performance and recognition memory in autism/PDD. *Journal of Child Psychology and Psychiatry*, **37**: 865–872.

Briskman, J., Happé, F., Frith, U. (2001). Exploring the cognitive phenotype of autism: Weak 'central coherence' in parents and siblings of children in autism: II. Real-life skills and preferences. *Journal of Child Psychology and Psychiatry*, **42**: 309–316.

Brosnan, M., Daggar, R., Collomosse, J. (2010). The relationship between systemising and mental rotation and the implications for the extreme male brain theory of autism. *Journal of Autism and Developmental Disorders*, **40**: 1–7.

Brown, R., Hobson, R., Lee, A., Stevenson, J. (1997). Are there 'autistic-like' features in congenitally blind children? *Journal of Child Psychology and Psychiatry*, **38**: 693–703.

Bruner, J., Feldman, C. (1993). Theories of mind and the problem of autism. In *Understanding other Minds: Perspectives from Autism*. Oxford: Oxford University Press, pp. 267–291.

Burgess, P.W. (1997). Theory and methodology in executive function research. In *Methodology of Frontal and Executive Function*. Hove, UK: Psychology Press, pp. 81–116.

Burnette, C.P., Mundy, P.C., Meyer, J.A., *et al.* (2005). Weak central coherence and its relations to theory of mind and anxiety in autism. *Journal of Autism and Developmental Disorders*, **35**: 63–73.

Carlson, S.M., Moses, L.J. (2001). Individual differences in inhibitory control and children's theory of mind. *Child Development*, **72**: 1032–1053.

Carlson, S.M., Mandell, D.J., Williams, K. (2004a). Executive function and theory of mind: Stability and prediction from ages 2 to 3. *Developmental Psychology*, **40**: 1105–1122.

Carlson, S.M., Moses, L.J., Claxton, L.J. (2004b). Individual differences in executive functioning and theory of mind: An investigation of inhibitory control and planning ability. *Journal of Experimental Child Psychology*, **87**: 299–319.

Caron, M-J., Mottron, C., Berthiaume, C., Dawson, M. (2006). Cognitive mechanisms, specificity and neural underpinnings of visuo-spatial peaks in autism. *Brain*, **129**: 1789–1802.

Carruthers, P. (1996). Autism as mind-blindness: An elaboration and partial defence. In *Theories of Theories of Mind*. Cambridge: Cambridge University Press, pp. 257–273.

Castelli, F., Frith, C., Happé, F., Frith, U. (2002). Autism, Asperger syndrome and brain mechanisms for the attribution of mental states to animated shapes. *Brain*, **125**: 1839–1849.

Charman, T., Baron-Cohen, S. (1992). Understanding drawings and beliefs: A further test of the metarepresentation theory of autism: A research note. *Journal of Child Psychology and Psychiatry*, **33**: 1105–1112.

Christ, S.E., Holt, D.D., White, D.A., Green, L. (2007). Inhibitory control in children with autism spectrum disorder. *Journal of Autism and Developmental Disorders*, **37**: 1155–1165.

Clark, P., Rutter, M. (1981). Autistic children's responses to structure and to interpersonal demands. *Journal of Autism and Developmental Disorders*, **11**: 201–217.

Colle, L., Baron-Cohen, S., Hill, J. (2007). Do children with autism have a theory of mind? A non-verbal test of autism versus specific language impairment. *Journal of Autism and Developmental Disorders*, **37**: 716–723.

Dahlgren, S.O., Trillingsgaard, A. (1996). Theory of mind in non-retarded children with autism and Asperger's syndrome: A research note. *Journal of Child Psychology and Psychiatry*, **37**: 759–763.

Damasio, A.R., Maurer, R.G. (1978). A neurological model for childhood autism. *Archives of Neurology*, **35**: 777–786.

Dawson, G., Adams, A. (1984). Imitation and social responsiveness in autistic children. *Journal of Abnormal Child Psychology*, **12**: 209–225.

Dawson, G., Meltzoff, A.N., Osterling, J., Rinaldi, J. (1998). Neuropsychological correlates of early symptoms of autism. *Child Development*, **69**: 1276–1285.

Dawson, G., Munson, J., Estes, A., *et al.* (2002). Neurocognitive function and joint attention ability in young children with autism spectrum disorder versus developmental delay. *Child Development*, **73**: 345–358.

Dennett, D. C. (1978). Beliefs about beliefs. *The Behavioral and Brain Sciences*, **4**: 568–570.

Diamond, A. (2002). Normal development of prefrontal cortex from birth to young adulthood: Cognitive functions, anatomy, and biochemistry. In *Principles of Frontal Lobe Function*. London: Oxford University Press, pp. 466–503.

Diamond, A. (2006). The early development of executive functions. In *Lifespan Cognition: Mechanisms of Change*. NY: Oxford University Press, pp. 70–95.

Eisenmajer, R., Prior, M. (1991). Cognitive linguistic correlates of 'theory of mind' ability in autistic children. *British Journal of Developmental Psychology*, **9**: 351–364.

Eslinger, P.J., Biddle, K.R., Grattan, L.M. (1997). Cognitive and social development in children with prefrontal cortex lesions. In *Development of the Prefrontal Cortex: Evolution, Neurobiology, and Behavior*. Baltimore, MD: Paul H. Brookes, pp. 295–335.

Eslinger, P.J., Grattan, L.M., Damasio, H., Damasio, A.R. (1992). Developmental consequences of childhood frontal lobe damage. *Archives of Neurology*, **49**: 764–769.

Farran, E.K., Jarrold, C. Gathercole, S.E. (2001). Block design performance in the Williams syndrome phenotype: a problem with mental imagery? *Journal of Child Psychology and Psychiatry*, **42**: 719–739.

Fisher, N., Happé, F., Dunn, J. (2005). The relationship between vocabulary, grammar, and false belief task performance in children with autistic spectrum disorders and children with moderate learning difficulties. *Journal of Child Psychology and Psychiatry*, **46**: 409–419.

Flynn, E., O'Malley, C., Wood, D. (2004). A longitudinal, microgenetic study of the emergence of false belief understanding and inhibition skills. *Developmental Science*, **7**: 103–115.

Frith, U. (1970). Studies in pattern detection II: Reproduction and production of colour sequences. *Journal of Experimental Child Psychology*, **10**: 120–135.

Frith, U. (1972). Cognitive mechanisms in autism: Experiments with colour and tone sequence production. *Journal of Autism and Childhood Schizophrenia*, **2**: 160–173.

Frith, U. (1989). *Autism: Explaining the Enigma*. Oxford, UK: Blackwell Publishers.

Frith, U., Frith, C.D. (2003). Development and neurophysiology of mentalising. *Philosophical Transactions of the Royal Society of London, Series B*, **358**: 459–473.

Frith, U., Happé, F. (1994). Autism: Beyond 'theory of mind'. *Cognition*, **50**: 115–132.

Frith, U., Hermelin, B. (1969). The role of visual and motor cues for normal, subnormal and autistic children. *Journal of Child Psychology and Psychiatry*, **10**: 153–163.

Frith, U., Morton, J., Leslie, A.M. (1991). The cognitive basis of a biological disorder: Autism. *Trends in Neurosciences*, **14**: 433–438.

Frith, U., Happé, F., Siddons, F. (1994). Autism and theory of mind in everyday life. *Social Development*, **3**: 108–124.

Frye, D., Zelazo, P.D., Palfai, T. (1995). Theory of mind and rule-based reasoning. *Cognitive Development*, **10**: 483–527.

Gilotty, L., Kenworthy, L., Sirian, L., Black, D.O., Wagner, A.E. (2002). Adaptive skills and executive function in autism spectrum disorders. *Child Neuropsychology*, **8**: 241–248.

Goodman, R. (1989). Infantile autism: A syndrome of multiple primary deficits? *Journal of Autism and Developmental Disorders*, **19**: 409–424.

Gottesman, I.I., Gould, T.D. (2003). The endophenotype concept in psychiatry: Etymology and strategic intentions. *American Journal of Psychiatry*, **160**: 636–645.

Green, S., Pring, L., Swettenham, J. (2004). An investigation of first-order false belief understanding of children with congenital profound visual impairment. *British Journal of Developmental Psychology*, **22**: 1–17.

Griffith, E.M., Pennington, B.F., Wehner, E.A., Rogers, S.J. (1999). Executive functions in young children with autism. *Child Development*, **70**: 817–832.

Guerts, H.M., Verté, S., Oosterlaan, J., Roeyers, H., Sergeant, J.A. (2004). How specific are executive functioning deficits in attention deficit hyperactivity disorder and autism? *Journal of Child Psychology and Psychiatry*, **45**: 836–854.

Guerts, H.M., **Corbett, B.**, **Solomon, M.** (2009). The paradox of cognitive flexibility in autism. *Trends in Cognitive Sciences*, **13**: 74–82.

Happe, F. (1993). Communicative competence and theory of mind in autism: A test of Relevance Theory. *Cognition*, **48**: 101–119.

Happé, F. (1999). Understanding assets and deficits in autism: Why success is more interesting than failure. *Psychologist*, **12**: 540–546.

Happé, F.G. (1994a). An advanced test of theory of mind: Understanding of story characters' thoughts and feelings by able autistic, mentally handicapped, and normal children and adults. *Journal of Autism and Developmental Disorders*, **24**: 129–154.

Happé, F.G. (1994b). Annotation: Current psychological theories of autism: The 'Theory of Mind' account and rival theories. *Journal of Child Psychology and Psychiatry*, **35**: 215–229.

Happé, F.G. (1994c). Wechsler IQ profile and theory of mind in autism: A research note. *Journal of Child Psychology and Psychiatry*, **35**: 1461–1471.

Happé, F.G. (1995). The role of age and verbal ability in the theory of mind task performance of subjects with autism. *Child Development*, **66**: 843–855.

Happé, F.G. (1997). Central coherence and theory of mind in autism: Reading homographs in context. *British Journal of Developmental Psychology*, **15**: 1–12.

Happé, F., **Booth, R.** (2008). The power of the positive: Revisiting weak coherence in autism spectrum disorders. *Quarterly Journal of Experimental Psychology*, **61**: 50–63.

Happé, F., **Frith, U.** (2006). The weak coherence account: detail-focused cognitive style in autism spectrum disorders. *Journal of Autism and Developmental Disorders*, **36**: 5–25.

Happé, F., **Ronald, A.** (2008). 'Fractionable autism triad': A review of evidence from behavioural, genetic, cognitive and neural research. *Neuropsychology Review*, **18**: 287–304.

Happé, F., **Ehlers, S.**, **Fletcher, P.**, *et al.* (1996). 'Theory of mind' in the brain: Evidence from a PET scan study of Asperger syndrome. *Neuroreport*, **8**: 197–201.

Happé, F., **Booth, R.**, **Charlton, R.**, **Hughes, C.** (2006a). Executive function deficits in autism spectrum disorders and attention-deficit/hyperactivity disorder: Examining profiles across domains and ages. *Brain and Cognition*, **61**: 25–39.

Happé, F., **Ronald, A.**, **Plomin, R.** (2006b). Time to give up on a single explanation for autism. *Nature Neuroscience*, **9**: 1218–1220.

Heaton, P., **Wallace, G.L.** (2003). Annotation: The savant syndrome. *Journal of Child Psychology and Psychiatry*, **45**: 899–911.

Hermelin, B. (2001). *Bright Splinters of the Mind. A Personal Story of Research with Autistic Savants*. London: Jessica Kingsley.

Hermelin, B., **O'Connor, N.** (1967). Remembering of words by psychotic and subnormal children. *British Journal of Psychology*, **58**: 213–218.

Hermelin, B., **O'Connor, N.** (1970). *Psychological Experiments with Autistic Children*. New York: Penguin Books.

Hill, E.L. (2004). Evaluating the theory of executive dysfunction of autism. *Developmental Review*, **24**: 189–233.

Hill, E.L., Bird, C.M. (2006). Executive processes in Asperger syndrome: Patterns of performance in a multiple case series. *Neuropsychologia*, **44**: 2822–2835.

Hill, E.L., Frith, U. (2003). Understanding autism: Insights from mind and brain. *Philosophical Transactions of the Royal Society of London Part B*, **358**: 281–289.

Hobson, R.P. (1989). Beyond cognition: A theory of autism. In *Autism: Nature, Diagnosis, and Treatment*. New York: The Guilford Press, pp. 22–48.

Hobson, R.P. (1993). Understanding persons: The role of affect. In *Understanding Other Minds: Perspectives from Autism*. Oxford: Oxford University Press, pp. 204–227.

Hobson, R.P. (2002). *The Cradle of Thought*. London: Pan Macmillan.

Holroyd, S., Baron-Cohen, S. (1993). Brief report: How far can people with autism go in developing a theory of mind? *Journal of Autism and Developmental Disorders*, **23**: 379–385.

Hughes, C. (1996). Control of action and thought: Normal development and dysfunction in autism: A research note. *Journal of Child Psychology and Psychiatry*, **37**: 229–236.

Hughes, C. (1998a). Executive function in preschoolers: Links with theory of mind and verbal ability. *British Journal of Developmental Psychology*, **16**: 233–253.

Hughes, C. (1998b). Finding your marbles: Does preschoolers' strategic behavior predict later understanding of mind? *Developmental Psychology*, **34**: 1326–1339.

Hughes, C. (2001). Executive dysfunction in autism: Its nature and implications for the everyday problems experienced by individuals with autism. In *The Development of Autism: Perspectives from Theory and Research*. Mahwah, NJ: Lawrence Erlbaum Associates, pp. 255–275.

Hughes, C., Ensor, R. (2005). Theory of mind and executive function in two-year-olds: A family affair? *Journal of Developmental Neuropsychology*, **28**: 645–665.

Hughes, C., Ensor, R. (2007). Executive functions and theory of mind: Predictive relations from 2 to 4. *Developmental Psychology*, **43**: 1447–1459.

Hughes, C., Graham, A. (2002). Measuring executive functions in childhood: Problems and solutions? *Child and Adolescent Mental Health*, **7**: 131–142.

Hughes, C., Leekam, S. (2004). What are the links between theory of mind and social relations? Review, reflections and new directions for studies of typical and atypical development. *Social Development*, **13**: 590–619.

Hughes, C., Russell, J. (1993). Autistic children's difficulty with mental disengagement from an object: Its implications for theories of autism. *Developmental Psychology*, **29**: 498–510.

Hughes, C., Russell, J., Robbins, T.W. (1994). Evidence for executive dysfunction in autism. *Neuropsychologia*, **32**: 477–492.

Hughes, C., Soares-Boucaud, I., Hochmann, J., Frith, U. (1997). Social behaviour in pervasive developmental disorders: Effects of informant, group and 'theory of mind'. *European Child and Adolescent Psychiatry*, **6**: 191–198.

Jarrold, C., Russell, J. (1997). Counting abilities in autism: Possible implications for central coherence theory. *Journal of Autism and Developmental Disorders*, **27**: 25–37.

Jarrold, C., Butler, D.W., Cottington, E.M., Jimenez, F. (2000). Linking theory of mind and central coherence bias in autism and in the general population. *Developmental Psychology*, **36**: 126–138.

Jolliffe, T., Baron-Cohen, S. (1997). Are people with autism and Asperger syndrome faster than normal on the Embedded Figures Test? *Journal of Child Psychology and Psychiatry*, **38**: 527–534.

Joseph, R.M., Tager-Flusberg, H. (2004). The relationship of theory of mind and executive functions to symptom type and severity in children with autism. *Development and Psychopathology*, **16**: 137–155.

Joseph, R.M., McGrath, L.M., Tager-Flusberg, H. (2005). Executive dysfunction and its relation to language ability in verbal school-age children with autism. *Developmental Neuropsychology*, **27**: 361–378.

Kanner, L. (1943). Autistic disturbances of affective contact. *Nervous Child*, **2**: 217–250.

Karmiloff-Smith, A. (1998). Development itself is the key to understanding developmental disorders. *Trends in Cognitive Sciences*, **2**: 389–398.

Karmiloff-Smith, A., Scerif, G., Thomas, M. (2002). Different approaches to relating genotype to phenotype in developmental disorders. *Developmental Psychobiology*, **40**: 311–322.

Klin, A. (2000). Attributing social meaning to ambiguous visual stimuli in higher-functioning autism and Asperger syndrome: The social attribution task. *Journal of Child Psychology and Psychiatry*, **41**: 831–846.

Klin, A., Volkmar, F. (1993). The development of individuals with autism: Implications for the theory of mind hypothesis. In *Understanding Other Minds: Perspectives from Autism*. Oxford: Oxford University Press, pp. 317–331.

Klin, A., Volkmar, F.R., Sparrow, S.S. (1992). Autistic social dysfunction: Some limitations of the theory of mind hypothesis. *Journal of Child Psychology and Psychiatry*, **33**: 861–876.

Klin, A., Jones, W., Schultz, R., Volkmar F. (2003). The Enactive Mind – from actions to cognition: Lessons from autism. *Philosophical Transactions of the Royal Society: Biological Sciences*, **358**: 345–360.

Lawson, J., Baron-Cohen, S., Wheelwright, S. (2004). Empathizing and systemizing in adults with and without Asperger Syndrome. *Journal of Autism and Development Disorders*, **34**: 301–310.

Leekam, S.R., Perner, J. (1991). Does the autistic child have a metarepresentational deficit? *Cognition*, **40**: 203–218.

Leslie, A.M. (1987). Pretense and representation: The origins of 'theory of mind'. *Psychological Review*, **94**: 412–426.

Leslie, A.M. (1991). The theory of mind impairment in autism: Evidence for a modular mechanism of development? In *Natural Theories of Mind: Evolution, Development and Simulation of Everyday Mindreading*. Oxford: Blackwell, pp. 63–78.

Leslie, A.M., Frith, U. (1988). Autistic children's understanding of seeing, knowing and believing. *British Journal of Developmental Psychology*, **6**: 315–324.

Leslie, A.M., Happé, F. (1989). Autism and ostensive communication: The relevance of metarepresentation. *Development and Psychopathology*, **1**: 205–212.

Leslie, A.M., Thaiss, L. (1992). Domain specificity in conceptual development: Neuropsychological evidence from autism. *Cognition*, **43**: 225–251.

Lezak, M. D. (1995). *Neuropsychological Assessment*, 3rd ed. New York: Oxford University Press.

Liss, M., Fein, D., Allen, D., *et al.* (2001). Executive functioning in high-functioning children with autism. *Journal of Child Psychology and Psychiatry*, **42**: 261–270.

López, B., Leekam, S.R. (2003). Do children with autism fail to process information in context? *Journal of Child Psychology and Psychiatry*, **44**: 285–300.

López, B., Hadwin, J., Donnelly, N., Leekam, S. (2004). Face processing in high-functioning adolescents with autism: Evidence for weak central coherence? *Visual Cognition*, **11**: 673–688.

Lopez, B. R., Lincoln, A. J., Ozonoff, S., Lai, Z. (2005). Examining the relationship between executive functions and the restricted, repetitive symptoms of autistic disorder. *Journal of Autism and Developmental Disorders*, **35**: 245–260.

Lord, C., Rutter, M., Le Couteur, A. (1994). Autism Diagnostic Interview–Revised: A revised version of a diagnostic interview for caregivers of individuals with possible pervasive developmental disorders. *Journal of Autism and Developmental Disorders*, **24**: 659–685.

Lord, C., Risi, S., Lambrecht, L., *et al.* (2000). The Autism Diagnostic Observation Schedule–Generic: A standard measure of social and communication deficits associated with the spectrum of autism. *Journal of Autism and Developmental Disorders*, **30**: 205–223.

Luria, A.R. (1966). *Higher Cortical Functions in Man.* New York: Basic Books.

Mandy, W.P., Skuse, D.H. (2008). Research review: what is the association between the social-communication element of autism and repetitive interests, behaviours and activities? *Journal of Child Psychology and Psychiatry*, **49**: 795–808.

McEvoy, R.E., Rogers, S.J., Pennington, B.F. (1993). Executive function and social communication deficits in young autistic children. *Journal of Child Psychology and Psychiatry*, **34**: 563–578.

Miller, C.A. (2001). False belief understanding in children with specific language impairment. *Journal of Communication Disorders*, **34**: 73–86.

Minshew, N.J., Goldstein, G., Muenz, L.R., Payton, J.B. (1992). Neuropsychological functioning in nonmentally retarded autistic individuals. *Journal of Clinical and Experimental Neuropsychology*, **14**: 749–761.

Minshew, N.J., Goldstein, G., Siegel, D.J. (1997). Neuropsychologic functioning in autism: Profile of a complex information processing disorder. *Journal of the International Neuropsychological Society*, **3**: 303–316.

Minter, M., Hobson, R., Bishop, M. (1998). Congenital visual impairment and 'theory of mind'. *British Journal of Developmental Psychology*, **16**: 183–196.

Miyake, A., Friedman, N.P., Emerson, M.J., Witzki, A.H., Howerter, A. (2000). The unity and diversity of executive functions and their contributions to complex 'frontal lobe' tasks: A latent variable analysis. *Cognitive Psychology*, **41**: 49–100.

Morgan, B., Maybery, M., Durkin, K. (2003). Weak central coherence, poor joint attention, and low verbal IQ: Independent deficits in early autism. *Developmental Psychology*, **39**: 646–656.

Wimmer, H., Perner, J. (1983). Beliefs about beliefs: Representation and constraining function of wrong beliefs in young children's understanding of deception. *Cognition*, **13**: 103–128.

Wing, L., Wing, J.K. (1971). Multiple impairments in early childhood autism. *Journal of Autism and Childhood Schizophrenia*, **1**: 256–266.

Witkin, H.A., Oltman, P.K., Raskin, E., Karp, S. (1971). *A Manual for the Embedded Figures Test*. Palo Alto, CA: Consulting Psychologists Press.

Yerys, B.E., Hepburn, S.L., Pennington, B.F., Rogers, S.J. (2007). Executive function in preschoolers with autism: Evidence consistent with a secondary deficit. *Journal of Autism and Developmental Disorders*, **37**: 1068–1079.

Yirmiya, N., Solomonica-Levi, D., Shulman, C., Pilowsky, T. (1996). Theory of mind abilities in individuals with autism, Down syndrome, and mental retardation of unknown etiology: The role of age and intelligence. *Journal of Child Psychology and Psychiatry*, **37**: 1003–1014.

Yirmiya, N., Erel, O., Shaked, M., Solomonica-Levi, D. (1998). Meta-analyses comparing theory of mind abilities of individuals with autism, individuals with mental retardation, and normally developing individuals. *Psychological Bulletin*, **124**: 283–307.

Zelazo, P.D., Burack, J., Benedetto, E., Frye, D. (1996). Theory of mind and rule use in individuals with Down Syndrome: A test of the uniqueness and specificity claims. *Journal of Child Psychology and Psychiatry*, **37**: 479–484.

Ziatas, K., Durkin, K., Pratt, C. (1998). Belief term development in children with autism, Asperger syndrome, specific language impairment, and normal development: Links to theory of mind development. *Journal of Child Psychology and Psychiatry*, **39**: 755–763.

8

Cognitive flexibility in autism: a social-developmental account

PETER HOBSON AND JESSICA HOBSON

There are important social-developmental contributions to the acquisition of flexible, generative, context-sensitive thinking and engagement with the world. We highlight how among individuals with autism, limitations in the propensity to identify with the attitudes of other people might lead to a paucity of movement across alternative 'takes' on the world, and with this, specific forms of cognitive restriction and rigidity.

8.1 Introduction

Consider this condensed version of a classic description of a person with autism called L (Scheerer *et al.* 1945). L was first seen at the age of 11 with a history of severe learning difficulties. He was said never to have shown interest in his social surroundings. Although he had an IQ of only 50 on a standardised test of intelligence, L could recount the day and date of his first visit to a place, and could usually give the names and birthdays of all the people he met there. He could spell forwards and backwards.

L's background history included the fact that in his fourth and fifth years he rarely offered spontaneous observations or reasons for any actions or perceived event. Nor would he imitate an action of others spontaneously. He was unable to understand or create an imaginary situation. He did not play with toys, nor did he show any conception of make-believe games. He was unable to converse in give-and-take language. He barely noticed the presence of other children, and was said to have 'little emotionality of normal depth and coherence'.

Researching the Autism Spectrum: Contemporary Perspectives, ed. I. Roth and P. Rezaie. Published by Cambridge University Press.

Up to 15 years of age, L was unable to define the properties of objects except in terms relating to his own use of the objects or to specific situations. For example, he defined orange as 'that I squeeze with', and an envelope as 'something I put in with'. He could neither grasp nor formulate similarities, differences or absurdities, nor could he understand metaphor. At the age of 15 he defined the difference between an egg and a stone as 'I eat an egg and I throw a stone'. Once, when the doctor said 'Goodbye my son', L replied: 'I am not your son'. When asked 'What would happen if you shot a person?', L replied: 'He goes to the hospital'. He showed no shame in parading naked through the house.

We begin with this case description, for two reasons. First, it captures something of the quality of rigid thinking that typifies autism – a 'stuckness' that does not extend to all kinds of thought. Second, it sets L's cognitive limitations in a broader context (also Kanner, 1943). Not only do we see that there is specificity to L's impairments, indeed that in some respects he has exceptional cognitive abilities as well as disabilities, but also our attention is drawn to aspects of L's communicative and social-emotional relations that might bear an intimate relation to the nature of his thinking disorder. For example, L would rarely see someone else's actions and make those his own through imitation, he seemed not to engage with others' feelings or perspectives in either verbal or non-verbal give-and-take exchanges, and he seemed unselfconscious. If we were to focus too narrowly on data from children's performance on standardised cognitive tests, revealing though these can be for what is characteristic of children, we might overlook developmentally important links among the children's impairments across different domains of functioning.

It remains the case that a hallmark of the syndrome of autism is the children's lack of flexibility in acting, thinking and relating to the world. Why should this be? It is not self-evident why individuals who are limited in their engagement with other people should also be restricted in thinking about things in one way and then another, nor that they should appear insensitive to context in adjusting their thought and language, nor that they should become preoccupied with certain narrow topics to the exclusion of others. If we could explain these coincidences in the case of autism – and we shall suggest the explanation is not far beneath the surface of case descriptions such as that of L – then this might lead us to deeper understanding of the foundations for and/or implications of thinking itself.

Our aim in this chapter, then, is not to present a comprehensive account of the sources of inflexibility in thinking among persons with autism. Partly this is because there may be several causes (both aetiological and developmental) to this aspect of the disorder, some of which operate in only a proportion of affected children. Yet despite such heterogeneity, we consider that one important source of restrictions in thinking among most if not all individuals with autism is their difficulty in engaging with, and being moved by, the bodily expressed attitudes of other people towards a shared world. If, as Vygotsky (1978, p. 57) argued, 'All the higher functions originate as actual relations between human individuals', then no wonder if the children's failure to interiorise their experience of other people's relatedness to the environment leads to impoverishment in their own ability to generate and adopt multiple 'takes' on the world.

At present, evidence for or against the thesis we shall be propounding is inconclusive. Indeed, one reason we believe it may be worthwhile to articulate our position on these matters is that this may provoke researchers to seek evidence that it is mistaken. Yet our hunch is that it will prove to be important in explaining cognitive deficits that characterise autism.

8.2 Frameworks of understanding

In the spirit of developmental psychopathology, the challenge of understanding why children with autism are limited in the flexibility of their thinking is linked with another challenge, namely that of characterising the nature and basis of flexible thinking among children who do not have autism. From a complementary perspective, if we can both conceptualise and account for the development of thinking among typically developing children, this should stand us in good stead when we try to pinpoint factors that impair the development of thinking in the atypical case. Indeed, the way we think about thinking makes a big difference to the probability of success in explaining its development and pathology. Here it may be helpful to consider two contrasting approaches to the cognitive abnormalities in autism, presented in oversimplified but not unfamiliar guises for the sake of argument.

8.2.1 A 'hardware' approach

One might start by considering paradigmatic cases of flexible thinking among adults as manifest in tests of executive functioning, and then note how neurological conditions such as frontal lobe pathology can interfere with such performance (see Hill, 2004 and Pellicano (Chapter 7) this volume, for detailed discussion and overview of studies we shall not be citing here). In this case there seems to be little problem in identifying what is 'cognitive', and every reason to analyse how localised neurological dysfunction – problems with the hardware needed for thinking – can compromise cognitive abilities. Then we can transpose similar principles to the case of children with autism, and examine their abilities on appropriately styled tests of executive functioning from a neuropsychological perspective.

Yet this strategy is not without its hazards. Early in the life of typically as well as atypically developing children, the organisation of cognitive abilities such as those entailed in executive function tests, as well as the organisation of the brain subserving the abilities in question, may be quite different to what pertains in adulthood. Moreover, autism is a developmental disorder with early onset. This means that even in comparison with typically developing young children, the basis and organisation of affected children's cognitive and/or neurological functioning may be unusual.

In order to establish that when children with and without autism achieve similar levels of performance on particular tests, this reflects similar underlying mental processes, one needs to accumulate evidence that the patterning of these abilities in relation to other abilities and disabilities is also similar. Evidence for unusual profiles of executive ability among children with autism (reviewed in Geurts *et al.* 2009; Hill, 2004; also Lind and Williams, 2010), for improvements in performance when tests are administered by computers rather than human beings (Kenworthy *et al.* 2008) and for a *lack* of expected dysfunction among those who are very young (e.g. Griffith *et al.* 1999) has punctured early enthusiasm for explaining executive dysfunction in autism as the product of primary frontal lobe disorder. Such evidence highlights the need to justify both the ascription of 'executive dysfunction' (as commonly understood) to children with autism – without such justification, it is difficult to see how the approach has the status of a major cognitive theory of autism (Hill and Frith, 2003) – and the assumption that it maps on to specific brain pathology.

If one were to establish a correlation between an autism-specific atypicality in neurological functioning and a pattern of cognitive dysfunction, it would remain open to question whether the neurological side of the correlation is primary and not secondary to abnormality in thinking. Brains are structured by experience and by neural functioning earlier in life, so we should not presume that neurofunctional atypicalities detected among, say, adolescents with autism, play a causative role in determining their profiles of psychological disability. Although a hardware approach is going to feature in any valid explanation of autism, then, for the present purposes the critical question is whether it explains the children's inflexibility in thinking – and if so, whether it does so without the need for further levels of psychological, and developmental, explanation.

8.2.2 *A 'software' approach*

A 'software' approach to cognitive dysfunction in autism does not dispense with the idea that neuropathology is important in causing very many cases of the syndrome (perhaps not all, as we shall illustrate with the case of congenital blindness), nor does it underestimate the need for a neurodevelopmental story to complement and interpenetrate an account of the children's atypical psychological development. In the present context, what it may offer is a way of seeing how those qualities of cognitive inflexibility that characterise autism could arise out of the children's limitations in social experience. The software analogy is meant to capture how *even to the extent that the brain regions subserving cognitive flexibility might be intact* (in the sense of available for performing the relevant functions, at least early in development), still children with autism might be at risk for thinking in rigid, context-insensitive ways. To repeat: This approach still admits that in most cases, neurological disorder will feature as a necessary part of the explanation of the children's dysfunction. It is the level at which this operates that is critical. In particular, neurological disorder (perhaps of various kinds) might explain impairments in the children's social-affective relations, and such impaired social relatedness account for their partial failure to develop flexible thinking.

We have suggested that the very concept of thinking may need revisiting. So where is our point of embarkation for a more detailed specification of a software approach? It is with typically developing infants, and with the construction of the means (software) to think according to one perspective and then another, with sensitivity to context. It is with a theory that grounds creative, generative thinking in communication between and among persons. Communication arises on the basis of modes of interpersonal engagement and role-shifting that are non-inferential and affectively configured (which does not make them 'non-cognitive'). From this starting-point, we distinguish between those forms of thinking that depend upon *social* perspective-taking, and those forms of (prototypically, sensorimotor) thinking for which social role-taking is relatively unimportant. We arrive at a view of the cognitive impairments characteristic of autism in which the children's *relative* failure to engage with the psychological stances of other people is critical for their own limited abilities to generate fresh context-sensitive ideas, as well as their difficulties in shifting from one communicative stance to another.

At this point, an aside is in order. It may be considered that much of the previous paragraph goes over ground already covered by 'theory of mind' approaches to the communicative and cognitive deficits of autism (e.g. as articulated in Baron-Cohen *et al.* 2000). We acknowledge that our account, first presented some years ago (especially Hobson, 1989; 1993), has points of overlap with theory of mind theorising, and there is no doubt that research from a theory of mind perspective has been fruitful and important in furthering our understanding of the relations among communication, interpersonal understanding and thought (e.g. Baron-Cohen, 2000; Frith, 2003; Happé, 1995; Tager-Flusberg, 2000). Yet there are many fundamental contrasts between the two theoretical perspectives (e.g. Hobson, 1990; 1991). A bedrock of theory of mind theorising has been children's mental representations of people's mental states, and computations that are performed upon these postulated units of psychological functioning. We stress how such representations are a developmental achievement founded upon 'qualities of relatedness' between the growing child and his or her social and non-social environment. These social relations have affective and motivational as well as cognitive aspects. Aspects are not components, and if basic forms of personal relatedness are not decomposable into cognitive, affective and motivational parts out of which they are constructed (Hobson, 2008), then it may be a mistake to divorce the foundations of 'thinking about' from (for example) 'feeling towards' objects, events and people.

We can illustrate what this means by considering the development of symbolic functioning. According to at least one influential theory of mind account, that of Leslie (e.g. Leslie, 1987), symbolising takes place through the operation of a computational mechanism that comes on line in the second year of life. Our view is that the kinds of symbolic representation and symbolic functioning that are impaired among children with autism, as well as the kinds of pragmatic linguistic adjustment that are compromised, are those that have a developmental grounding in affectively configured relations and non-verbal communication between a child and other people (e.g. Hobson, 2000). One implication is that creative symbolising bears the stamp of the social-relational matrix out of which it has emerged. In particular, the creativity, flexibility and context-sensitivity of symbolising reflect the creativity, flexibility and context-senstivity of engaging with, relating to and moving among person-anchored perspectives. By 'person-anchored' perspectives we mean not the perspectives of particular other people, even though adopting the mental orientations of actual people sets this form of role-taking in motion, but perspectives taken from the position of 'virtual' stances in the mind – where those stances are created as 'software' for the hardware of the brain through an infant identifying with the attitudes of other embodied people. As Vygotsky (1978) described, what happens between people – in this case, adopting the stances and orientations of others towards a shared world – is interiorised to become a feature of the individual's own propensity to move through alternative stances all by him/herself. So . . . how does this happen?

8.3 A social-developmental account of flexible, creative symbolic thinking

Over the first two-thirds or so of the first year of life, infants relate with persons on the one hand, and things on the other (Trevarthen, 1979). Then towards the end of the first year, in what Trevarthen and Hubley (1978) called the stage of secondary intersubjectivity, they relate to others' relations towards a shared world, for example in episodes of joint attention in which they bring objects to show to someone else, apparently with the aim of sharing experiences (Bretherton *et al.* 1981; Carpenter *et al.* 1998). Yet it is only in the middle of the second year of life that the child, now moving out of infancy, comes to conceptualise self and other as separate individuals who have their own takes on the world. This is manifest in toddlers' growing propensity to comply and co-operate with others, and to engage in co-ordinated role-responsive interactions (e.g. Kaler and Kopp, 1990). From around the age of 18 months, moreover, toddlers not only make self-descriptive utterances such as 'my book' or 'Mary eat' (Kagan, 1982), but they also show silly or coy behavior in front of a mirror (Lewis and Brooks-Gunn, 1979) – and there is evidence that personal pronoun usage and self-recognition may reflect development in self-concepts that are also relevant for advanced pretend play (Lewis and Ramsay, 2004). More or less explicit forms of emotional understanding and self-reflective awareness, together with a capacity to symbolise, appear to have emerged hand-in-hand.

We suggest that critical for the transition to thinking of self and other as discrete persons who live in a shared world, and with this to thinking *about* the world from multiple points of view, is the fact that from around nine or ten months of age, infants are *moved* in responding to the attitudes of others. The nature of this movement is what matters. Take the case of social referencing, where an infant is confronted with an emotionally ambiguous object or event – in one well-known early study (Sorce *et al.* 1985), this was what seemed like a 'cliff' that prevented the child reaching a goal – and the infant looks towards and then responds to the affective expression of a parent, as this has directedness to the object or event in question. In the 'visual cliff' experiment, 14 out of 19 12-month-olds who perceived that their mothers were looking to the cliff with smiles tentatively proceeded towards their goal, whereas none of those who witnessed their mothers showing fear did so. Here we see how the infant is able to identify with the attitudes of the other as 'other' – which also accounts for why the infant shows things to others, and is interested in the other's reactions – such that the world comes to have meaning according-to-oneself-as-identified-with-the-other, and therefore (potentially at least) a new meaning-according-to-oneself.

Such movements in affective stance establish a framework within which a child can, over the next nine months or so of life, come to conceptualise – that is, think about – how different persons have different takes on the same shared world. The critical element in this is that in the child's own experience, even prior to conceptualizing another person as a person, some of the otherness of the other-person-anchored attitude is registered. The structure of such social co-orientation in relation to a given object or event is such as to establish the possibility of the infant coming to differentiate how two person-anchored attitudes can be brought to bear on the same object or event in the environment. In addition, from around the end of the first year the infant begins to adopt the stance of the other towards his or her own attitudes, which as Mead (1934) described, is important for at least some forms of reflective self-awareness. The reversibility of communication – that what X means when you use it to communicate something to me is what X means when I use it to communicate to you – and the emancipation of meanings from the objects in which those meanings reside paves the way for symbolic thought.

Therefore we propose that among typically developing human beings from infancy onwards – but not in the same way for most children with autism – there is a natural propensity to *identify with* other people's attitudes, and that this plays a pivotal role in shaping subsequent cognitive as well as social development. It is critical that this process cannot be classified as simply affective, nor as simply motivational, nor as simply cognitive; rather, it is a process with affective, motivational and cognitive aspects. We are drawn to identify with others, identifying-with is a feature of our affective responsiveness, and the social-communicative transactions configured by identification are critical for the acquisition of special qualities of thinking. So, too, according to our account, much of the flexibility, creativity and fecundity of thinking *derive from* these characteristics of the social relations on the basis of which symbolic thinking (of a particular kind) is founded. As Vygotsky (1962, p. 8) wrote, what we need to envisage is '. . . a dynamic system of meaning in which the affective and the intellectual unite. It shows that every idea contains a transmuted affective attitude toward the bit of reality to which it refers'.

8.4 Studies in autism: flexibility in attitude and stance

It is well known that children with autism have limitations in joint attention and other kinds of person-with-person engagement well before they could be expected to conceptualise minds (e.g. Charman *et al.* 1997). Perhaps most relevant for the present purposes, they are atypical in their relative lack of engaging in 'sharing' forms of joint attention and in social referencing (Sigman *et al.* 1992). All this makes it plausible that, as one of us argued some years ago (e.g. Hobson, 1989; 1990; 1993), it is in the children's limited engagement with other people's attitudes, both in one-to-one mutual exchanges and in person-person-world interactions such as those of joint attention and social referencing, that we find the *source* of later deficits in interpersonal understanding (so-called Theory of Mind). More specifically, we propose, the final common pathway to autism is a limitation in the children's propensity to identify with the attitudes of others (originally Hobson, 1993, but more recently Hobson, 2002; Hobson *et al.* 2006; 2008; Hobson and Hobson, 2007; Hobson and Lee, 1999; Hobson *et al.* 2007).

What is the evidence in support of this thesis and how does it bear on the issue of cognitive flexibility? One part of what it means to identify with someone else is that one individual apprehends and responds to the other-person-centred source of attitudes. In other words, one is affectively engaged with and cares about the other person's feelings *as* the other's. In a recent programme of research on social emotions among children and adolescents with autism (Hobson *et al.* 2006), we interviewed parents of matched children with and without autism. Parents felt they could recognise in their children with autism not only emotions such as anger and fear and emotional responsiveness to other people's mood states, but also pride and jealousy. Yet in contrast with parents of children without autism, rarely were they able to report that their children with autism showed more person-focused emotions or qualities of relatedness, for example guilt or empathic concern. Several remarked on the absence of specifically person-directed displays of pride, even though they felt confident their children could feel proud. This points to a specific impairment in the children's abilities not only to think about other people's emotional states, but also to feel for and relate to the people whose states they are.

Here we can see that what it means to understand minds involves more than thought. If to think were enough to cause a sea-change in personal relations, then children's acquisition of seemingly coherent thoughts about people's feelings, wishes, and so on – and many children with autism do acquire such thoughts – would be the harbinger of radical changes in clinical features of autism. Yet such alterations are often modest. The fact is that feelings are constitutive of the kinds of thought about minds (or more fundamentally, persons) that really make a difference. Here is one particular, and particularly important, expression of cognitive flexibility – movement to thinking about other people as centres of consciousness.

Now consider a study of communication that focuses upon the kind of immediate, unreflective (and arguably, unconceptualised) role-taking that characterises the process of identifying with the attitudes of someone else. Hobson and Meyer (2005) presented a 'sticker test' in which children needed to communicate to another person where on her body she should place her sticker-badge. The majority of children without autism pointed to a site on their own bodies to indicate the tester's body, that is, anticipating that the other person would identify with their act of identifying with her body. The children with autism rarely communicated in this way; instead, most pointed to the body of the investigator to indicate where the sticker should be placed. Although it is possible that this style of flexible self-other communication depends upon thinking or understanding other people's minds, we consider it more likely that such seemingly effortless and natural stance-shifting reflects a more basic form of self-other connectedness and differentiation that has a cognitive aspect – not as a cause, but as an essential property of such relations – and affective and motivational aspects, too.

Affective as well as motivational concomitants to what might be considered 'cognitive' communication were brought out in a further study. Hobson *et al.* (2007) created a setting in which participants had the task of observing an investigator who demonstrated an action, and then communicating to another tester who only subsequently entered the room that he should complete the same action. There were six actions demonstrated, and for each in turn, the demonstrator's instruction was: 'Get Pete to do this'. Three actions involved goal-directed use of objects (e.g. using a mechanical arm to place a cloth frog into a waste-bin), two were non-goal-directed involving the body (e.g. raising hands above head), and three included a form of expressive style (e.g. placing hands on hips in proud, assertive stance). As predicted, the results were that participants with autism contrasted with matched participants without autism in showing lesser degrees of (a) emotional engagement with the testers, (b) joint attention that implicated sharing of experiences, (c) communication of expressive styles of action and (d) role-shifting from that of the learner to that of the teacher. When these measures were combined in a composite index of identifying with someone else, the two groups were almost completely distinct. Apart from a single individual with autism who achieved a score equal to the lowest-scoring three participants without autism, there was complete separation of the two groups.

The question arises whether in one-to-one interpersonal communicative exchanges – the kinds of exchange familiar between typically developing young infants and their caregivers – the structure of communication is shaped by processes of identification. Hobson and Hobson (2007) invited independent raters to watch videotapes of participants interacting (one at a time) with an adult whose actions they had been asked to imitate, and to judge the quality of each look they made to the adult's face. The actions could be imitated either as seen from the participant's point of view, or as adopted from the point of view of the demonstrator (Meyer and Hobson, 2004). There was a significant group difference, in that participants with autism were less likely to adopt the tester's orientation-to-herself as an orientation-to-themselves. For example, if they saw the tester rolling a wheel far-from-herself and close-to-participant, they were less likely than participants without autism to roll the wheel far-from-themselves and close-to-tester. More important for the issue of sharing was that those participants who imitated the tester's self/other-orientation (a relatively rare event among those with autism) *also* tended to be those most likely to manifest 'sharing looks' towards the tester in the imitation task itself. This relation did not hold for looks in which participants were judged to be checking out, or responding to prompts from, the tester. The result applied within each group of participants, and had been predicted on the basis that both the imitation of self/other-orientation, and qualities of person-with-person engagement reflected in sharing looks, are structured by processes of identification. Once again, to *think* about other human beings' states of mind and to adjust communication in relation to those states implicates *feelings* in relation to those others, and it is also to be *motivated* (or 'moved') to act and communicate accordingly. This is hardly surprising, if such thinking is a developmental implication of identifying with others.

8.5 Symbolic thinking in autism

Symbolic play is an especially clear manifestation of children's ability knowingly to apply alternative meanings to materials that do not usually have these meanings. There is substantial evidence that children with autism are limited in their creative representational play, especially in their spontaneous play (e.g. Lewis and Boucher, 1988; Ungerer and Sigman, 1981; Wing *et al.* 1977). On the other hand, many children with autism do achieve some ability to make one thing stand for another, so it is difficult to argue that as a group, they completely lack the ability to 'represent representations'. The really important question here is whether the developmental underpinnings of the play they achieve, and therefore the qualities and creativity of this play, are the same as in the case of typically developing children.

Again we encounter a debate in the literature (Jarrold *et al.* 1993), as to whether the children have limited potential to engage in symbolic play, or whether they are less motivated to do so. According to the present approach, the reason they are less motivated is the same reason that their ability to engage in symbolic play is restricted: lacking the usual interpersonal sources of symbolic functioning, they also lack the kinds of motivation and investment that come with engaging with other people's stances. Just as they are limited in their propensity to be moved among alternative person-anchored perspectives, so, too, they are limited in the spontaneous impetus to move among alternative symbolic meanings. From the complementary viewpoint of typical early development, the pull for children to adopt this and then that perspective is derived from the pull, through identification, to take other-person-centred stances.

Is there evidence in support of such a thesis? In a recent study we compared two matched groups of children, one with and one without autism, for their ability to engage in symbolic play (Hobson *et al.* 2009). As it turned out, these two groups were similar in the mechanics of play, that is, on ratings of whether they were able to make one thing stand for another, or represent absent properties, or pretend that something was present when it was not. Yet there were significant group differences insofar as in 'subjective' judgements that had acceptable inter-rater reliability, the children with autism were rated as showing less creativity and fun, they were less invested in the new meanings of the play, and they were less aware of themselves as initiators of the new meanings. Of course, these results might be interpreted as demonstrating that the children with autism were perfectly able to symbolise in play, but as a separate matter, they showed little affective and motivational investment. In our view, by contrast, these very qualities of affective and motivational investment betrayed what it meant for the children *without* autism to symbolise. The investment and fun that accompanied their play was intrinsic to their symbolic thinking, and reflected the interpersonal transactions from which this form of thinking was derived.

8.6 The case of congenital blindness

Features of autism are prevalent among congenitally blind children. Brown *et al.* (1997) reported that approximately one half of such children between the ages of 4 and 8 in special schools for the blind (this was not an epidemiological study) who were without obvious neurological impairment met the criteria for the full syndrome of autism, and many of those who did not have the diagnosis displayed some features of autism. This at-risk status had been predicted on the basis of reasoning that children who are congenitally blind are deprived of being moved by the attitudes of embodied other people towards a visually specified world, in such a way as to be lifted out of their own viewpoint and to experience 'takes' on the world that are registered as having their source in someone else. An extension of this study by Hobson *et al.* (1999) confirmed that the syndrome of autism among blind children was closely comparable to that manifest in matched sighted children with autism, except that among the former group, the social impairment tended to be less severe.

What is most important about this for the present purposes is that congenitally blind children show restriction in creative symbolic play, and manifest other forms of restricted communication and activity that appear to have similarities with those seen among sighted children with autism (e.g. Hobson and Bishop, 2003). In a study specifically concerned with symbolic play among congenitally blind children who did not have the syndrome of autism (Bishop *et al.* 2005), we compared socially impaired with more socially able children who were matched for mental age and chronological age. This matching procedure meant that group differences in play could not be attributed to disparities in general intellectual functioning. The results were that the socially impaired children were limited in the attribution of symbolic meanings to play materials, the ascription of individual roles to play figures, and the anchorage of play in the scenario as presented by the adult. Within this at-risk sample, therefore, those children who were able to establish interpersonal engagement (the principal criterion for social ability) were also those who showed more elaborate symbolic play – as we had predicted on the basis of a hypothesis concerning the social-developmental bases for this kind of flexible thinking.

8.7 Executive dysfunction reconsidered

In this chapter we have chosen to focus upon a particular way of approaching the topic of cognitive flexibility, as well as limitations in flexibility in the thinking of individuals with autism. We have not reviewed, nor attempted to reinterpret, the substantial evidence that has accrued from administering tests of executive functioning and/or creativity to children, adolescents and adults with autism (for such reviews, see Geurts *et al.* 2009; Kenworthy *et al.* 2008; Hill, 2004). However, it may be appropriate to illustrate how this might be achieved by citing two important studies in this tradition, and returning to the case of L with which we began.

Minshew *et al.* (2002) administered a battery of executive function tests to 90 individuals with autism and of normal IQ, and over 100 control participants without autism. Through a factor analysis of the data, they were led to the conclusion that the participants with autism were relatively able to complete tests of concept identification such as the Halstead Category Test of rule-following, or the Wisconsin Card Sorting Test where groupings were inherent in the test materials and the task was to identify attributes such as form or colour. When it came to tests of concept formation, on the other hand, for example the Gold-Scheerer object sorting test or the 20 Questions Task, when alternative, self-generated shifts in sorting strategy were needed, they were far less able. In an overview of these and other results, the authors suggested that there is a changing pattern of deficits among the children with autism, depending upon levels of ability: 'the most impaired individuals with autism have neither rule learning nor concept formation abilities, less impaired individuals have rule learning abilities but inflexibility in applying them, and the highest ability individuals can discern and flexibly apply rules but not formulate original concepts' (Minshew *et al.* 2002; page 327). The authors' interpretation of these findings was neuropsychological, for example in their suggestion that individuals with autism might have abnormalities in the neural processes involved in self-initiating a schema for problem solving, but this is not the only theoretical option for explaining the results.

Before considering an alternative perspective, we turn to a second study in which Craig and Baron-Cohen (1999) administered the Torrance Creativity Tests to groups of children with autism and Asperger syndrome, and others showing typical development. The results were that the former two groups tended to generate fewer novel ideas of changes to objects when asked to do so, and most interestingly, they also generated more reality-based suggestions for what ambiguous shapes could be, rather than coming up with the kinds of imaginative idea (especially those involving ascriptions of animacy) that were frequent among typically developing children. As the authors considered from a theory of mind perspective (citing Leslie, 1987), this imaginative deficit among the individuals with autism and Asperger syndrome was more than a matter of failing to generate ideas, and might reflect a difficulty in representing mental attitudes towards a proposition, as in 'I can pretend that . . . '. We fully agree that this form of creativity and flexibility is grounded in imaginative activity that arises from self-conscious shifting among alternative attitudes and 'takes' on the world – but of course, we also believe that this has a developmental grounding in a child's affectively configured engagement with others.

At this point it may be worth returning to the original passage in which Scheerer *et al.* (1945) summarised what they meant by L's impairment in abstract attitude (a formulation which Minshew *et al.* 2002 cited with approval), in order to see whether one might encompass their formulation within a social-developmental account. These authors considered the abstract attitude to be a 'common functional basis' for the following (amongst other things): 'to behold simultaneously different aspects of the same situation or object, to shift from one aspect to another; to understand a general frame of reference, a symbolic meaning as relation between a given specific percept and a general idea; to evolve common denominators, to reason in concepts, categories, principles; to assume different mental states . . . to plan ahead ideationally . . . to behave symbolically (e.g. demonstrating, make belief, etc); to reflect upon oneself, giving verbal account of acts; to detach one's ego from a given situation or inner experience; to think in terms of the "mere possible", to transcend the immediate reality and uniqueness of a given situation, a specific aspect or sense impression' (Scheerer *et al.* 1945; page 37).

It is our contention that the forms of abstract attitude and 'detachment' that are missing in autism are precisely those for which appropriately patterned intersubjective experience is necessary. Note how in the formulation by Scheerer *et al.*, as well as in the case illustration of L with which we began, there is a close connection between aspects of self-reflective awareness and thinking. In particular, L had difficulty reflecting on himself, detaching himself from a situation or inner experience, and transcending immediate reality. The story we have sketched about young children's conceptual development in differentiating between self and other with their distinct and yet connected attitudes to a shared world is also a story about the growth in infants' understanding of the differentiation between people's takes and attitudes towards objects or events, and those objects or events as foci for such attitudes. In accordance with the ideas of Mead (1934) as well as Werner and Kaplan (1984), the achievement of self-reflective awareness and the ability to think about self and other appears to be one side of a coin, of which the other face is the ability to grasp how symbols can function as the means to thought. One could not think about self and other without symbols, but one could not achieve the requisite ability to use symbols without grasping how symbolic vehicles and their referents are linked and yet differentiated – something that requires an understanding of what it means to take alternative person-anchored perspectives on a shared world.

Self/other awareness and role-shifting, with the movement among alternative perspectives that these entail, are intrinsic to a certain mode of flexibility in thinking. We have suggested that these features of mental functioning are structured and motivated by the social-developmental process of identifying with other people's attitudes. If certain forms of difficulty in generating ideas are linked with communicative impairments in autism (and see Bishop and Norbury, 2005, for additional evidence), this may be explained by the importance of communicative transactions for establishing the capacity to generate new perspectives within an individual's own mind. If this is so, then it is not difficult to see why children with autism, with their profound impairments in engaging and identifying with the attitudes of others, can also become stuck in one orientation within their own minds, and thereby constrained in generating and applying alternative perspectives in a flexible and context-sensitive manner.

8.8 Acknowledgement

This chapter was written while the authors were receiving project grant support on social dimensions of cognitive flexibility from the Wellcome Trust.

8.9 References

Baron-Cohen, S. (2000). Theory of mind and autism: a fifteen year review. In *Understanding Other Minds: Perspectives from Developmental Cognitive Neuroscience*. New York: Oxford University Press, pp. 3–20.

Baron-Cohen, S., Tager-Flusberg, H., Cohen, D.J. (2000). *Understanding Other Minds: Perspectives from Developmental Cognitive Neuroscience*. New York: Oxford University Press.

Bishop, D.V.M., Norbury, C.F. (2005). Executive functions in children with communication impairments, in relation to autistic symtomatology. I: Generativity. *Autism*, **9**: 7–27.

Bishop, M., Hobson, R.P., Lee, A. (2005). Symbolic play in congenitally blind children. *Development and Psychopathology*, **17**: 447–465.

Bretherton, I., McNew, S., Beeghly-Smith, M. (1981). Early person knowledge as expressed in gestural and verbal communication: When do infants acquire a 'theory of mind'? In *Infant Social Cognition: Empirical and Theoretical Considerations*. Hillsdale, NJ: Erlbaum, pp. 333–373.

Brown, R., Hobson, R.P., Lee, A., Stevenson, J. (1997). Are there 'autistic-like' features in congenitally blind children? *Journal of Child Psychology and Psychiatry*, **38**: 693–703.

Carpenter, M., Nagell, K., Tomasello, M. (1998). Social cognition, joint attention, and communicative competence from 9 to 15 months of age. *Monographs of the Society for Research in Child Development*, Volume **63**.

Charman, T., Swettenham, J., Baron-Cohen, S., *et al.* (1997). Infants with autism: An investigation of empathy, pretend play, joint attention, and imitation. *Developmental Psychology*, **33**: 781–789.

Craig, J., Baron-Cohen, S. (1999). Creativity and imagination in autism and Asperger syndrome. *Journal of Autism and Developmental Disorders*, **29**: 319–326.

Frith, U. (2003). *Autism: Explaining the Enigma*, 2nd edn. Oxford: Blackwell.

Geurts, H.M., Corbett, B., Solomon, M. (2009). The paradox of cognitive flexibility in autism. *Trends in Cognitive Sciences*, **13**: 74–82.

Griffith, E.M., Pennington, B.F., Wehner, E.A., Rogers, S.J. (1999). Executive functions in young children with autism. *Child Development*, **70**: 817–832.

Happé, F. (1995). *Autism: An Introduction to Psychological Theory*. Cambridge, MA: Harvard University Press.

Hill, E.L. (2004). Evaluating the theory of executive dysfunction in autism. *Developmental Review*, **24**: 189–233.

Hill, E.L., Frith, U. (2003). Understanding autism: insights from mind and brain. *Philosophical Transactions of the Royal Society of London Part B*, **358**: 281–289.

Hobson, J.A., Harris, R., García-Pérez, R., Hobson, R.P. (2008). Anticipatory concern: A study in autism. *Developmental Science*, **12**: 249–263.

Hobson, J.A., Hobson, R.P. (2007). Identification: The missing link between joint attention and imitation? *Development and Psychopathology*, **19**: 411–431.

Hobson, R.P. (1989). Beyond cognition: A theory of autism. In *Autism: Nature, Diagnosis, and Treatment*. New York: Guilford Press, pp. 22–48.

Hobson, R.P. (1990). On acquiring knowledge about people and the capacity to pretend: Response to Leslie. *Psychological Review*, **97**: 114–121.

Hobson, R.P. (1991). Against the theory of 'Theory of Mind'. *British Journal of Developmental Psychology*, **9**: 33–51.

Hobson, R.P. (1993). *Autism and the Development of Mind*. Hove, Sussex: Erlbaum.

Hobson, R.P. (2000). The grounding of symbols: A social-developmental account. In *Reasoning and the Mind*. Hove, UK: Psychology Press, pp. 11–35.

Hobson, R.P. (2002). *The Cradle of Thought*. London: Pan Macmillan, and New York: Oxford University Press.

Hobson, R.P. (2008). Interpersonally situated cognition. *International Journal of Philosophical Studies*, **6**: 377–397.

Hobson, R.P., Bishop, M. (2003). The pathogenesis of autism: insights from congenital blindness. *Philosophical Transactions of the Royal Society of London Part B*, **358**: 335–344.

Hobson, R.P., Lee, A. (1999). Imitation and identification in autism. *Journal of Child Psychology and Psychiatry*, **40**: 649–659.

Hobson, R.P., Lee, A., Brown R. (1999). Autism and congenital blindness. *Journal of Autism and Developmental Disorders*, **29**: 45–56.

Hobson, R.P., Meyer, J.A. (2005). Foundations for self and other: A study in autism. *Developmental Science*, **8**: 481–491.

Hobson, R.P., Chidambi, G., Lee, A., Meyer, J. (2006). Foundations for self-awareness: An exploration through autism. *Monographs of the Society for Research in Child Development*, Serial number 284: **71**.

Hobson, R.P, Lee, A., Hobson, J.A. (2007). Only connect? Communication, identification, and autism. *Social Neuroscience*, **2**: 320–335.

Hobson, R.P., Lee, A., Hobson, J.A. (2009). Qualities of symbolic play among children with autism: A social-developmental perspective. *Journal of Autism and Developmental Disorders*, **39**: 12–22.

Jarrold, C., Boucher, J., Smith, P. (1993). Symbolic play in autism: A review. *Journal of Autism and Developmental Disorders*, **23**: 281–307.

Kagan, J. (1982). The emergence of self. *Journal of Child Psychology and Psychiatry*, **23**: 363-381.

Kanner, L. (1943). Autistic disturbances of affective contact. *Nervous Child*, **2**: 217–250.

Kaler, S.R., Kopp, C.B. (1990). Compliance and comprehension in very young toddlers. *Child Development*, **61**: 1997–2003.

Kenworthy, L., Yerys, B.E., Anthony, L.G., Wallace, G.L. (2008). Understanding executive control in autism spectrum disorders in the lab and in the real world. *Neuropsychological Review*, **18**: 320–338.

Leslie, A.M. (1987). Pretense and representation: The origins of 'Theory of mind'. *Psychological Review*, **94**: 412–426.

Lewis M., Brooks-Gunn, J. (1979). *Social Cognition and the Acquisition of Self*. New York and London: Plenum.

Lewis, M., Ramsay, D. (2004). Development of self-recognition, personal pronoun use, and pretend play during the second year. *Child Development*, **75**: 1821–1831.

Lewis, V., Boucher, J. (1988). Spontaneous, instructed and elicited play in relatively able autistic children. *British Journal of Developmental Psychology*, **6**: 325–339.

Lind, S.E., Williams, D.M. Behavioural, biopsychosocial, and cognitive models of Autism Spectrum Disorders. In *International Handbook of Autism and Pervasive Developmental Disorders*. New York: Springer, in press.

Mead, G.H. (1934). *Mind, Self, and Society*. Chicago: University of Chicago Press.

Meyer, J.A., Hobson, R.P. (2004). Orientation in relation to self and other: The case of autism. *Interaction Studies*, **5**: 221–244.

Minshew, N.J., Meyer, J.A., Goldstein, G. (2002). Abstract reasoning in autism: A dissociation between concept formation and concept identification. *Neuropsychology*, **16**: 327–334.

Scheerer, M., Rothmann, E., Goldstein, K. (1945). A case of 'idiot savant': an experimental study of personality organisation. *Psychological Monographs*, **58**: 1–63.

Sigman, M.D., Kasari, C., Kwon, J.H., Yirmiya, N. (1992). Responses to the negative emotions of others by autistic, mentally retarded, and normal children. *Child Development*, **63**: 796–807.

Sorce, J.F., Emde, R.N., Campos, J., Klinnert, M.D. (1985). Maternal emotional signaling: Its effect on the visual cliff behavior of 1-year-olds. *Developmental Psychology*, **21**: 195–200.

Tager-Flusberg, H. (2000). Language and understanding minds: connections in autism. In *Understanding Other Minds: Perspectives from Developmental Cognitive Neuroscience*. New York: Oxford University Press, pp. 124–149.

Trevarthen, C. (1979). Communication and cooperation in early infancy: a description of primary intersubjectivity. In *Before Speech: The Beginning of Human Communication*. London: Cambridge University Press, pp. 321–347.

Trevarthen, C., Hubley, P. (1978). Secondary intersubjectivity: Confidence, confiding and acts of meaning in the first year. In *Action, Gesture and Symbol: The Emergence of Language*. London: Academic Press, pp. 183–229.

Ungerer J.A., Sigman, M. (1981). Symbolic play and language comprehension in autistic children. *Journal of the American Academy of Child Psychiatry*, **20**: 318–337.

Vygotsky, L.S. (1962). *Thought and Language*. Cambridge, Massachusetts: MIT Press.

Vygotsky, L.S. (1978). Internalization of higher psychological functions. In *Mind in Society*. Cambridge, MA: Harvard University Press, pp. 52–57.

Werner, H., Kaplan, B. (1984). *Symbol Formation*. Hillsdale, NJ: Lawrence Erlbaum Associates Inc.

Wing, L., Gould, J., Yeates, S.R., Brierly, L.M. (1977). Symbolic play in severely mentally retarded and in autistic children. *Journal of Child Psychology and Psychiatry*, **18**: 167–178.

9

Language in autism spectrum disorders

JILL BOUCHER

Studies of structural language in individuals with autistic spectrum disorder (ASD) are reviewed, and theories of the causes of structural language anomalies and impairments in ASD are presented and discussed. It is concluded that the factors that may contribute to language impairment in individuals with ASD are many and various; that impaired mindreading is always implicated, but that some additional and critical causal factor remains to be conclusively identified.

9.1 Introduction

Languages, defined in formal or structural terms, are systems of mainly arbitrary items (e.g. sounds, signs or written letters; morphemes; words) with rules for combining items to convey meaning to others with shared knowledge of the language. Language can be analysed and characterised at the level of grammar (morphology and syntax) and meaning (semantics); and, in the case of spoken language, phonology[1].

Communication, on the other hand, involves the use of language in social interaction, whether directly in face-to-face talk, or indirectly as in, for example, a recorded phone message or a Last Will and Testament. Thus, language is a means, or method, of communicating. Non-linguistic, or non-verbal, signals including

[1] Expressive use of phonological knowledge is sometimes referred to as 'articulation'. 'Articulation' in this sense should not be confused with the ability to produce speech. Speech is the output channel for spoken language, just as writing is the output channel for written language, and hand, face and body postures and movements constitute the output channel for signed language.

Researching the Autism Spectrum: Contemporary Perspectives, ed. I. Roth and P. Rezaie. Published by Cambridge University Press.

facial expression, gesture, and body language also provide means, or methods, of communicating. Prosody, which involves the use of vocal tone, pitch, rhythm and inflexion during speech also comes under the heading of non-verbal communication. Factors influencing the communicative use of language and non-verbal communication signals in specific instances can be analysed and characterised in the study of pragmatics.

All individuals with an autistic spectrum disorder (ASD) have impaired communication, this being one of the necessary diagnostic features of all forms of ASD (American Psychiatric Association, 2000; World Health Organisation, 1992). Thus, all individuals with ASD have impaired pragmatics, and most also have impaired prosody. Some individuals with ASD also have clinically significant structural language impairments. Others, however, do not. This chapter is about structural language and language impairment in people with ASD; it is not centrally about communication[2]. The first part of the chapter describes and discusses the patterns of linguistic abilities, anomalies and impairments that occur across the spectrum. The second part of the chapter reviews theories of the causes of the patterns of linguistic strengths and weaknesses that have been described.

9.2 Patterns of language abilities and impairments across the spectrum

Patterns of language ability across the spectrum are discussed below under the following sub-headings:

- Asperger syndrome (AS – strictly defined in terms of ASD plus normal IQ and language with no history of language delay)
- Narrowly-defined High-Functioning Autism (HFA – referring to individuals with ASD, normal IQ and currently normal language following an early history of abnormality or delay)
- Broadly-defined High-Functioning Autism (referring to individuals with ASD, normal IQ and currently normal language regardless of early history, thus comprising individuals with a strict diagnosis of AS plus those with 'narrowly-defined HFA')
- Autistic Spectrum Disorder with Language Impairment (ASD-LI)

It is worth stressing that the terms do not identify mutually exclusive categories, but rather those 'different ways of cutting the cake' that have been used in studies designed to investigate different profiles of language ability that may emerge.

[2] Structural language, non-verbal communication signals including prosody, and pragmatics are indissolubly linked in reality. The sharp distinction made here is intended to focus attention solely on structural language in ASD, rather than to deny the interconnectedness of language, its expression and its uses.

9.2.1 *Asperger syndrome*

According to DSM-IV (American Psychiatric Association, 2000) and ICD-10 (World Health Organisation, 1992) criteria, Asperger syndrome should be diagnosed only in individuals with the triad of behavioural impairments characteristic of individuals with ASD who have normal intelligence and language, and no history of delay or abnormality of language development. Asperger syndrome thus represents the purest form of ASD, with the pathognomic behaviours occurring in the absence of intellectual or clinically significant linguistic impairment either past or present.

Asperger himself described the language used by the children he originally studied as being idiosyncratic and pedantic, but normal or superior in terms of breadth of vocabulary and grammatical correctness (Asperger, 1944; translated in Frith, 1991). So, for example, language used by an 11-year-old boy quoted by Asperger included the following: 'I can't do this orally, only headily' (meaning he knew what he wanted to say but couldn't express it); 'I wouldn't like to say I'm unreligious, but I just don't have any proof of God'. Other examples of idiosyncratic and pedantic language are: 'Missage' (meaning 'going to sleep when your favourite person is away'); 'fonding' (meaning 'affection'); and 'tammer' ('getting involved') used by an adult with AS (Tantam, 1991); and 'May I extract a biscuit from the container?' and 'I wish to thank you for the hospitality extended to me this afternoon' said by children with AS (Wing, 1996).

Asperger considered that the oddities of expressive language in the children he studied were associated with their social impairments, constituting a problem of the communicative use of language rather than of language itself. Subsequent studies of language comprehension in people with AS largely confirm this interpretation, demonstrating impaired ability to understand non-literal uses of language where the speaker's intention must be taken into account, as in the comprehension of irony, metaphor, sarcasm and some forms of humour (Happé, 1995; Martin and McDonald, 2004; Rajendran *et al.* 2005). An interpretation of linguistic anomalies in AS in terms of communication impairment is also consistent with the conspicuous abnormalities of pragmatics and of prosody that have been noted from Asperger onwards (Asperger, 1944; Baltaxe, 1977; McCann and Peppé, 2003; Shriberg *et al.* 2001).

There is, however, some evidence suggesting that people with AS process the structural components of language differently from neurotypical individuals. For example, Kamio *et al.* (2007) showed a relative lack of semantic priming effects for written words in a group of individuals with AS. Similarly, in a detailed single-case study, Worth and Reynolds (2008) showed that a boy with AS with normal language on most standardised measures performed strikingly poorly on a semantic decision-making task. Consistent with these observations, Ring *et al.* (2007) showed atypical EEG responses in a group of participants with AS when reading sentences containing semantic incongruities.

Language ability overall has also been shown to be somewhat below average in individuals with AS despite the impression given by the tendency to use pedantic words and phrases. Thus, Koning and Magill-Evans (2001) reported that language as measured by the Clinical Evaluation of Language Fundamentals – Revised (CELF-R) (Semel *et al.* 1987) was below average overall in a group of boys with AS, with a significant impairment of receptive language relative to a comparison group (see also Saalasti *et al.* 2008). Similarly, Howlin (2003) found below average language abilities in a group of young adults with AS, although scores were within the normal range.

In sum, most of the evidence is consistent with the broad statement that structural language is normal in individuals with AS. However, across groups of adolescents and young adults with AS, mean levels of spoken language are somewhat below average, especially in terms of comprehension. There is no evidence of impaired phonology, and little evidence of impaired grammar. There is, however, some evidence of anomalous semantic processing.

9.2.2 *Narrowly defined high functioning autism*

The issues to be considered in the present section concern whether or not language in individuals with narrowly defined HFA (see the second bullet point above) resembles language in AS, despite the difference in early history; and, related to this, whether or not language in people with narrowly defined HFA is, in fact, completely normal.

Three studies have shown that language in individuals with narrowly defined HFA normalises to levels comparable to those achieved by individuals with AS. Mayes and Calhoun (2001) compared expressive language in children between the ages of 2 years 8 months and 12 years 9 months, 24 of whom qualified for a diagnosis of AS whereas 23 had narrowly defined HFA. They found no significant differences between the expressive language abilities of the two groups. Similarly, Howlin (2003) assessed language in 76 young adults divided into two groups on the basis of whether or not they had a history of language delay. The groups were equated for age and non-verbal IQ. Howlin found no significant differences in language ability as assessed using vocabulary tests, and language was within the normal range in both groups, although slightly below average as noted above. Seung (2007) carried out more detailed assessment of language used by adolescents and adults with either AS or narrowly defined HFA, equated for age and non-verbal ability, and found no significant differences between language in the two groups, although some non-significant differences in uses of verb tense markers were reported. All three of these studies included, in addition to assessment of language, assessment of specifically ASD-related behaviours. No significant differences were found between individuals with AS or HFA in terms of ASD-related behaviours; nor were there differences in relationships between language and ASD-related behaviours in the groups studied.

People with narrowly-defined HFA also share with individuals with AS subclinical anomalies of semantic processing, as indicated by studies of brain activity. Dunn and Bates (2005) assessed brain activity using EEG in two groups of high-functioning children with currently normal language following initial delay, one aged 8–9 years and one aged 11–12 years. Children in both HFA groups performed similarly to age and ability matched comparison groups on the behavioural task, but showed atypical brain responses to semantically related as compared to unrelated words. Similarly, Gaffrey *et al.* (2007) assessed brain activity during a semantic decision task in two adult males with AS and eight with narrowly-defined HFA all of whom had clinically normal language, comparing findings in this combined group with findings on an age and non-verbal ability matched group of neurotypical males. Abnormal brain activity in the combined AS–HFA group was observed. No differences between the participants with a diagnosis of AS as opposed to a diagnosis of HFA were reported.

The above evidence all tends to show that the early language problems that may be used to differentiate narrowly-defined HFA from strictly defined AS tend to resolve leaving only subclinical abnormalities of lexical-semantic processing. In contrast, one study suggests that individuals diagnosed with AS or narrowly-defined HFA differ in terms of grammatical competence when assessed in adolescence (Ghaziuddin *et al.* 2000). The participants with AS in this study tended to produce longer sentences than the HFA group, and their sentences were significantly more complex and also more grammatically correct than those produced by the HFA group. The two latter findings remained significant when differences in verbal IQ were taken into account.

A longitudinal study by Bennett *et al.* (2008) also suggests that the persistence of grammatical impairments may be critical in determining where children with ASD and normal non-verbal IQ eventually fall on a continuum of language abilities, and therefore on a continuum of diagnostic or descriptive terms. Bennett *et al.* (2008) studied 19 children with AS and 45 high-functioning children with early language problems, from pre-school age (4–6 years) through to adolescence (15–17 years), assessing each child on five different occasions. All the children in the study had non-verbal IQ > 70 at the outset of the study, with mean quotients of 100 in the AS group and 87 in the group with early language delay. The children's grammatical abilities were assessed at Time 1 (4–6 years) and at Time 2 (6–8 years). At Times 3–5 broader outcome measures were used, subsuming structural language under the heading of 'communication'.

The main finding from this study was that the best predictor of outcome in terms of autism-related behaviours and general developmental attainments at Times 4 and 5 (up to late teenage) was grammatical competence at Time 2 (6–8 years). Notably, the presence or absence of grammatical impairments at Time 2 was a better predictor of outcome than either language impairments at Time 1, or the diagnosis of AS or HFA based on whether or not there was a reported history of language delay. Information is not given by Bennett *et al.* (2008) concerning structural language abilities at Times 4 and 5. However, the authors' suggestion that language abilities at age 6–8 years might be used diagnostically to distinguish between AS and 'autism' implies that children with significant grammatical impairments at this age remain language impaired, and only those with relatively normal grammar at this age fall into the narrowly-defined HFA subgroup in later childhood.

In sum, most studies of language in older children and adults with narrowly-defined HFA show that language attainment resembles that of individuals with AS in being within the normal range although slightly below average levels. Individuals with narrowly-defined HFA may also resemble those with AS in that semantic meaning may be mediated by non-typical brain systems. However, one study has reported that individuals with narrowly-defined HFA differ from those with AS in having poorer grammatical outcomes, and another study suggests that grammatical competence at age 6–8 years predicts whether a child with initial language delay may or may not at a later age be described as having narrowly-defined HFA, as opposed to ASD with language impairment, highlighting the possible significance of grammatical development.

9.2.3 *Broadly defined high functioning autism*

Results of studies such as those of Mayes and Calhoun (2001), Howlin (2003) and Seung (2007), cited in the previous section, are consistent with other evidence that has failed to find reliable behavioural differences between AS and narrowly-defined HFA (for reviews see Frith, 2004; Macintosh and Dissanayake, 2004; Prior, 2003; Volkmar and Klin, 2000). The accumulation of negative evidence is sometimes used to justify use of the term 'HFA' to refer to all individuals with the triad of impairments, normal intellectual ability and currently normal language (i.e. no distinction is made between individuals with a strict diagnosis of AS as opposed to those who may be described as having narrowly-defined HFA). Findings from studies of this undifferentiated group, referred to here as having 'broadly-defined HFA', are considered next.

A behavioural study by Kelley *et al.* (2006) of children with broadly-defined HFA strengthens the finding of Kamio *et al.* (2007) on children with AS (see above) showing that even high-functioning individuals with ostensibly 'normal' language, have subtle semantic processing impairments. Kelley *et al.* (2006) reported residual semantic impairments in the absence of any abnormalities of phonology or syntax in young children with an early diagnosis of ASD who were at the time of testing considered to be functioning normally.

These findings are consistent with some of the evidence from behavioural studies not designed to assess language directly, but rather to probe the acquisition and use of conceptual-semantic and lexical-semantic knowledge. For example, in addition to well-known demonstrations of failure to utilise semantic relatedness in tests of verbal memory (Bowler *et al.* 1997; Minshew *et al.* 1992; Tager-Flusberg, 1991; Toichi and Kamio, 2002) abnormalities of concept acquisition and categorical knowledge have been shown in some studies (Bott *et al.* 2006; Dunn *et al.* 1996) and impaired semantic priming in others (Kamio *et al.* 2007). However, other findings from this broad group of studies indicate relatively intact semantic abilities in high-functioning individuals with normal language (Hala *et al.* 2007; Toichi and Kamio, 2001; Walenski *et al.* 2008; Whitehouse *et al.* 2007a).

Dunn and Bates (2005) review this discrepant evidence and conclude that 'Although there is significant evidence that individuals with autism comprehend basic concepts and word meanings, they do not appear to extract and apply commonalities among category members'. Minshew and colleagues suggest that semantic impairments in individuals with broadly-defined HFA are restricted to tasks involving 'complex material' (Minshew *et al.* 1997; Williams *et al.* 2006). Toichi and Kamio (2001) suggested that discrepancies relating to semantic processing by people with broadly-defined HFA may be explained in terms of specific difficulties with spoken as opposed to written inputs. However, in a later publication Toichi (2008) suggests that the discrepant findings may be explained in terms of impaired relationships between episodic and semantic memory.

The above findings are consistent with the results of studies assessing brain activity during semantic processing. Thus, Dunn and Bates (2005) reported atypical patterns of EEG during semantic processing in children with broadly-defined HFA. Similarly, Harris *et al.* (2006) reported anomalous distribution of brain activity as assessed using fMRI in adult males with broadly-defined HFA, during semantic processing. The results of these studies are consistent with those of the studies by Ring *et al.* (2007) and by Gaffrey *et al.* (2007) cited in Sections 9.2.1 and 9.2.2 (on AS and on narrowly-defined HFA), respectively.

Numerous other studies of broadly-defined HFA have investigated anatomy and function of brain regions involved in language processing more generally, reporting a wide range of differences between HFA groups and neurotypical controls.

Many of these studies report abnormalities of language lateralisation. However, these abnormalities vary in kind, with reversed asymmetry being reported in some studies (e.g. Boucher *et al.* 2005; Herbert *et al.* 2002; 2005) and lack of the normal asymmetry in other studies (e.g. Schmidt *et al.* 2009). Other studies suggest that specific structures or brain regions mediating language in neurotypical populations develop and function differently in individuals with broadly defined HFA (for reviews see Groen *et al.* (2008); Herbert and Kenet (2007); Kleinhans *et al.* (2008)).

In sum, behavioural findings from studies of language in broadly defined HFA add to evidence already cited in the sections on language in AS and in narrowly-defined HFA, in that they indicate subtle anomalies in the processing of semantic meaning accompanied by atypical brain activity in individuals with clinically normal language. However, the observation of minor grammatical anomalies in cases of narrowly-defined HFA but not in children with AS, as reported by Ghaziuddin *et al.* (2000) (see above), suggests that it may be premature to conclude that grammar is completely unaffected in all individuals within the broadly-defined HFA group. In addition, the considerable body of evidence showing that language in this group is subserved by partially different, or differently lateralised, brain structures shows that language has been acquired differently, and is processed atypically, by this group. Nevertheless, the most striking observation, overall, is that despite the differences in brain representation, language in people with broadly-defined HFA is so very little affected.

9.2.4 *Autistic spectrum disorder with language impairment (ASD-LI)*

Until the early 1980s, 'early childhood autism' was diagnosed only in individuals with clinically significant language impairment, the large majority of whom were low-functioning, where low-functioning is taken to mean non-verbal IQ or full-scale IQ < 70. Much of what is known about structural language in ASD-LI comes from studies carried out during this early period, and these studies are reviewed first.

Early studies showed that 50–75% of the individuals with this diagnosis never acquired useful language in any modality (Rapin, 1991). With the expansion of the definition of ASD to include people with AS or HFA, the *proportion* of mute individuals within the group of all individuals with ASD has reduced. However, the *absolute* numbers of individuals with ASD who are non-verbal have not changed, even if they constitute a smaller proportion than previously of the total population diagnosed with ASD.

Most non-verbal individuals are severely or profoundly intellectually disabled, often with multiple handicaps. However, this is not invariably the case, some having adaptive abilities significantly in advance of their communication skills and discrepant with their complete lack of expressive language (Carter *et al.* 1998; Kraijer, 2000). Language in these individuals has been little researched except within the context of the intervention method known as Facilitated Communication, a method that has been widely criticised on the grounds that claimed 'miracle cures' are an artefact of the methods used (see Mostert, 2004 for a review). This is unfortunate in that it obscures the fact that research is needed to investigate the nature and causes of language impairment in mute individuals who are not overall profoundly intellectually disabled. If, for example, language comprehension were found to be only moderately impaired in some individuals with a complete lack of intentional communicative output, this would be of considerable theoretical and practical interest and importance.

Early studies of language in those individuals with ASD-LI who do acquire some useful language were widely interpreted as showing a pattern of delay rather than deviance, at least in the acquisition of phonology and grammar (see reviews by Swisher and Demetras, 1985 and Tager-Flusberg, 1981; 1989). In other words, it was concluded that although language development begins late and progresses slowly, reaching a plateau beyond which further development does not occur, the stages through which language develops resemble those observed in young typically developing children, and are mental-age appropriate.

For example, studies of articulation in children with ASD-LI demonstrated that articulatory errors were similar to those made by younger, typically developing children (Bartolucci *et al.* 1976) and comparable to errors made by children with intellectual disabilities without autism (Boucher, 1976a). A detailed study by Tager-Flusberg *et al.* (1990) appeared to demonstrate conclusively that grammatical competence is delayed, rather than deviant, settling a controversy concerning these children's acquisition of articles and verb tense endings (Bartolucci *et al.* 1980; Howlin, 1984; see also Bartak *et al.* 1975).

The area of language development that appeared to be more deviant than simply delayed concerned the acquisition of lexical meaning, as evident from tests of comprehension and also from the study of expressive uses of words and phrases by children with ASD-LI. Both Kanner (1943; 1946) and Asperger (1944) had noted a characteristic tendency amongst children across the whole spectrum of autism-related disorders to use stereotyped language, idiosyncratic words and phrases including neologisms, and to make errors in the use of personal pronouns. A detailed study by Rutter and colleagues comparing patterns of language impairments in children with ASD-LI and children with specific language impairment (SLI) underlined the fact that the major difference between the language of the two groups was in the area of unusual or bizarre utterances by the ASD-LI group (Bartak *et al.* 1975; 1977; Cantwell *et al.* 1978). However, these researchers also noted that comprehension impairment was more severe in the ASD-LI than in the SLI group despite the fact that both groups were selected using receptive language impairment as a criterion, and despite the fact that the groups were equated for single word picture-naming ability.

Other researchers emphasised the fact that echolalia is common and persistent in less able individuals with ASD-LI, associated with a tendency to reproduce whole sentences or phrases in contexts closely similar to those in which they were originally heard, and often with functional though idiosyncratic meaning (Fay and Schuler, 1980; Kanner, 1946; Prizant and Duchan, 1981). In their fascinating and insightful book on language in autism, Fay and Schuler (1980) remarked:

> If there is one pervasive theme in the study of the language of childhood autism it is *the permanence of the initial learning situation*. How can speech be brought into line with adult models if the *only associations are first associations* that are tenaciously stored and recycled as if they were cast in concrete?' (pp. 77–78; italics as in the original).

Fay and Schuler go on to suggest that as a result of the paucity and rigidity of the associations to words or phrases learned by a child with autism, language for these individuals denotes but does not connote. Thus, at least for young or less able individuals with limited language, words and phrases are used like proper names, having a single referent rather than having a rich and generalisable network of associations and meaning.

Evidence from some early experimental studies including those of Hermelin and O'Connor (1967) further suggested that the ability to utilise word meanings in, for example, tests of memory, is impaired. This kind of evidence led some influential researchers to propose that children with autism, as then diagnosed, have a fundamental impairment in the acquisition of conceptual knowledge and hence lexical-semantic meaning (Fay and Schuler, 1980; Hermelin and O'Connor, 1970; Menyuk, 1978; Menyuk and Quill, 1985). However, tests of knowledge of basic and superordinate categories failed to confirm this hypothesis, the children with autism performing appropriately for mental age (Tager-Flusberg, 1985; Ungerer and Sigman, 1987). These observations prefigured observations of a similar discrepancy in high functioning individuals with normal language (noted in a previous section) between unimpaired comprehension of basic concepts and word meanings but impaired use of semantic knowledge in cognitive tasks.

The view that language development in individuals with ASD-LI is predominantly delayed rather than deviant, and most commonly characterised by normal or mental age appropriate phonology and grammar, with oddities of word usage, remained current until the end of the last century (see for example the review by Lord and Paul, 1997). However, a rather different picture of the pattern of language impairment associated with ASD-LI began to emerge towards the end of the century, especially from some large-scale studies of younger children than those previously investigated.

Thus, through the 1990s Rapin and colleagues collected a wide variety of data on hundreds of children with ASD referred to specialist clinics for assessment, diagnosis and treatment. Data relating to language in the group as a whole were reported during the 1990s (Tuchman *et al.* 1991; Rapin, 1996) and findings on those children with clinically significant LI are summarised in a review by Rapin and Dunn (2003). The conclusions from this review were: that children with ASD-LI aged between 3 and 6 years invariably have impaired language comprehension; approximately 35% have the kind of 'higher order processing' problems that relate most clearly to linguistic meaning; while approximately 65% fall into the clinical category of 'mixed receptive/expressive language disorder' that includes grammatical and phonological impairments. In their most recent follow-up of language in the whole cohort, Rapin *et al.* (2009) report that by ages 7 to 9 years, 73% of those children with clinically significant LI had poor comprehension but intact phonology; and 27% had moderately or mildly impaired comprehension with 'severe and persistent' phonological impairments. Because most of the children in the latter subgroup were low-functioning, and a non-autistic low-functioning comparison group was not included, it is not possible to conclude whether or not the phonological impairments were typical of intellectually disabled children at this age, or autism-specific in kind.

Deviant rather than simply delayed language development was also reported in two large-scale studies of unselected groups of pre-school children with ASD, using information from parental report (Charman *et al.* 2003; Luyster *et al.* 2007). The children studied understood more words and phrases than they spontaneously used, following the normal pattern. However, whereas the discrepancy between comprehension and production is large in typically developing children, it was much smaller in the ASD groups in both studies, consistent with Rapin and Dunn's (2003) observation that comprehension is invariably and markedly impaired in young children with ASD-LI.

A smaller-scale but detailed study by Eigsti *et al.* (2007) confirmed Rapin and Dunn's report of significant impairments of productive morphology and syntax in young children with ASD and initial language delay. In this study spontaneous language used by a mixed ability group of 16 children with ASD aged 3–6 years was compared with spontaneous language produced by an ability-matched group of children with developmental delay without ASD and a group of younger typically developing children. The main findings were that the children with ASD had shorter mean length of utterance (MLU) than the developmentally delayed group, and somewhat shorter MLU than the younger typically developing group. The children with ASD were also significantly impaired in their use of various grammatical constituents and forms as measured using the Index of Productive Syntax (IPSyn) (Scarborough, 1990). Moreover the pattern of syntactic development in the ASD group differed from that in either of the other groups, and was thus deviant rather than simply delayed. Most strikingly, the abnormalities of grammatical development occurred in children the majority of whom had non-verbal IQ > 70 and single word comprehension within the normal range. Consistent with their relatively good lexical ability on single-word testing, the ASD group produced as many and as varied words as the two other groups. However, the ASD group produced significantly more jargon words than either of the other groups.

A study by Condouris *et al.* (2003) of 44 children who were somewhat older than those assessed in the studies described above also showed that children with ASD-LI have reduced MLU and impaired syntax as measured using the IPSyn. The number of different word roots used in spontaneous speech was also below age-related norms. The main purpose of this study was, however, to compare the results of language assessment based on spontaneous speech as compared with assessment based on the results of standardised clinical language tests. The two sets of measures were correlated in predicted ways: for example, scores on clinical tests of vocabulary correlated with the number of word roots used in spontaneous speech. However, measures of spontaneous speech, and especially the IPSyn, produced results indicative of a considerably greater degree of language impairment than did the standardised tests, an observation that is relevant to interpreting Eisgsti *et al.*'s (2006) findings described above. Subsequent experimental tests of verb tense marking by 19 of the ASD-LI children studied by Condouris *et al.* (2003) confirmed the presence of grammatical abnormalities similar to those originally reported in 1980 by Bartolucci *et al.* (Roberts *et al.* 2004).

All the above findings suggest that clinically significant grammatical and phonological impairments are more common in children with ASD-LI than was widely thought to be the case up until the late 1990s. Rapin and Dunn (2003) suggest two possible explanations of discrepancies between the results of earlier and later studies.

Their first suggestion was that earlier studies focused on relatively high functioning children excluding those with moderate or severe language impairment and significant intellectual disability, and that patterns of language impairment differ across lower- and higher-functioning language impaired groups. However, early studies did not, in fact, focus mainly on more able individuals with ASD-LI; moreover, many studies over several decades have shown that grammatical impairments can occur alongside higher-order lexical impairments in individuals with non-verbal IQ within the normal range, although significant phonological impairments are rarely noted (e.g. Bartak *et al.* 1975; Bennett *et al.* 2008; Eigsti *et al.* 2007; Kjelgaard and Tager-Flusberg, 2001).

Rapin and Dunn's (2003) second suggested explanation of the discrepancies between the traditional profile of language strengths and weaknesses and their own findings concerns the ages of the groups assessed. Rapin and Dunn point out that most early studies focused on older children and adolescents, whereas children included in the studies they reviewed were all below the age of 6 years. Children studied by Eigsti *et al.* (2007) (also by Charman *et al.* 2003, and by Luyster *et al.* 2007) were also below age 6.

Rapin and Dunn (2003) provide evidence consistent with this explanation, some of which is amplified in the latest evidence from follow-up assessments of children from the original cohort (Rapin *et al.* 2009, see above). In these reviews, Rapin and colleagues note that the prevalence of grammatical and especially phonological impairments declines with age, leaving a predominance of higher-order processing impairments marked in particular by impaired language comprehension. Nevertheless, a minority of predominantly low-functioning children have grammatical and especially phonological impairments that persist beyond the age of 6.

Twelve of the 19 children initially investigated by Bartak *et al.* (1975; 1977), and reported to have some phonological and syntactic immaturities were also reassessed in a follow-up study two years after their initial assessment (Cantwell *et al.* 1978). Detailed analysis of spontaneous language produced by these children, then aged between 6 and 11 years (mean age 9 years 2 months) showed 'generally correct usage' of a majority of grammatical forms (excluding personal pronouns). In addition, a reduced percentage of children had phonological errors. However, high rates of stereotypic or echolalic utterances remained. This trend towards reduced grammatical and phonological impairment with persistent abnormalities of word use and meaning brings the group profile closer to the traditional profile of linguistic strengths and weaknesses than had been the case two years previously.

Bartak *et al.*'s group was followed up again in early adulthood (Mawhood *et al.* 2000). Severe problems of language comprehension and production remained even on measures of single word comprehension and use. However, gains in absolute language levels had been made across the group as a whole, and eight individuals were judged to be using 'good sentence speech' and five individuals were described as having 'immature speech'. By contrast, six individuals were predominantly mute or echolalic. Thus the trend towards the more traditional profile of language abilities appears to continue into adulthood in a majority but not all individuals with ASD-LI, some of whom actually regress.

In sum, the discrepancy between the traditional picture of language impairments in children with ASD-LI and findings such as those reviewed by Rapin and Dunn (2003) cannot be explained in terms of differences in intellectual ability of the individuals studied. Indeed, the studies of language impairment in high functioning individuals reviewed above might suggest that this subset of individuals with ASD-LI is particularly prone to grammatical impairments (e.g. Bennett *et al.* 2008; Eigsti *et al.* 2007; Kjelgaard and Tager-Flusberg, 2001). However, the discrepancy between the older and more recent literatures may be at least partly explained in terms of differences in the ages of the children studied. Specifically, it appears that the phonological/articulatory impairments and grammatical impairments common in children with ASD-LI under the age of 6 years tend to decline with age, leaving a predominance of problems associated with the processing of lexical-semantic meaning. Phonological impairments persist only in a minority of less able children and may be mental age appropriate.

A study of spontaneous language produced by adults with ASD-LI underlines the pervasiveness and persistence of lexical-semantic abnormalities in ASD-LI (Perkins *et al.* 2006). In this study, seven adults with ASD-LI, only one of whom was high-functioning and none of whom lived independently, but who were all described by their carers as 'quite voluble', were recorded in one-to-one conversation with a familiar adult. Corpora of language from each participant were analysed linguistically and it was concluded that all seven adults were relying to an abnormal extent on using certain preferred lexical items, phrases or grammatical frames within their conversation, and in some cases on reproducing words or phrases recently used by the interlocutor. It also became clear that the words and phrases used by these adults were not always understood by them. For example, two individuals used specific words apparently appropriately within their conversation, asking shortly afterwards what the words meant.

The conclusion from this study was that imitation, repetition and formulaicity are utilised by these relatively voluble adults to maintain discourse to the best of their ability, but often in the absence of comprehension even of the language they themselves are using. Perkins *et al.* (2006) suggest that the language used by individuals with ASD-LI does not accurately represent the individual's conceptual knowledge. This conclusion is reminiscent of Fay and Schuler's (1980) comments regarding the narrowed meaning of 'language set in concrete'. It is also consistent with a comment by Lord and Paul (1997, p. 212) that individuals with ASD-LI have 'limited ability to integrate linguistic input with real-world knowledge'. In a detailed account of the speech, syntax and discourse of the adults studied by Perkins *et al.* (2006), Dobbinson (2000) reported that articulatory errors occurred only in the less able participants (thus associated with mental age rather than with ASD). However, grammatical errors occurred in all the participants studied. These did not affect word order, but consisted generally of truncations, omissions, or substitutions especially of 'closed class' words such as conjunctions, articles or pronouns.

Summarising findings on language in individuals with ASD-LI is not easy, not least because of the paucity of research, especially recent research investigating language in low-functioning people with ASD-LI. Compared with the number of recent studies on perceptual abilities, executive functions and social skills including communication, recent studies of language in ASD-LI are rare. Moreover, such studies as exist tend to focus on individuals with normal non-verbal IQ. Early studies, which were relatively more common and which did include low-functioning participants, seldom used large groups, and the methods used may have lacked rigour by contemporary standards (Lord and Paul, 1997; Tager-Flusberg *et al.* 2005). Attempting to draw some meaningful picture from the available research is also difficult because there are many different facets of language to be assessed including comprehension and expression, articulation, multiple grammatical forms and rules, meaning and conceptual knowledge. In addition, the methods that have been used to collect and analyse linguistic data are very varied, including parental report, standardised clinical tests, experimental investigation, and the collection and analysis of corpora of spontaneous language, each method having some unique influence on the findings reported. This makes comparisons across studies difficult. It is in any case unlikely that a single ASD-LI phenotype exists, even when the effects of deprivation, hearing impairment or other co-morbid conditions have been excluded as influences on language outcomes (as has generally been the case in studies referred to above).

Given all the above limitations, it might be wiser not to try to summarise the findings at all. However, a few generalisations – ignoring the considerable individual variation that exists – can be made with reasonable confidence, as follows:

1. Language impairment in ASD-LI is non-modality-specific, acquisition of written or signed language being generally as much affected as the acquisition of spoken language.
2. Semantics is universally and persistently affected, being strikingly deviant in the most severely language-impaired individuals. Deviancy is most obvious in the oddities of language production which, though varying with age and ability, is characterised by narrowed and idiosyncratic (non-shared) meaning and repetitiveness. However, impaired semantics has more severe effects on comprehension (where the language to be understood is not under the individual's control) than on production. Impaired lexical semantics and also impairments in the use of semantic knowledge in some cognitive tasks might suggest that the semantic meaning-base (networks of conceptual knowledge) is abnormal in content and/or organisation. However, this is unproven.

3. Grammar is also impaired in individuals with ASD-LI, especially in young children. Syntax (in the sense of word order) may be less affected than morphology (grammatical forms and rules for their use). It is unclear whether morphological impairments reflect delayed and incomplete development, or deviant development. The tendency for grammatical impairments to decline with age might argue for the former. On the other hand, evidence for unevenness in grammatical development and for the persistence of certain kinds of morphological errors is more indicative of deviant development.
4. Phonology ('articulation') is least likely to be impaired, especially in older children and adults with ASD-LI; and if impaired is probably mental age appropriate, rather than deviant in ways that are autism-specific.
5. Non-verbal ability within the normal range does not protect an individual from language impairment. However, verbal IQ and language level generally covary and (a point not made above) the more severe the language impairment the greater the discrepancy between verbal and non-verbal IQ, generally speaking, with non-verbal IQ the better preserved (see for example Lord and Paul, 1997).
6. The preceding generalisations relating to language in individuals with ASD-LI mirror the distribution of subclinical language anomalies in individuals with Asperger syndrome or high functioning ASD with currently normal language. Specifically, anomalies of semantic processing are common if not universal in these groups; mild, subclinical grammatical impairments have occasionally been noted in individuals whose language has normalised following initial delay; but clinically significant phonological impairments are never noted in group studies of people with Asperger syndrome or of people whose language has normalised following initial delay.

9.3 Causes of language impairment across the spectrum

There are undoubtedly numerous contributory causes of linguistic anomalies and impairments, whether subclinical or clinically significant, in individuals with ASD. There are, for example, numerous medical conditions that co-occur with ASD more often than can be explained by chance, and which have varied and specific effects on language acquisition. Such conditions include hearing loss, visual impairment, Down syndrome, Fragile-X syndrome, Turner's syndrome and epilepsy, to name a few. Children with ASD are also as vulnerable as other children to psychosocial deprivation or diseases occurring sporadically, with effects on language acquisition. The fact that co-morbidities are very common in association with ASD undoubtedly helps to explain why language is so often impaired, and why language profiles are so heterogeneous, especially in unselected groups (i.e. those where no exclusion criteria have been applied).

The aim of this section of the chapter is to present and discuss theories that try to account for such homogeneity as may be observed in individuals without significant sensory impairment or other co-morbid medical condition with known effects on language, as represented by the generalisations listed at the end of the previous section. Theories to be discussed fall into two groups: those that implicate social impairments and those that implicate cognitive impairments.

9.3.1 *Explanations invoking social deficits*

Impaired 'mindreading' (Baron-Cohen, 1995) undoubtedly affects the way in which language is acquired by people with ASD (Bloom, 2000; Hobson, 1993). Typically developing infants routinely infer the speaker's intention when forming an association between a novel object or action and a novel word – something that children with autism do not generally do (Baron-Cohen *et al.* 1997; Parish-Morris *et al.* 2007; Preissler, 2008). Moreover, impaired social attention (Bopp *et al.* 2009) and especially joint attention (Siller and Sigman, 2008) are predictive of delayed language development. It can be assumed, therefore, that impaired mindreading contributes to the abnormalities of lexical-semantic meaning that occur across the spectrum, and especially to the tendency to use words and phrases with idiosyncratic (i.e. unshared) meaning. Impaired mindreading can also explain the problems that younger and less able individuals have in understanding and using deictic terms, the meaning of which depends on the identity of the speaker ('you'/'me'), or the speaker's location in space ('here'/'there') or in time ('now', 'then'). Impaired mindreading also helps to explain why comprehension of others' current speech is invariably impaired, since not only does the person with ASD have a narrow, idiosyncratic meaning-base, but they also fail to take account of other people's knowledge, thoughts and feelings in interpreting heard speech. Thus comprehension impairments derive in part from pragmatic or use-of-language impairments that are closely allied to semantic impairments in structural language.

However, as pointed out by Bloom (2000), impaired mindreading cannot offer a sufficient explanation of clinically significant language impairments co-occurring with ASD. This is because individuals with AS or other form of high functioning ASD without language impairment have impaired mindreading abilities but nevertheless develop clinically normal language without early delay. As Bloom argues, there must be other prerequisites for language acquisition that are available to these able individuals (but not to individuals with ASD who do not acquire normal language), and that are sufficient for the acquisition of ostensibly normal language.

In sum, impaired mindreading may explain some of the semantic anomalies observed in the language of high-functioning individuals with intact language, but cannot by itself explain the clinically significant structural language impairments in people with ASD-LI. By contrast, mindblindness and the plethora of social difficulties associated with it is the major cause of impaired communication, including use of language, in people with ASD.

9.3.2 *Explanations invoking cognitive deficits*

When 'early childhood autism' was conceptualised as invariably involving impaired language, it was suggested by various researchers that the condition was, at root, a particularly severe type of developmental language disorder with secondary effects on social behaviour and behavioural flexibility (Churchill, 1972; Rutter, 1968; Rutter *et al.* 1971; but see Boucher, 1976b). Attempts to identify the cause or causes of the language impairment were therefore given high priority. Explanations that were proposed at the time included impaired ability to form semantic categories that are integrated into an underlying conceptual system (Fay and Schuler, 1980; Menyuk, 1978; Tager-Flusberg, 1981); impaired ability to form symbols (Ricks and Wing, 1975); difficulties in processing transient sequential inputs (Rutter, 1983; Tanguay, 1984); and (related to this) impaired ability to segment heard speech into its constituent components (Prizant, 1983). None of these hypotheses was reliably confirmed or disconfirmed at the time. They are not necessarily mutually exclusive, and all remain of potential interest especially in terms of how they may or may not fit in with current theories, as considered next.

An implication of the early suggestion that autism results from a severe developmental language disorder was that language impairment in ASD-LI constitutes a type of specific language impairment (SLI). Rutter and his colleagues investigated this hypothesis in the set of longitudinal studies that has been described above (Bartak *et al.* 1975; 1977; Cantwell *et al.* 1978; Howlin *et al.* 2000; Mawhood *et al.* 2000). The aim of this set of studies was to compare not only language profiles but also cognitive, social and behavioural characteristics of individuals with ASD-LI and individuals with receptive-expressive developmental language disorder, a subtype of SLI. Had substantial overlap been found, especially in terms of linguistic profiles, then it might have been inferred that the causes of language impairment in ASD-LI and in SLI were at least partly the same. In the event, discriminant analyses using either linguistic or cognitive measures differentiated the two groups reliably when the children were first seen, again two years later, and again (though less reliably) in early adulthood. In addition, successive assessments revealed different developmental trajectories in the two groups.

Several recent studies have, however, revived interest in the theory that an important cause of language impairment in ASD-LI is co-morbid SLI. Evidence from these studies concerns common features within linguistic profiles and shared cognitive 'markers' in the two conditions; some possibly shared abnormalities of brain structure and function; and some possibly shared genetic factors. This evidence is reviewed by Williams *et al.* (2008) who conclude the following. First, although there is some overlap in linguistic profiles in the two conditions, especially in younger children, there are also significant differences. Most obviously, phonological impairments are common and relatively persistent in prototypical forms of SLI, whereas persistent phonological impairments are rare in ASD-LI. Second, although certain impairments that are reliable diagnostic markers of SLI – namely impaired non-word repetition and sentence repetition, and certain errors of verb tense marking – also occur in individuals with ASD-LI, there is evidence to suggest that the overlap is superficial and differently caused in the two conditions. Third, neither the evidence from brain studies nor from genetic studies is robust. Williams *et al.*'s (2008) overall conclusion is that the 'ASD-LI = ASD + SLI' theory remains unproven, at least in terms of its capacity to explain most or all cases of ASD-LI (when non-specific factors such as co-morbid sensory impairment have been excluded).

Tager-Flusberg and her colleagues, whose research has done much to revive interest in the suggestion that co-morbid SLI is the major cause of ASD-LI (Kjelgaard and Tager-Flusberg, 2001; Tager-Flusberg, 2004; 2006) have, however, assumed that the evidence of behavioural overlap is sufficiently strong to warrant a hypothesis concerning shared causes. Accordingly, Walenski *et al.* (2005) propose that both SLI and ASD-LI result at least in part from deficits of procedural memory. This hypothesis builds on Ullman's (2001) model of the cognitive prerequisites for language acquisition in which it is argued that phonological and grammatical development are largely dependent on procedural memory, whereas lexical development is dependent on declarative memory. Walenski *et al.*'s (2005) hypothesis also builds on a paper by Ullman and Pierpoint (2005) in which it is argued that procedural memory deficits cause the phonological and grammatical impairments in prototypical SLI. Walenski *et al.* (2005) argue that procedural memory deficits cause the grammatical impairments in ASD-LI and some problems of word retrieval. However, they argue in addition that mindblindness is the major cause of lexical-semantic impairments in ASD-LI, and that problems of linguistic meaning are more marked in ASD-LI than in SLI because children with SLI do not have major mindreading difficulties.

Whereas the latter part of Walenski *et al.*'s explanatory theory is empirically supported (see above), empirical evidence of procedural memory impairments in ASD is either negative or lacking (see Boucher and Mayes (in press), for a review of studies of memory in ASD). Moreover, studies of language in ASD-LI (reviewed above) do not suggest that grammatical – let alone phonological – impairments are the most prominent or persistent kind of impairment characteristic of ASD-LI.

The procedural memory deficit explanation of SLI is only one of several competing explanations of that disorder. Assuming for the moment that language impairment in ASD-LI generally results from co-morbid SLI, is there any other theoretical explanation of SLI that might apply to language impairments in ASD?

Several longstanding theoretical explanations of SLI focus on impairments in the sensory-perceptual processing of heard speech (see Leonard and Deevy (2006) for a review of theories). Deficits in auditory (speech) perception are consistent with increasing evidence of anomalies and impairments in auditory processing and perception in individuals with ASD generally, and in low-functioning and language impaired individuals in particular (e.g. Cardy *et al.* 2008; Tecchio, 2003). These findings are additional to well-established findings that children with ASD lack the normal preferential responses to speech as opposed to non-speech sounds (Klin, 1991; Lepisto *et al.* 2005). However, sensory or perceptual problems confined to the auditory modality cannot explain why language impairment in ASD-LI is non-modality specific (see generalisation (1) above). If, on the other hand, findings of impaired auditory processing were shown to be representative of non-modality-specific sensory-perceptual impairments, then they might help to explain language impairments in ASD-LI. In this case, however, the causes of language impairments in ASD-LI and SLI would diverge, because language impairments in SLI have predominant effects on spoken language only.

Another strongly argued theory identifies problems of phonological short term and working memory as a critical cause of SLI (Gathercole, 2006; Gathercole and Baddeley, 1990). However, this theory seems unlikely to offer an explanation of language impairment in ASD-LI because immediate verbal recall of unrelated words or digits is relatively unimpaired (Boucher and Mayes, in press). Moreover, although non-word repetition is impaired in individuals with ASD-LI as well as those with SLI (Kjelgaard and Tager-Flusberg, 2001; Whitehouse *et al.* 2007b), there is evidence to suggest that the impairment stems from different causes in the two conditions (Whitehouse *et al.* 2008).

In sum, the theory that language impairment in ASD-LI generally results from co-morbid SLI is contraindicated by differences in presenting profiles in most individuals, and also by differences in the developmental trajectories in the two disorders (Howlin *et al.* 2000; Rapin and Dunn, 2003). This conclusion holds even when the additional effects of social impairments on language development in ASD but not in SLI are taken into account (Williams *et al.* 2008). However, there is sufficient evidence to suggest that ASD and SLI are loosely related in some way not yet identified.

In the first place, in their comparison of language in children with SLI and children with high-functioning ASD-LI, Bartak *et al.* (1975) identified 'mixed' cases of autism and SLI in approximately 15% of potential participants. Although studies carried out many years ago may be questioned on grounds of differences in diagnostic criteria or other methodological detail, differences in criteria mainly concern the presence of structural language impairment; moreover, this particular study was methodologically exemplary. The finding of mixed cases should not, therefore, be discounted. In the second place, and as already noted, findings from numerous studies over recent years have been interpreted as indicative of possible links between ASD and SLI at aetiological, neurobiological and behavioural levels of description. Although it has been argued that this evidence is not robust and that the case for a meaningful link between SLI and ASD-LI is unproven (Williams *et al.* 2008), it must also be concluded that the case *against* such a meaningful link is unproven.

A third and quite different source of evidence is sufficient grounds by itself for keeping an open mind concerning the relationship between ASD and SLI. This concerns the occurrence of forms of language and communication disorder that are intermediate between prototypical forms of SLI and ASD-LI. Initially, children with these kinds of intermediate difficulties were described as having 'higher order language processing' problems affecting semantics and pragmatics (Allen, 1989; Rapin and Allen, 1983). Because communication was affected in these children in addition to semantic aspects of structural language, there was considerable discussion as to whether 'semantic-pragmatic disorder' was a form of ASD or a subtype of SLI (Bishop, 1989; Boucher, 1998; Brook and Bowler, 1992). However, subsequent research has established that pragmatic language impairments can occur independently of both significant structural language impairments (including semantic impairment) such as define SLI, and of the social impairments characteristic of ASD. Pragmatic language impairment (PLI) is therefore now treated as a rare 'stand-alone' condition intermediate between SLI and ASD (Bishop and Norbury, 2002; Botting and Conti-Ramsden, 1999; 2003).

It could be the case that language-related impairments in SLI, PLI and ASD-LI are all subtly different in kind and differently caused. However, there is both an orderliness and a relatedness amongst patterns of language impairment that occur in subtypes of SLI through PLI to ASD-LI that suggests otherwise. The orderliness concerns the fact that combinations of impairments along different dimensions of language co-occur only along 'adjacent' dimensions of language, whether in SLI or in ASD-LI, as illustrated in Table 9.1. The relatedness concerns the fact that in SLI language is most commonly impaired within the dimensions of phonology and grammar, less commonly involving semantics, and least commonly involving pragmatics, whereas the exact opposite is the case in ASD-LI. This is also

Table 9.1 *Schematic representation of the orderliness of patterns of spared and impaired abilities across linguistic dimensions in SLI through PLI to ASD, and of the symmetry of these patterns across the three disorders*

SLI profiles	Phonological impairment	Grammatical impairment	Semantic impairment	Pragmatic impairment
1				
2				
3				
4				
5				
6				
PI				
ASD profiles				
1				
2				
3				
4				

Key

- Linguistic dimension most likely to be significantly impaired.
- Linguistic dimension second most likely to be significantly impaired.
- Linguistic dimension third most likely to be significantly impaired.
- Linguistic dimension least likely to be significantly impaired.
- No significant impairment.

illustrated in Table 9.1. This orderliness and symmetry seems unlikely to be a chance occurrence, although not easy to explain (but see Boucher, 2000 for an attempted explanation)[3].

[3] This explanation focused on the different frequencies at which temporal analysis must be carried out during the acquisition of different facets of structural language including the rules and conventions contributing to pragmatics. Thus, acquisition of phonology requires very high frequency temporal analysis (putatively impaired in prototypical forms of SLI, spared in ASD); acquisition of syntactic and morphological rules requires somewhat less high frequency temporal analysis (putatively impaired in most individuals with SLI; somewhat affected in ASD); the acquisition of conceptual knowledge, word meaning, and the rules and convention of pragmatics such as require temporal analysis of ongoing events (as opposed to syllables, or phrases, clauses and sentences), require a slower rate of temporal analysis (less affected in prototypical forms of SLI but significantly impaired in PLI and ASD). Neurophysiological timing mechanisms are genetically determined, and it may be assumed that related genes contribute to the development of timing mechanisms at the rates hypothesised to be differentially affected across various forms of SLI and ASD-LI.

Boucher *et al.* (2008a) have proposed an explanation that accepts, or partly accepts, some of the theories discussed above, but that goes beyond them in one critical respect. Boucher *et al.* (2008a) agree with numerous others that impaired mindreading contributes to the semantic anomalies characteristic across the spectrum. They also accept a role for co-morbid SLI, as proposed by Tager-Flusberg and various colleagues. However, Boucher *et al.* argue that co-morbid SLI probably affects a minority of individuals with ASD-LI – (perhaps the 15% identified as 'mixed' cases in the Bartak *et al.* 1975 study) – including those high-functioning individuals in whom grammatical impairments are most prominent. Boucher *et al.*'s main argument, however, is that language impairment in lower-functioning individuals with ASD-LI can best be explained by a combination of impaired declarative memory, with intact procedural memory and also immediate and working memory.

Declarative memory can be subdivided into episodic and semantic memory. The latter form of declarative memory is known to be impaired across the spectrum (see Chapter 10) and can have subtle effects on the acquisition of word meanings (Holdstock *et al.* 2002), contributing to the subclinical semantic anomalies observed even in individuals with AS. Boucher *et al.* (2008a) hypothesise that semantic memory as well as episodic memory is impaired in lower-functioning individuals with ASD, constituting a more pervasive impairment of declarative memory than that which occurs in high-functioning individuals. According to Ullman's (2001) model, declarative memory is essential for the acquisition of lexical items. These include not only open class words such as nouns, adjectives and verb stems, but also closed class words with grammatical functions, such as articles, prepositions and conjunctions; also irregular grammatical forms such as irregular past tense forms or plurals. Thus, a pervasive declarative memory impairment would have predominant effects on semantics, but would also affect certain facets of grammar. At the same time, intact immediate memory would be used compensatorily in ways that can help to explain the repetitiveness and formulaicity of autistic language. Equally, intact procedural memory (in those individuals without co-morbid SLI) would help to ensure relatively normal acquisition of phonology, and also of regular, rule-based aspects of grammar. Finally, a pervasive impairment of declarative memory would limit the ability to acquire factual knowledge both directly (via semantic memory) and indirectly (via language based learning). Thus, this component of Boucher *et al.*'s (2008a) overall explanation of language impairments across the spectrum can explain why language and learning impairments are so closely linked in lower-functioning individuals with ASD-LI.

The declarative memory hypothesis is in the early stages of empirical testing (see Boucher *et al.* (2008b) for a preliminary report). This hypothesis therefore takes its place alongside other untested explanations of language impairment in ASD-LI, as outlined earlier in this section.

9.4 Summary

Structural language acquisition varies from clinically normal to absent across the autistic spectrum. However, even individuals with clinically normal language have oddities of semantic usage and atypical brain activity during semantic processing tasks. Brain regions involved in language processing more generally are also structurally and functionally atypical in this group. It is uncertain whether or not initial language delay in high-functioning individuals with ASD and clinically normal language predicts language outcomes. Most available evidence suggests not, but there is some slight contrary evidence.

Individuals with ASD and some useful, though clinically impaired, language (ASD-LI) may have significant phonological and grammatical output problems in early childhood, additional to poor comprehension and limited semantic knowledge. Over time, phonological impairments tend to resolve to mental-age appropriate levels (but short of normalising in low-functioning individuals), and expressive grammatical impairments become less prominent (but still present), leaving receptive language and higher order semantic processing as the predominant language impairment. Various explanations of ASD-LI have been proposed. Leaving aside the many non-specific factors that may impair language acquisition in individual cases (e.g. co-morbid hearing loss, Down syndrome, environmental deprivation), it is agreed that impaired mindreading and associated impairments of social interaction invariably contribute. The role of co-morbid SLI is controversial, some recent theorists claiming a major role for this factor. It is argued here that co-morbid SLI probably contributes to language impairment in a minority of individuals with ASD-LI, including those cases where clinically significant LI occurs in otherwise high-functioning individuals. It is proposed instead that the major factor underlying LI and also intellectual disability in lower-functioning individuals is a pervasive impairment of declarative memory involving semantic as well as episodic memory difficulties, but leaving other memory systems mainly intact.

9.5 References

American Psychiatric Association. (2000). *Diagnostic and Statistical Manual: 4th Edn, Text Revised (DSM IV-TR)*. New York: American Psychiatric Association.

Allen, D. (1989). Developmental language disorders in preschool children: Clinical subtypes and syndromes. *School Psychology Review*, **18**: 442–451.

Asperger, H. (1944). Die 'autistichen psychopathen' im kindersalter. *Archive für Psychiatrie und Nervenkrankenheiten*, **117**: 76–136. (Reprinted in *Autism and Asperger Syndrome*, by U. Frith, editor, 1991, Cambridge UK: Cambridge University Press).

Baltaxe, C. (1977). Pragmatic deficits in the language of autistic adolescents. *Journal of Pediatric Psychology*, **2**: 176–180.

Baron-Cohen, S. (1995). *Mindblindness: An Essay on Autism and Theory of Mind*. London: MIT Press.

Baron-Cohen, S., Baldwin, D., Crowson, M. (1997). Do children with autism use the speaker's direction of gaze (SDG) strategy to crack the code of language? *Child Development*, **68**: 48–57.

Bartak, L., Rutter, M., Cox, A. (1975). Comparative study of infantile autism and specific developmental receptive language disorder 1: Children. *British Journal of Psychiatry*, **126**: 127–145.

Bartak, L., Rutter, M., Cox, A. (1977). Comparative study of infantile-autism and specific developmental receptive language disorders 3: Discriminant function analysis. *Journal of Autism and Developmental Disorders*, **7**: 383–396.

Bartolucci, G., Pierce, S., Streiner, D., Eppel, P. (1976). Phonological investigation of verbal autistic and mentally retarded subjects. *Journal of Autism and Developmental Disorders*, **6**: 303–316.

Bartolucci, G., Pierce, S., Streiner, D. (1980). Cross-sectional studies of grammatical morphemes in autistic and mentally retarded children. *Journal of Autism and Developmental Disorders*, **10**: 39–50.

Bennett, T., Szatmari, P., Bryson, S., *et al.* (2008). Differentiating autism and Asperger syndrome on the basis of language delay or impairment. *Journal of Autism and Developmental Disorders*, **38**: 616–625.

Bishop, D.V.M. (1989). Autism, Asperger's syndrome and semantic-pragmatic disorder: Where are the boundaries? *British Journal of Disorders of Communication*, **24**: 107–121.

Bishop, D.V.M., Norbury, C.F. (2002). Exploring the borderlands of autistic disorder and specific language impairment: A study using standardised diagnostic instruments. *Journal of Child Psychology and Psychiatry*, **43**: 917–929.

Bloom, P. (2000). *How Children Learn the Meanings of Words*. Cambridge, MA: MIT Press.

Bopp, K., Mirenda, P., Zumbo, B. (2009). Behaviour predictors of language development over 2 years in children with autism spectrum disorders. *Journal of Speech, Language, and Hearing Research*, **52**: 1106–1120.

Bott, L., Brock, J., Brockdorff, N., Boucher, J., Lamberts, K. (2006). Perceptual similarity in autism. *Quarterly Journal of Experimental Psychology*, **59**: 1237–1254.

Botting, N., Conti-Ramsden, G. (1999) Pragmatic language impairment without autism: The children in question. *Autism*, **3**: 371–396.

Botting, N., Conti-Ramsden, G. (2003). Autism, primary pragmatic difficulties, and specific language impairment: can we distinguish them using psycholinguistic markers? *Developmental Medicine and Child Neurology*, **45**: 515–524.

Boucher, J. (1976a). Articulation in early childhood autism. *Journal of Autism and Developmental Disorders*, **6**: 297–302.

Boucher, J. (1976b). Is autism primarily a language disorder? *British Journal of Disorders of Communication*, **11**: 135–143.

Boucher, J. (1998). SPD as a distinct diagnostic entity: Logical considerations and directions for future research. *International Journal of Language and Communication Disorders*, **33**: 71–108.

Boucher, J. (2000). Time parsing, normal language acquisition, and language-related developmental disorders. In *New Directions in Language Development and Disorders*. London: Kluwer Academic/Plenum Publishers, pp. 13–23.

Boucher, J., Mayes, A. Memory. In *The Neuropsychology of Autism*. Oxford: Oxford University Press, in press.

Boucher, J., Cowell, P., Howard, M., *et al.* (2005). A combined clinical neuropsychological and neuroanatomical study of adults with high-functioning autism. *Cognitive Neuropsychiatry*, **10**: 165–214.

Boucher, J., Mayes, A., Bigham, S. (2008a). Memory, language and intellectual ability in low functioning autism. In *Memory in Autism*. Cambridge: Cambridge University Press, pp. 268–289.

Boucher, J., Bigham, S., Mayes, A., Muskett, T. (2008b). Recognition and language in low functioning autism. *Journal of Autism and Developmental Disorders*, **38**: 1259–1269.

Bowler, D.M. Matthews, N., Gardiner, J. (1997). Asperger's syndrome and memory: Similarity to autism but not amnesia. *Neuropsychologia*, **35**: 65–70.

Brook, S.L., Bowler, D.M. (1992). Autism by another name? Semantic and pragmatic impairments in children. *Journal of Autism and Developmental Disorders*, **22**: 61–81.

Cantwell, D., Baker, L., Rutter, M. (1978). Comparative study of infantile autism and specific developmental receptive language disorder 4: Analysis of syntax and language function. *Journal of Child Psychology and Psychiatry*, **19**: 351–362.

Cardy, J., Flagg, E., Roberts, W., Roberts, T. (2008). Auditory evoked fields predict language ability and impairment in children with autism. *International Journal of Psychophysiology*, **68**: 170–175.

Carter, A.S., Volkmar, F., Sparrow, S., *et al.* (1998). The Vineland Adaptive Behaviour Scales: Supplementary norms for individuals with autism. *Journal of Autism and Developmental Disorders*, **28**: 287–302.

Charman, T., Drew, A., Baird, C., Baird, G. (2003). Measuring early language development in preschool children with autism spectrum disorder using the MacArthur Communicative Development Inventory (Infant Form). *Journal of Child Language*, **30**: 213–236.

Churchill, D. (1972). The relation of infantile autism and early childhood schizophrenia to developmental languge disorders of childhood. *Journal of Autism and Childhood Schizophrenia*, **2**: 182–197.

Condouris, K., Meyer, E., Tager-Flusberg, H. (2003). The relationship between standardized measures of language and measures of spontaneous speech in children with autism. *American Journal of Speech-Language Pathology*, **12**: 349–358.

Dobbinson, S. (2000). Repetitiveness and productivity in the language of adults with autism. Unpublished PhD thesis, University of Sheffield.

Dunn, M., Bates, J. (2005). Developmental change in neutral processing of words by children with autism. *Journal of Autism and Developmental Disorders*, **35**: 361–376.

Dunn, M., Gomes, H., Sebastian, M. (1996). Prototypicality of responses of autistic, language disordered, and normal children in a word fluency task. *Child Neuropsychology*, **2**: 99–108.

Eigsti, I.M., Bennetto, L., Dadlani, M.B. (2007). Beyond pragmatics: morphosyntactic development in autism. *Journal of Autism and Developmental Disorders*, **37**: 1007–1023.

Fay, W., Schuler, A. (1980). *Emerging Language in Autistic Children*. Baltimore: Edward Arnold.

Frith, U. (1991). *Autism and Asperger Syndrome*. Cambridge: Cambridge University Press.

Frith, U. (2004). Confusions and controversies about Asperger syndrome. *Journal of Child Psychology and Psychiatry*, **45**: 672–687.

Gaffrey, M., Kleinhans, N., Haist, F., *et al.* (2007). Atypical participation of visual cortex during word processing in autism: An fMRI study of semantic decision. *Neuropsychologia*, **45**: 1672–1684.

Gathercole, S.E. (2006). Nonword repetition and word learning: The nature of the relationship. *Applied Psycholinguistics*, **27**: 513–543.

Gathercole, S., Baddeley, A. (1990). Phonological memory deficits in language disordered children: is there a causal connection? *Journal of Memory and Language*, **29**: 336–360.

Ghaziuddin, M., Thomas, P., Napier, E., *et al.* (2000). Brief Report: Brief syntactic analysis in Asperger syndrome: A preliminary study. *Journal of Autism and Developmental Disorders*, **30**: 67–70.

Groen, W., Zwiers, M., Van Der Gaag, R-J., Buitelaar, J. (2008). The phenotype and neural correlates of language in autism: An integrative review. *Neuroscience and Biobehavioural Reviews*, **32**: 1416–1425.

Hala, S., Pexman, P., Glenwright, M. (2007). Priming the meaning of homographs in typically developing children and children with autism. *Journal of Autism and Developmental Disorders*, **37**: 329–340.

Happé, F. (1995). Understanding minds and metaphors: Insights from the study of figurative language in autism. *Metaphor and Symbol*, **10**: 275–295.

Harris, G.J., Chabris, C.F., Clark, J., *et al.* (2006). Brain activation during semantic processing in autism spectrum disorders via functional magnetic resonance imaging. *Brain and Cognition*, **61**: 54–68.

Herbert, M.R., Kenet, T. (2007). Brain abnormalities in language disorders and autism. *Pediatric Clinics of North America*, **54**: 563–583.

Herbert, M.R., Harris, G.J., Adrien, K.T., *et al.* (2002). Abnormal asymmetry in language association cortex in autism. *Annals of Neurology*, **52**: 588–596.

Herbert, M.R., Ziegler, D.A., Deutsch, C.K., *et al.* (2005). Brain asymmetries in autism and developmental language disorder: A nested whole-brain analysis. *Brain*, **128**: 213–226.

Hermelin, B., O'Connor, N. (1967). Remembering of words by psychotic and subnormal children. *British Journal of Psychology*, **58**: 213–218.

Hermelin, B., O'Connor, N. (1970). *Psychological Experiments with Autistic Children*. Oxford: Plenum Press.

Hobson, R.P. (1993). *Autism and the Development of Mind*. Hove: Lawrence Erlbaum Associates.

Holdstock, J., Mayes, A., Isaac, C., Gong, Q, Roberts, N. (2002). Differential involvement of the hippocampus and temporal lobe cortices in rapid and slow learning of new semantic information. *Neuropsychologia*, **40**: 748–768.

Howlin, P. (1984). The acquisition of grammatical morphemes in autistic children: A critique and replication of the finding of Bartolucci, Pierce, and Streiner, 1980. *Journal of Autism and Developmental Disorders*, **14**: 127–136.

Howlin, P. (2003). Outcome in high-functioning adults with autism with and without early language delays: Implications for the differentiation between autism and Asperger syndrome. *Journal of Autism and Developmental Disorders*, **33**: 3–13.

Howlin, P., Mawhood, L., Rutter, M. (2000). Autism and developmental receptive language disorder – a follow-up comparison in early adult life. II: Social, behavioural, and psychiatric outcomes. *Journal of Child Psychology and Psychiatry*, **41**: 561–578.

Kamio, Y., Robins, D., Kelley, E., Swainson, B., Fein, D. (2007). Atypical lexical/semantic processing in high-functioning autism spectrum disorders without early language delay. *Journal of Autism and Developmental Disorders*, **37**: 1116–1122.

Kanner, L. (1943). Autistic disturbances of affective contact. *Nervous Child*, **2**: 217–250.

Kanner, L. (1946). Irrelevant and metaphorical language in early infantile autism. *Journal of Pediatrics*, **25**: 211–217.

Kelley, E., Paul, J., Fein, D., Naigles, L. (2006). Residual language deficits in optimal outcome children with a history of autism. *Journal of Autism and Developmental Disorders*, **36**: 807–828.

Kjelgaard, M.M., Tager-Flusberg, H. (2001). An investigation of language impairment in autism: implications for genetic subgroups. *Language and Cognitive Processes*, **16**: 287–308.

Kleinhans, N., Axel-Muller, R., Cohen, D., Courchesne, E. (2008). Atypical functional lateralisation of language in autistic spectrum disorders. *Brain Research*, **1221**: 115–125.

Klin, A. (1991). Young autistic children's listening preferences in regard to speech: A possible characterization of the symptom of social withdrawal. *Journal of Autism and Developmental Disorders*, **21**: 29–42.

Koning, C., Magill-Evans, J. (2001). Social and language skills in adolescent boys with Asperger syndrome. *Autism*, **5**: 23–36.

Kraijer, D. (2000). Review of adaptive behaviour studies in mentally retarded persons with autism/pervasive developmental disorder. *Journal of Autism and Developmental Disorders*, **30**: 39–48.

Leonard, L., Deevy, P. (2006). Cognitive and linguistic issues in the study of children with specific language impairment. In *Handbook of Psycholinguistics*, 2nd edn. New York: Elsevier/Academic Press.

Lepisto, T., Kujala, T., Vanhala, R., Alku, P., Huotilainen, M., Näätänen, R. (2005). The discrimination of and orienting to speech and non-speech sounds in children with autism. *Brain Research*, 1066: 147–157.

Lord, C., Paul, R. (1997). Language and communication in autism. In *Handbook of Autism and Pervasive Developmental Disorders*, 1st edn. New York: Wiley and Sons, pp. 195–225.

Luyster, R., Lopez, K., Lord, C. (2007). Characterising communicative development in children referred for autism spectrum disorders using the MacArthur-Bates Communicative Development Inventory (CDI). *Journal of Child Language*, **34**: 623–654.

Macintosh, K., Dissanayake, C. (2004). The similarities and differences between autistic disorder and Asperger's disorder: A review of the empirical evidence. *Journal of Child Psychology and Psychiatry*, **45**: 421–434.

Martin, I., McDonald, S. (2004). An exploration of causes of non-literal language problems in individuals with Asperger syndrome. *Journal of Autism and Developmental Disorders*, **34**: 311–328.

Mawhood, L., Howlin, P., Rutter, M. (2000). Autism and developmental receptive language disorder – a comparative follow-up in early adult life I: Cognitive and language outcomes. *Journal of Child Psychology and Psychiatry*, **41**: 547–559.

Mayes, S.D., Calhoun, S. (2001). Non-significance of early speech delay in children with autism and normal language and implications for DSM-IV Asperger disorder. *Autism*, **5**: 81–94.

McCann, J., Peppé, S. (2003). Prosody in autism spectrum disorders: A critical review. *International Journal of Language and Communication Disorders*, **38**: 325–350.

Menyuk, P. (1978). The language of autistic children: What's wrong and why. In *Autism: A Reappraisal of Concepts and Treatment*. New York: Plenum Press, pp. 105–116.

Menyuk, P., Quill, K. (1985). Semantic problems in autistic children. In *Communication Problems in Autism*. New York: Plenum Press, pp. 127–145.

Minshew, N., Goldstein, G., Muenz, L., Payton, J. (1992). Neuropsychological functioning in non-mentally retarded autistic individuals. *Journal of Clinical and Experimental Neuropsychology*, **14**: 749–761.

Minshew, N., Goldstein, G., Siegel, D. (1997). Neuropsychologic functioning in autism: Profile of a complex information processing disorder. *Journal of the International Neuropsychological Society*, **3**: 303–317.

Mostert, M. (2004). Facilitated communication since 1995: A review of published studies. *Journal of Autism and Developmental Disorders*, **31**: 287–313.

Parish-Morris, J., Hennon, E.A., Hirsch-Pasek, K., Golinkoff, R.M., Tager-Flusberg, H. (2007). Children with autism illuminate the role of social intention in word learning. *Child Development*, **78**: 1265–1287.

Perkins, M., Dobbinson, S., Boucher, J., Bol, S., Bloom, P. (2006). Lexical knowledge and lexical use in autism. *Journal of Autism and Developmental Disorders*, **36**: 795–805.

Preissler, M. (2008). Associative learning of words and pictures in low-functioning children with autism. *Autism*, **12**: 231–248.

Prior, M. (2003). *Learning and Behaviour Problems in Asperger Syndrome*. New York: Guilford Press.

Prizant, B. (1983). Gestalt language and gestalt processing in autism. *Topics in Language Disorders*, **3**: 16–23.

Prizant, B., Duchan, J. (1981). The functions of immediate echolalia in autism children. *Journal of Speech and Hearing Disorder*, **46**: 241–249.

Rajendran, G., Mitchell, P., Rickards, H. (2005). How do individuals with Asperger syndrome respond to nonliteral language and inappropriate requests in computer-mediated communication? *Journal of Autism and Developmental Disorders*, **35**: 429–443.

Rapin, I. (1991). Autistic children: Diagnosis and clinical features. *Pediatrics*, **87**: 751–760.

Rapin, I. (1996). *Preschool Children With Inadequate Communication*. London: Mac Keith Press.

Rapin, I., Allen, D. (1983). Developmental language disorders: Nosological considerations. In *Neuropsychology of Language, Reading and Spelling*. New York: Academic Press, pp. 155–184.

Rapin, I., Dunn, M. (2003). Update on the language disorders of individuals on the autistic spectrum. *Brain and Development*, **25**: 166–172.

Rapin, I., Dunn, M., Allen, D., Stevens, M., Fein, D. (2009). Subtypes of language disorders in school-age children with autism. *Developmental Neuropsychology*, **34**: 66–84.

Ricks, D.M., Wing, L. (1975). Languge, communication, and the use of symbols in normal and autistic children. *Journal of Autism and Developmental Disorders*, **5**: 191–221.

Ring, H., Sharma, S., Wheelwright, S., Barrett, G. (2007). An electrophysiological investigation of semantic incongruity processing by people with Asperger's syndrome. *Journal of Autism and Developmental Disorders*, **37**: 281–290.

Roberts, J.A., Rice, M.L., Tager-Flusberg, H. (2004). Tense marking in children with autism. *Applied Psycholinguistics*, **29**: 429–448.

Rutter, M. (1968). Concepts of autism: A review of research. *Journal of Child Psychology and Psychiatry*, **9**: 1–25.

Rutter, M. (1983). Cognitive deficits in the pathogenesis of autism. *Journal of Child Psychology and Psychiatry*, **24**: 513–531.

Rutter, M., Bartak, L., Newman, S. (1971). Autism – a central disorder of cognition and language? In *Infantile Autism: Concepts, Characteristics, and Treatment*. London: Churchill Livingstone.

Saalasti, S., Lepisto, T., Toppila, E., *et al.* (2008). Language abilities in children with Asperger syndrome. *Journal of Autism and Developmental Disorders*, **38**: 1574–1580.

Scarborough, H. (1990). Index of productive syntax. *Applied Psycholinguistics*, **11**: 1–22.

Schmidt, G., Rey, M., Oram Cardy, J., Roberts, T. (2009). Absence of M100 source asymmetry in autism associated with language functioning. *Neuroreport*, **20**: 1037–1041.

Semel, E., Wiig, E., Secord, W. (1987). *Clinical Evaluation of Language Fundamentals-R*. San Antonio: The Psychological Corporation.

Seung, H.K. (2007). Linguistic characteristics of individuals with high functioning autism and Asperger syndrome. *Clinical Linguistics and Phonetics*, **21**: 247–259.

Shriberg, L., Paul, R., McSweeny, J., Klin, A., Cohen, D. (2001). Speech and prosody characteristics of adolescents and adults with high-functioning autism and Asperger syndrome. *Journal of Speech, Language, and Hearing Research*, **44**: 1097–1115.

Siller, M., Sigman, M. (2008). Modeling longitudinal change in the language abilities of children with autism: Parent behaviors and child characteristics as predictors of change. *Developmental Psychology*, **44**: 1691–1704.

Swisher, L., Demetras, M. (1985). Expressive language characteristics of autistic children. In *Communication Problems in Autism*. New York: Plenum Press, pp. 147–162.

Tager-Flusberg, H. (1981). On the nature of linguistic functioning in early infantile autism. *Journal of Autism and Developmental Disorders*, **11**: 45–56.

Tager-Flusberg, H. (1985). The conceptual basis for referential word use in children with autism. *Child Development*, **56**: 1167–1178.

Tager-Flusberg, H. (1989). A psycholinguistic perspective on language development in the autistic child. In *Autism: New Directions in Diagnosis, Nature and Treatment*. New York: Guilford Press, pp. 92–115.

Tager-Flusberg, H. (1991). Semantic processing in the free recall of autistic children: Further evidence of a cognitive deficit. In *Autism: Nature, Diagnosis, and Treatment*. New York: Guilford Press, pp. 92–109.

Tager-Flusberg, H. (2004). Do autism and specific language impairment represent overlapping language disorders. In *Developmental Language Disorders*. Hove, UK: Psychology Press, pp. 31–52.

Tager-Flusberg, H. (2006). Defining phenotypes in autism. *Clinical Neuroscience Research*, **6**: 219–224.

Tager-Flusberg, H., Calkins, S., Nolin, T., *et al.* (1990). A longitudinal study of language acquisition in autistic and Down syndrome children. *Journal of Autism and Developmental Disorders*, **20**: 1–21.

Tager-Flusberg, H., Lord, C., Paul, R. (2005). Language and communication in autism. In *Handbook of Autism and Pervasive Developmental Disorders*, 3rd edn. Hoboken, NJ: John Wiley and Sons, pp. 335–364.

Tanguay, P. (1984). Towards a new classification of serious psychopathology in children. *Journal of the American Academy of Child Psychiatry*, **23**: 378–384.

Tantam, D. (1991). Asperger syndrome in adulthood. In *Autism and Asperger Syndrome*. Cambridge: Cambridge University Press, pp. 147–183.

Tecchio, F. (2003). Auditory sensory processing in autism: A magnetoencephalographic study. *Biological Psychiatry*, **54**: 647–654.

Toichi, M. (2008). Episodic memory, semantic memory and self-awareness in high-functioning autism. In *Memory in Autism: Theory and Evidence*. Cambridge: Cambridge University Press, pp. 143–165.

Toichi, M., Kamio, Y. (2001). Verbal association for simple common words in high-functioning autism. *Journal of Autism and Developmental Disorders*, **31**: 483–490.

Toichi, M., Kamio, Y. (2002). Long-term memory and levels-of-processing in autism. *Neuropsychologia*, **40**: 964–969.

Tuchman, R., Rapin, I., Shinnar, S. (1991). Autistic and dysphasic children. *Pediatrics*, **88**: 1211–1218.

Ullman, M. (2001). The declarative/procedural model of lexicon and grammar. *Journal of Psycholinguistic Research*, **30**: 37–69.

Ullman, M., Pierpoint, E. (2005). Specific language impairment is not specific to language: The procedural deficit hypothesis. *Cortex*, **41**: 399–433.

Ungerer, J., Sigman, M. (1987). Categorisation skills and receptive language development in autistic children. *Journal of Autism and Developmental Disorders*, **17**: 3–16.

Volkmar, F., Klin, A. (2000). Diagnostic issues in Asperger syndrome. In *Asperger Syndrome*. New York: Guilford Press, pp. 25–71.

Walenski, M., Tager-Flusberg, H., Ullman, M. (2005). In *Understanding Autism: From Basic Neuroscience to Treatment*. New York: Taylor and Francis, pp. 175–203.

Walenski, M., Mostofsky, S., Gidley-Larson, J., Ullman, M. (2008). Brief Report: Enhanced picture naming in autism. *Journal of Autism and Developmental Disorders*, **38**: 1395–1399.

Whitehouse, A.J., Barry, J.G., Bishop, D.V. (2007a). The broader language phenotype of autism: a comparison with specific language impairment. *Journal of Child Psychology and Psychiatry*, **48**: 822–830.

Whitehouse, A.J., Maybery, M.T, Durkin, K. (2007b). Evidence against poor semantic encoding in individuals with autism. *Autism*, **11**: 241–254.

Whitehouse, A.J., Barry, J.G., Bishop, D.V. (2008). Further defining the language impairment of autism: is there a specific language impairment subtype? *Journal of Communication Disorders*, **41**: 319–336.

Williams, D.L., Goldstein, G., Minshew, N.J. (2006). Neuropsychologic functioning in children with autism: Further evidence for disordered complex information-processing. *Child Neuropsychology*, **12**: 279–298.

Williams, D., Botting, N., Boucher, J. (2008). Language in autism and specific language impairment: Where are the links? *Psychological Bulletin*, **134**: 944–963.

Wing, L. (1996). *The Autistic Continuum*. London: Constable.

World Health Organisation. (1992). *International Classification of Mental and Behavioural Disorders: Clinical Descriptions and Diagnostic Guidelines*, 10th edn. (ICD-10). Geneva: World Health Organisation.

Worth, S., Reynolds, S. (2008).The assessment and identification of language impairment in Asperger's syndrome: A case study. *Child Language, Teaching and Therapy*, **24**: 55–71.

10

Memory in autism: binding, self and brain

DERMOT BOWLER, SEBASTIAN GAIGG AND SOPHIE LIND

Memory can be thought of as the capacity of an organism to utilise past experience in order to direct current and future behaviour. Such a capacity entails the registering and recording – the encoding – of that experience in such a way as to enable its subsequent retrieval. Retrieval can be either voluntary or involuntary and the resultant information may or may not form part of conscious awareness. The processes of encoding and retrieval are the result of a range of psychological processes and are in turn influenced by other factors both psychological and physiological. In this respect, study of the patterning of memory processes and the factors that influence their operation can give clues to the wider psychological functioning of the individual. It is in this last respect that the study of memory can enhance our understanding of people with Autism Spectrum Disorder (ASD). ASD is not 'caused by' difficulties in memory, but the patterning of memory seen in individuals with ASD can provide clues to underlying cognitive and neuropsychological atypicalities as well as giving us a window onto their inner experiences of the world.

10.1 Preliminary remarks

Any discussion of memory in ASD must first emphasise the heterogeneous nature of the conditions that comprise the autism spectrum. An important aspect of this diversity is the distinction between ASD with accompanying intellectual disability (often referred to as 'low-functioning ASD' or LFA) and ASD without it (often termed 'high-functioning ASD' or HFA), a group that, as here defined, also

Researching the Autism Spectrum: Contemporary Perspectives, ed. I. Roth and P. Rezaie. Published by Cambridge University Press.

includes individuals with Asperger's disorder. Intellectual disability in itself has consequences for memory (see Bray *et al.* 1997 and Wyatt and Conners, 1998 for reviews), but we should be careful about assuming that these consequences operate similarly in individuals with co-occurring ASD. Nor should we assume that atypical memory patterns identified in individuals with HFA necessarily hold for those from the lower functioning parts of the spectrum. Similar arguments hold for the distinction between individuals who have good language and communication skills and those whose language capabilities are diminished or absent. At present, systematic investigations into how these dimensions affect memory in the context of ASD are thin on the ground, so readers need to be aware of potential difficulties of interpretation when drawing conclusions from research that has been limited to particular subgroups of people within the ASD population.

The same caveat applies to the topic of memory. Although at first it appears to be a straightforward process – the recollection of something that happened in the past – a moment's reflection throws up quite considerable complexity. 'Memory' is always *of* something and is assessed using particular procedures, often with a particular aim or purpose in mind. The writing of this chapter entails the recollection of words (verbal memory) and concepts (semantic memory) that have to be organised in a way that takes into account (however, imperfectly) the minds of potential readers. Some of the information comes into the author's mind through a deliberate act of recollection (albeit prompted by the various cues that nudge authors to complete manuscripts on time) while other ideas are engendered by the reading of source texts. And all of these ideas are sorted and edited, accepted or rejected, in the light of the overall aim of the exercise. Even this anecdotal scenario highlights the complexities that begin to emerge when considering where to draw boundaries for the concept of 'memory'. We need to be clear about the kinds of material that are being remembered, whether the memory involves unsupported recollection, prompted recollection or simply recognition that we had encountered something previously. We also need to decide whether the remembered material was learned very recently or some time (maybe even years) ago. The topics of recollection, prompting or recognition have engendered some of the principal test measures used in laboratory and clinical studies of memory. Recollection is usually tested by *free recall*, in which participants study lists of words and then recall as many as they can in any order. The prompt here is minimal, usually involving a request from the experimenter to recall the words just studied. *Cued recall* provides more concrete and specific hints to aid recall. These hints may be phonological (e.g. words that rhyme with . . . ; words that begin with . . .) or semantic (e.g. there were flowers, items of furniture, etc.) in nature. Recognition involves studying long lists of items and then presenting these again, interspersed with non-studied items, asking the participant to indicate whether or not they had seen the item at study. Recognition may also be tested by presenting participants with a studied and a new word and asking them to indicate which they had seen before.

In parallel with material and procedural issues is the question of how we conceptualise what is going on in the brain and the mind during the operation of memory. New information must be encoded, which implies some kind of storage system, or a system that marks already-stored information in a way that links it to the study episode. For example, when we see the word CAT in a list of items presented in a memory experiment, we mark our existing representation of 'cat' in a way that informs us that it was one of the studied items. Subsequent retrieval implies its own system or set of processes (for a fuller exposition of these topics, see Gardiner, 2008). Some theorists argue that memory can be divided into two distinct sets of processes, those that operate over the very short term (e.g. working memory, Baddeley and Hitch (1974)), and which are distinct from the processes that subtend long-term memory. Others (e.g. Bjork and Whitten (1974) and Crowder (1976)) argue for an undivided memory system that may vary in its particular characteristics depending on when retrieval happens. Advocates of both positions generally argue that memory (or long-term memory, in the case of advocates of multi-store models) can be divided into *procedural* and *declarative* memory systems. Procedural memory involves skills such as riding a bicycle or playing a musical instrument; declarative memory involves the conscious retrieval of facts or events and can be further subdivided into sub-systems and processes. For reasons of space, our discussion here will be limited to declarative memory in ASD. More detail on short-term and working memory in ASD can be found in Poirier and Martin (2008), on procedural memory in Mostofsky *et al.* (2000) and on implicit memory in Bowler *et al.* (1997), Gardiner *et al.* (2003), Roediger and McDermott (1993) and Schacter and Tulving (1994).

Declarative memory is memory that is generally accessible to conscious awareness (Eichenbaum, 1999), different kinds of which are used by many theorists to delineate separate memory sub-systems and processes. Tulving (2001) posits several systems, each associated with a characteristic type of conscious awareness. The first of these systems is the *semantic memory system*, which is one's store of general knowledge or what Tulving calls 'timeless facts', the recall of which is accompanied by *noetic conscious awareness*, which is the experience one has when recalling items of general knowledge that are unaccompanied by any contextual detail or re-experiencing of the time at which they were learned. The second is the *episodic memory system*, which comprises recollection of personally experienced events and involves the self engaging in mental time travel to re-experience the spatio-temporal context of the recollected episode. It is this experience of the self re-experiencing the past that he terms *autonoetic conscious awareness* and regards as being the hallmark of episodic memory. To a similar end, Jacoby (1991) contrasts *familiarity*, a non-effortful process, and *recollection*, which involves active, conscious control by the participant. On this view, the quality of the conscious recollective experience depends on the relative contributions of familiarity and recollection to a particular memory. Across all these different systems and processes memory is affected by the depth of processing (Craik and Lockhart, 1972) called for by different kinds of material and by different memory tasks. For example, focusing on phonological aspects of words is thought of as entailing shallower levels of processing than does working out meaningful relations among them. All these different theoretical positions are tested experimentally using manipulations of the procedures outlined earlier. It is important to bear in mind that the results of a given experiment can often be interpreted in the light of different theoretical perspectives.

10.2 Empirical findings

10.2.1 *Standard experimental procedures*

Amongst the earliest studies of memory in ASD were ones concerned with memory span, a classic measure of short-term memory, which is determined by the number of items that a participant can correctly recall in the order in which they were presented. Initial reports showed that individuals with ASD exhibited relatively undiminished performance on such tasks by comparison with mental-age matched participants without ASD (Boucher, 1978; Hermelin and O'Connor, 1967). However, as Poirier and Martin (2008) observe, these early studies are compromised by the fact that groups were often matched on psychometric measures of digit span, which equates groups on their ability to recall the order of a series of numbers. When matching was based on non-span measures and when more demanding measures of span were utilised, Martin *et al.* (2006) found marginally diminished span in adults with HFA. More specifically, even though the absolute numbers of items recalled was undiminished, there was a significantly higher number of order errors in the recall of the HFA participants. These findings show that although the maximum number of items that individuals with ASD can recall is not different from that recalled by typical individuals, they have difficulties in recalling the precise order of the items, at least after a single exposure.

Free recall of longer lists of words – supra-span lists – without the requirement to preserve the order of the studied words has a number of characteristic features in typical individuals. The first few and the last few items in a list are more likely to be recalled than the middle items, yielding the classic *serial position curve* in free recall (Murdock, 1962). Recall of the last few items – the recency effect – is thought, by advocates of multi-store theories, to reflect the contents of a short-term store, whereas recall of the first few items – the primacy effect – is thought to result from processing of information into long-term memory. Another characteristic of supra-span list recall is that typical individuals tend to cluster (i.e. recall in sequence) items that are drawn from the same semantic category (Bousfield, 1953), and this clustering usually yields higher overall recall than for uncategorised lists. If the same list is presented repeatedly over several trials, then recall on each trial increases (*free recall learning*), and if the list is uncategorised, then participants will typically impose their own *subjective organisation* on the material, irrespective of the organisation of the studied list (Tulving, 1962). Assessments of phenomena such as these in ASD have yielded a characteristically distinct pattern of observations.

Free recall of uncategorised material in individuals with ASD is usually undiminished (Bowler *et al.* 1997; Minshew and Goldstein, 1993; 2001; Tager-Flusberg, 1991) unless there is concomitant intellectual disability (see Boucher and Lewis, 1989; Boucher and Warrington, 1976). In terms of the classic serial position effect, individuals with LFA tend to show diminished primacy and enhanced recency effects compared with typical controls (Boucher, 1978; 1981; O'Connor and Hermelin, 1967; Renner *et al.* 2000) whereas HFA individuals generally show typical serial position effects (Bowler *et al.* 2000b; Toichi and Kamio, 2002). The latter finding, however, needs to be interpreted with some caution since a recent study by Bowler *et al.* (2009) showed that the primacy effect of HFA participants shows a slower improvement over successive trials than that of typical individuals. This raises the possibility that the primacy effect observed on a single trial, although superficially similar between typical and HFA participants, may be mediated by qualitatively different processes.

The idea that memory operates in a qualitatively different manner in ASD and typical individuals is also evident in other memory phenomena. For instance, on later trials of multi-trial list learning, adults with HFA show slower rates of learning (Bennetto *et al.* 1996; Bowler *et al.* 2008a). Diminished learning is often a sign that participants fail to subjectively organise material for effective recall but surprisingly, individuals with ASD engage in such organisation to a similar extent as do typical participants (Bowler *et al.* 2008a). Individuals with ASD do, however, seem to engage in qualitatively different forms of subjective organisation. More specifically, while typical participants tend to converge in the way in which they organise a repeatedly presented list of words during their recall attempts (for example, by grouping items semantically or associatively), participants with ASD do not, indicating that their subjective organisation follows a rather idiosyncratic pattern. Differences in how memory operates in typical and ASD individuals are even more obvious when the to-be-remembered material is semantically interrelated. Typical individuals consistently exhibit a memory advantage for more meaningful information but in ASD this phenomenon seems to depend on the nature of the task. Failure to use semantic aspects of study lists to aid free recall has long been known to be a feature of memory in LFA and HFA (Bowler *et al.* 1997; 2000b; Hermelin and O'Connor, 1970; Tager-Flusberg, 1991; but see Leekam and Lopez, 2003). Moreover, individuals from all parts of the autism spectrum are less likely to cluster semantically related items together in recall (Bowler *et al.* 2010; Hermelin and O'Connor, 1967). When category-cued recall or recognition procedures are employed, however, individuals with ASD often exhibit a relatively typical memory advantage for semantically interrelated materials (Boucher and Warrington, 1976; Bowler *et al.* 2008b; Mottron *et al.* 2001; Tager-Flusberg, 1991; Toichi and Kamio, 2002). These more supported test procedures generally seem to prove less difficult for individuals with ASD (e.g. Bennetto *et al.* 1996; Bowler *et al.* 1997; Gardiner *et al.* 2003; Tager-Flusberg, 1991), suggesting that whatever processes are involved in free recall situations pose a particular difficulty for them. Individuals with ASD are, nonetheless, susceptible to associatively induced illusions using the Deese, Roediger, McDermott DRM paradigm (Deese, 1959; Roediger and McDermott, 1995) regardless of whether recognition or free recall procedures are employed. During the DRM paradigm, participants study a series of strong semantic associates of a non-studied word (e.g. *bed*, *snooze*, *blanket*, *pillow*, *night*... all of which are strong associates of *sleep*), which often leads them to falsely recall or recognise the non-studied associate during a test phase. Two out of three studies (Bowler *et al.* 2000b; Hillier *et al.* 2007) found that adults with HFA were as likely as typical participants to falsely recognise the non-studied associate and in the Bowler *et al.* (2000b) study the authors also failed to find significant group differences in a free recall test. The third study (Beversdorf *et al.* 2000), using a slightly different method from the standard DRM paradigm, reported increased discrimination of non-studied items in adults with ASD as did Hillier *et al.* (2007) when pictorial stimuli were used.

The final source of evidence, which suggests that memory operates differently in ASD, stems from a series of recent studies that have investigated whether individuals with ASD, like typical participants, remember emotionally significant information better than emotionally neutral information (see Reisberg and Hertel, 2004 and Uttl *et al.* 2006 for reviews). The first study to investigate this phenomenon in ASD (Beversdorf *et al.* 1998) asked adults with and without ASD to try to remember a series of emotionally charged and neutral statements (e.g. 'He talks about death' vs. 'He is talking with his roommate') for a subsequent free recall test. The results showed that only the typical comparison group recalled the emotionally charged statements significantly better than the neutral ones despite the fact that groups did not differ in terms of their recall of sentences and paragraphs that varied in terms of their syntactic and conceptual coherence. Recent studies have extended this finding. In one of these, Gaigg and Bowler (2008) presented participants with a list of words containing emotionally charged and neutral words and asked them to rate how emotionally intense they felt about them. During study, skin conductance responses, which index the extent to which participants are physiologically stimulated by the study material, were also measured. After participants had seen all the words, their free recall was tested at three points in time – immediately after they had seen the words, again after an hour and once more after at least one day. The findings showed that while groups did not differ in terms of their ratings of the words, their skin conductance responses to the words or their free recall performance on the immediate test, forgetting rates of emotional words over time were different in the ASD group. In a second experiment, Gaigg and Bowler (2009) employed a variant of the DRM illusion task developed by Pesta *et al.* (2001) in order to determine the extent to which it would be possible to induce false memories of emotionally charged words in individuals with ASD. Unlike typical participants who were far less likely to falsely recognise emotionally charged as compared to neutral words, those with ASD falsely recognised emotional and neutral words at roughly the same frequency. Finally, Deruelle *et al.* (2008) have recently shown that memory for pictorial stimuli is also atypically modulated by emotional factors in ASD. In that study individuals were asked to remember a series of positive, negative and neutral images and on a subsequent yes/no recognition test only the typical comparison group exhibited enhanced memory for the emotionally charged pictures. Only one study to date has failed to demonstrate differences between ASD and typical participants in their memories for emotionally charged stimuli and interestingly this study also employed a recognition test procedure albeit for verbal rather than pictorial stimuli (South *et al.* 2008). Recognition procedures generally pose few difficulties for individuals with ASD (Barth *et al.* 1995; Bennetto *et al.* 1996; Bowler *et al.* 2000a; 2000b; 2007; Minshew *et al.* 2001; but see Bowler *et al.* 2004)[1] and, in the context of verbal material, use of recognition procedures has been found to attenuate group differences in the use of semantic relations among study words to facilitate memory (e.g. Bowler *et al.* 2008b). Thus, the absence of group differences in the South *et al.* (2008) study may not

[1] Individuals with LFA sometimes do exhibit difficulties on tests of recognition (Ameli *et al.* 1988; Barth *et al.* 1995; Summers and Craik, 1994) although this seems to depend on the precise nature of the recognition procedure used. What is needed to settle this question is a systematic evaluation of the effects of procedural and participant characteristics on recognition memory.

necessarily indicate preserved influences of emotional factors on memory in ASD. In fact, Gaigg and Bowler's (2008) observation of preserved memory enhancement for emotional words in ASD on immediate but not delayed free recall procedures suggests that quantitative similarities between ASD and typical individuals may be mediated by qualitatively different processes in the two groups.

The findings outlined above show that the memory difficulties experienced by individuals with ASD are relatively subtle, and are present on tasks where minimal clues are given for recall and where information has to be manipulated or processed in some way. Before the broader implications of these observations are discussed, we need to present a further, and rather paradoxical set of findings centred on the fact that relatively spared recognition memory in ASD hides a subtle but persistent difficulty in episodic memory.

10.2.2 *Episodic memory*

Despite recognition being an aspect of memory that poses few difficulties, at least for individuals with HFA, recent research has shown that this spared capacity conceals an important difficulty with episodic memory. One of the hallmarks of human memory is the ability to re-experience oneself at the heart of the spatio-temporal context of a previously experienced episode. The ability to do this involves an awareness of self that is continuous through past, present and future, as well as an ability to recollect not only that a particular event took place but also the context in which it happened. Some of the research on memory in ASD discussed above is consistent with a prediction that individuals on the autism spectrum might have atypicalities of episodic memory. Their relatively greater difficulties on recall-based compared to recognition-based tasks points to episodic difficulties. In addition, their diminished recall of incidentally encoded context (Bennetto *et al.* 1996; Bowler *et al.* 2004; 2008b) – sometimes referred to as source memory – constitutes another strand of evidence, and the presence of frontal lobe-related executive function difficulties in ASD (see Hill, 2004a; 2004b), together with the finding of episodic memory difficulties in frontal lobe patients (Wheeler and Stuss, 2003), is a third. More indirect support comes from a theoretical perspective of Perner and colleagues (see Perner, 2001), who argue that the cardinal characteristic of episodic memory – the re-experiencing of the self at the heart of a personally experienced episode – depends on the ability to represent oneself as an experiencer of events, and to evoke that representation in memory. This *metarepresentational ability*[2] develops during the child's fourth and fifth years and according

[2] What is described here is Perner's conception of the term 'metarepresentation' (see Perner, 1991), which differs radically from that used by Leslie (e.g. Leslie, 1987), and which is also used in the context of 'theory of mind' in ASD.

to Perner, also underlies the ability to understand the behavioural consequences of false belief in others. Difficulties with false belief understanding are seen in at least some manifestations of ASD (Baron-Cohen *et al.* 1985; but see Bowler, 2007), and on Perner's arguments they should, as a consequence, experience diminished episodic remembering.

A widely used test of episodic memory is the 'Remember/Know' (R/K) procedure developed by Tulving (1985). Participants are asked to study a supra-span list of words for a later memory test. At test, they are presented with single words, half of which comprise the earlier-studied items, and are asked whether or not they had seen the word at study. If they answer 'yes', they are then asked to make either a 'remember' (R) judgement, where they can clearly recollect the episode of having studied the word, or a 'know' (K) judgement, where they simply know that they studied the item without any recollection of details of the study episode. Bowler *et al.* (2000a) utilised this procedure with adults with ASD and normal intelligence and found that the ASD group showed diminished R but not K responses by comparison with typical individuals matched on age and verbal IQ. In order to assess whether the R responses that the ASD participants did produce were the result of similar underlying processing to that of the comparison group, Bowler *et al.* (2000a) included in the study list words that are encountered in English either frequently or infrequently. Low frequency words typically yield more R responses in the R/K paradigm, and a similar pattern in the ASD group would suggest that although diminished in quantity, their R responses would be similar in quality to those of typical individuals. This is what Bowler *et al.* (2000a) found, and in a further series of studies that manipulated other factors known to affect levels of R and K responses in typical individuals, Bowler *et al.* (2007) found that adults with ASD and normal IQ responded to these manipulations in a similar manner to matched typical comparison participants. Dividing attention at study diminished R but left K responding unaffected, emphasising a perceptual set at study by asking participants to look out for blurred letters increased K responses but left R responses unaffected, and increasing number of study episodes increased R but not K responses.

The picture that emerges from the studies of Bowler *et al.* (2000a, 2007) is that individuals with ASD show quantitatively diminished but qualitatively similar experiences of episodic recollection. What remains to be established is whether this is the result of problems in re-constructing the spatio-temporal aspects of the recollected episode or in imagining the self at the heart of such recollection or of difficulties in both these factors. We will now discuss the research relating to both these possibilities as well as on the related issue of the ordering of elements of experience in time.

10.2.3 *Re-creating the spatio-temporal context of an episode*

Individual episodes are characterised by the co-occurrence of elements of experience (e.g. meeting a particular friend at a particular time of day in a particular place, etc.) that may form part of other, distinct episodes. What defines an individual episode is the combination of attributes that are unique to it. For an episode to be successfully retrieved, its elements need to be marked in such a way as to enable their subsequent retrieval as a bound unit. Bowler *et al.* (unpublished data) showed that this *relational binding* capacity is diminished in individuals with ASD. They replicated a study of Chalfonte and Johnson (1996) who asked older and younger typical adults to study sets of objects located in the cells of a grid. The objects were presented in non-canonical colours (e.g. a blue banana or a pink leaf). Participants' recognition of individual features (location, item, colour) and combinations of these features (item + location, item + colour) were then tested. Whereas older participants showed undiminished recognition of features, they were significantly poorer on recognition of combinations. Bowler *et al.* (unpublished data) found similar intact feature and diminished combination recognition in a group of HFA adults, demonstrating that they too had difficulties in recognising episodically defined bindings of elements of experience. They also found that this difficulty survived co-varying out performance on the Colour Trails Test, which is a measure of executive functioning. These findings were particularly surprising in that they demonstrate binding difficulties on a memory task – recognition – that does not usually pose problems for individuals with ASD.

It can be argued that an intact ability to re-construct the combinations of features unique to an episode and the development of an accurate sense of the temporal order of events are intimately and necessarily related. It follows from this that difficulties with the relational binding needed to recollect an episode should be accompanied by difficulties in temporal aspects of memory. There are several strands of evidence from the ASD literature that support the conjecture that this is the case in ASD. Bennetto *et al.* (1996) demonstrated diminished performance on an adaptation of the Corsi task in adolescents with ASD. This task presents participants with sequences of concrete words or line drawings. From time to time, a yellow card accompanied by a pair of previously presented items is presented and participants have to decide which of the two items had been presented more recently. Diminished performance was also reported in a serial order recall task in which Martin *et al.* (2006) asked adults with ASD to recall lists of digits that are close to their memory span. Although the number of items correctly recalled was similar to that of comparison participants, the ASD group made more order errors in recall, suggesting that they have difficulty recalling which items preceded and succeeded each recalled item. Theorists such as Brown *et al.* (2007) argue that sensitivity to such micro-contextual detail underlies successful serial recall, and its diminution in ASD further reinforces the idea that this population experiences particular difficulty in the accurate recall of the context of remembered material. The occurrence of the phenomenon in serial recall further supports the idea that accurate recall of context is needed for accurate temporal memory.

Individuals with ASD have also been shown to have difficulties in reconstructing the order of occurrence of a set of items. Gaigg *et al.* (unpublished data) asked adults with ASD and matched typical comparison participants to re-order alphabetically presented lists of seven historical figures either into their actual chronological order or into a pseudo-random order that had been studied just beforehand. Whereas performance on the first task was comparable between the two groups, the ASD participants were significantly worse on the second task, indicating that they had particular difficulty in encoding an episodically determined ordering of the studied material. Difficulty in temporally ordering recall of material is also reflected in poor performance on narrative tasks. Reported difficulties include poor narrative organisation (Losh and Capps, 2003), diminished story recall (Williams *et al.* 2006) and reduced use of temporal referential devices in narrative (Colle *et al.* 2008). In a series of tests of diachronic thinking (the ability to reason about the unfolding of events over time), Boucher *et al.* (2007) found poorer performance in children with ASD compared to matched typical children.

All these findings reinforce the long-held view (see Boucher, 2001; O'Connor and Hermelin, 1978) that individuals with ASD experience difficulties with remembering the temporal ordering of experience. The argument is made here that this problem is a consequence of difficulties with the binding together of elements of experience in episodic memory and which may have repercussions for the development of self-awareness. In a later section, we outline how such binding difficulties might have wider application to difficulties with semantic organisation as well as to episodic memory. First, we need to consider the other key aspect of episodic memory: the role of self awareness.

10.2.4 *The self and memory in ASD*

Memory and the self are thought to be intimately related. For example, it has been argued that the encoding of *autobiographical* (i.e. self-relevant) episodic memories presupposes a sufficiently elaborate self-concept (Howe and Courage, 1993). Likewise, autobiographical episodic memory allows one to re-experience past states of self, further enriching the self-concept (e.g. Conway and Pleydell-Pearce, 2000).

It is established that individuals with ASD have diminished autobiographical episodic memory (e.g. Crane and Goddard, 2008). Although such a diminution may potentially be accounted for in terms of difficulties with relational binding, it is also possible that such difficulties stem from an under-elaborated self-concept (see Lind, 2010, for a review). Although studies of mirror self-recognition (e.g. Ferrari and Matthews, 1983) and delayed video self-recognition (Lind and Bowler, 2009) indicate that individuals with ASD do possess explicit self-concepts, there is also evidence to suggest that their self-concepts may be under-elaborated in certain respects.

For example, individuals with ASD appear to have diminished awareness of their own mental states (e.g. Williams and Happé, 2009), emotional states (Ben Shalom *et al.* 2006; Gaigg and Bowler, 2008; Hill *et al.* 2004) and autistic traits (Johnson *et al.* 2009). Each of these sources of evidence suggests that individuals with ASD have reduced self-knowledge and hence under-elaborated self-concepts. More directly, using a self-understanding interview, Lee and Hobson (1998) found that individuals with ASD showed diminished self-knowledge in the social and psychological domains.

Studies of self-referential memory also shed light on these issues. Such studies typically involve asking participants to encode personality trait adjectives under self-referential (e.g. asking whether the words describe them) and non-self-referential (e.g. asking whether the words contain seven or more letters) conditions. Typical participants generally show a self-reference effect – i.e. an advantage for words encoded in the self-referential condition – and this is attributed to the fact that the self-concept is thought to act as an effective elaborative and organisational structure for memory encoding. Lombardo *et al.* (2007) and Henderson *et al.* (2009) found that individuals with ASD showed a reduced self-reference effect and this suggests that individuals with ASD have self-concepts that are under-elaborated and less effective as elaborative and organisational structures for memory encoding.

Thus, although there is no direct evidence for a causal connection between under-elaborated self-concepts and impaired autobiographical episodic memory in ASD, it is at least a plausible hypothesis. Irrespective of the underlying cause of autobiographical episodic memory impairments in ASD, the fact that such impairments exist suggests that individuals with ASD have difficulties with re-experiencing past states of self. Such a reduced awareness of past states of self implies that individuals with ASD have a diminished sense of personal history and a diminished temporally extended self (see Lind, 2010).

10.3 Wider conceptual themes

The findings reviewed so far show relatively subtle memory difficulties that tend to centre on manipulation of information in memory rather than the memory for the information itself. These difficulties tend to have greater repercussions on measures that provide less support at test (e.g. free recall) than those that do not (e.g. recognition). From the perspective of dual-store or working memory models, the findings both of span studies and on serial position effects show that difficulties seem to lie less with any of the memory storage systems and more with the central executive of the working memory system (Baddeley, 1986). Research also shows that there is particular difficulty in manipulating material in ways that enable the detail of past episodes to be re-constructed and that this interacts in some way with the 'mental time travel' that is needed for the operation of episodic recollection. And finally, the way in which memory is modulated by emotional factors operates atypically in ASD. In the following two sections, we will tease out some implications of these patterns of memory performance in an attempt to elucidate underlying processes that give rise to them. In a final section, we attempt to reconcile the empirical findings and theoretical speculations with a brain-based account.

10.3.1 *Task support*

The research reviewed so far paints a picture of difficulties in recalling material, especially when recall entails some effort, such as elucidating and manipulating semantic aspects of the material or when recall has to be enhanced over repeated trials. By contrast, fewer difficulties are seen on tasks that provide more explicit support for retrieval, such as cued recall or recognition. This particular pattern was first noted by Boucher (Boucher, 1981; Boucher and Warrington, 1976) and again by Bowler *et al.* (1997) and led to the coining of the term *Task Support Hypothesis* (TSH) by Bowler *et al.* (2004). As well as describing the patterning of memory performance across tasks in ASD, the TSH has proved to have considerable heuristic value. It has highlighted a parallel between the patterning of memory performance seen in typical ageing (Craik and Anderson, 1999) and in frontal lobe damage (Schacter, 1987) and has helped to account for some apparently contradictory findings in the literature. For example, Bennetto *et al.* (1996) reported diminished source memory in adolescents with ASD, whereas Farrant *et al.* (1998) reported no difficulties in a younger, lower-functioning group. The first study defined source memory as the number of intrusions from an earlier-learned list into the recall of a later list, whereas the second defined it in terms of children's capacity to indicate whether they themselves or the experimenter had spoken a given word at study. Bowler *et al.* (2004) noticed that the first study involved an unsupported measure of source, whereas the second involved a supported test. On this basis, they devised two experiments in which HFA participants studied lists of words, which were either presented in one of four ways, or which the participant had to manipulate in one of four ways. At test, participants were given a yes/no recognition test and if they said 'yes' to a test word, were asked either to select the means of presentation or the kind of action from a list on the screen (supported test), or else simply to recall what it was (unsupported test). The results showed no HFA-comparison group difference on the supported test, but diminished performance in the ASD group on the unsupported test, thus extending to source memory the view that memory is particularly difficult for people with ASD when unsupported test procedures are used. A similar role for task support on memory for incidentally encoded context was demonstrated by Bowler *et al.* (2008b). Participants with and without HFA studied a series of words on a screen. Each word was surrounded by a red rectangle, outside of which was another word that was either strongly or not at all associated with the word inside the frame. Participants were told to ignore the words outside the frame. Later testing used either a free recall or a four-option forced-choice procedure. In each case, participants were told to try to remember all words they had seen, whether inside or outside the frame. The results showed that associative relatedness between studied and incidentally encoded words (those inside and outside the frame respectively) benefitted both groups' recognition but enhanced recall only in the typical group. Both these studies show that supported test procedures yield better memory than unsupported procedures for incidentally encoded context as well as for incidentally encoded item–context relations.

The TSH paints a picture of memory in ASD as being heavily influenced by the here-and-now. This would suggest less 'top-down' processing in which stored representations influence how incoming information is interpreted. The diminished use of semantic structure to aid recall described earlier, together with demonstrations of diminished top-down processing in visual perception (see Mitchell and Ropar, 2004 for review) provide converging evidence that individuals with ASD store information in ways that are less likely to influence the processing of later, new information. The question now arises of why stored information is less effective in modulating the processing of incoming information in ASD, thus yielding a behavioural reliance on task support.

10.3.2 *Relational processing difficulties*

Research on episodic memory in people with ASD strongly supports the idea that they experience difficulty in processing relations among elements of experience. Understanding this difficulty can be enhanced by a more detailed consideration of the parallel problem that they sometimes experience in utilising semantic relations among studied items in order to enhance their recall. As we have already seen, failure to use meaning to aid recall has long been known to be a characteristic of ASD (Bowler *et al.* 1997; 2000a; Hermelin and O'Connor, 1970; Smith *et al.* 2007; Tager-Flusberg, 1991; but see Leekam and Lopez, 2003), yet performance on other tasks that rely on semantic processing seems relatively unimpaired. We have already mentioned that people with ASD perform as well as typical individuals on category-cued recall (Boucher and Warrington, 1976; Mottron *et al.* 2001; Tager-Flusberg, 1991; Toichi and Kamio, 2002), suggesting some ability to use meaningfulness to aid memory. One way to account for these apparently contradictory findings is to invoke the TSH, since semantic relatedness appears to be a problem only when less supported test procedures are used. This argument is further supported by Bowler *et al.*'s (2008b) observation that whereas relatedness between studied words and context enhanced recognition and recall of studied items for typical individuals, it enhanced only recognition for ASD adults of normal IQ. Thus, we can see that the requirement to engage in semantic processing is more likely to adversely affect memory in individuals with ASD when unsupported task procedures are utilised.

This account is problematic in that it merely describes and does not explain *why* support is needed for semantic processing. It may simply be that the two phenomena are opposite sides of the same coin. One way to go beyond description is to invoke the distinction between *item-specific processing* and *relational processing*. Item-specific processing refers to a tendency to focus on individual items of information without reference to relations among them. Item-specific processing has been shown to contribute heavily to performance on tests of recognition (Anderson and Bower, 1972), on which individuals with ASD perform well. Their pattern of performance on depth-of-processing tasks (for example, where memory is enhanced if studied words have to be rated on deeper, often semantic aspects such as asking if it is a fruit, rather than on shallower features such as number of vowels) also suggests that they perform as well as comparison participants on deeper processing tasks and better on shallower processing tasks (Toichi and Kamio, 2002; Toichi, 2008). The pattern of performance on the two processing levels suggests that individuals with ASD, unlike typical individuals, process words in the two conditions in a similar manner, one, moreover, at which they are highly proficient. It can be argued that this is likely to be an item-specific strategy, since it is difficult to see how shallow tasks could be accomplished by recourse to a relational strategy. More direct evidence on this question comes from a study by Gaigg *et al.* (2008), who adopted a procedure developed by Hunt and Seta (1984) in which participants studied lists of words drawn from a number of different categories. Some categories were represented by only 2 exemplars, whereas others had 4, 8, 12 or 16. Whereas typical comparison participants recalled similar proportions of items from small as from large categories, adults with ASD recalled far fewer items from the smaller categories. Following Hunt and Seta (1984), Gaigg *et al.* (2008) argue that this is because identification of exemplars from smaller categories requires alertness to semantic relations among items. By contrast, ability to recall individual exemplars from large (i.e. frequently represented) categories requires alertness to the unique features of each item. Moreover, Gaigg *et al.* (2008) found that whereas provision of a relational orienting task (sorting words into categories) enhanced the recall of the typical individuals, it did so for the ASD group to a lesser extent. Provision of an item-specific orienting task (rating word pleasantness) had similar effects on recall for both groups. Gaigg *et al.*'s findings are consistent with the view that whereas typical individuals have both relational and item-specific processing strategies at their disposal when performing memory tasks, individuals with ASD are dependent to a greater extent on item-specific processing alone. This would explain not only the patterning of performance across tasks described at the start of this chapter but also the greater reliance on task support seen in ASD. A focus on individual items of information diminishes relational semantic information available to aid recall, and diminishes the amount of related contextual information that can be drawn on to re-create episodic recollections and their associated self-involved states of conscious awareness.

Two caveats are in order concerning the foregoing account. The first is that we should be wary in attributing an *absence* of relational processing in ASD. It may simply be the case that the balance between the two types of processing is different in this population. The second, more serious concern, is that there exist tasks that appear to involve relational processing (deeper levels-of-processing manipulations, susceptibility to associatively generated memory illusions) that are, nevertheless, relatively unproblematic for individuals with ASD. To avoid inconvenient, *post hoc* attempts to accommodate these findings, we need a more principled theoretical account of the relational processing difficulties seen in ASD.

A speculative, yet empirically testable way to explain why relational processing difficulties are more likely to be seen on some tasks but not on others is through a detailed analysis of the demands that different memory tasks place on participants. When participants engage in free recall of a categorised list, in order for them to become aware of the categorical nature of the studied items, they have to consider each in relation to other words on the list (e.g. *cat with dog* or *apple*) and then to relate this comparison to higher order category labels (*animal*, *fruit*). Contrast this with the situation in a classic memory illusions experiment (e.g. Bowler *et al.* 2000b) described in an earlier section. Here, when participants study associates of a non-studied word, they are highly likely to remember the non-studied associate because it is activated by each of the studied items (e.g. bed-*sleep*, night-*sleep*, pillow-*sleep*, . . .). The operations required of the participant in the case of recall of the categorised list involve three-way processing between pairs of words and their hierarchical categories, whereas the illusory memories require only two-way processing between a studied item and its associate. On this analysis, what seems to pose particular difficulty for individuals with ASD is the complexity of the memory task. Task complexity in relation to typical children's development has been explored in detail by Halford (1992) who argues that cognitive development proceeds from a stage where individual items are processed in isolation (*unary relations*) followed by the processing of items in a pair-wise fashion (*binary relations*) and finally by the ability to process three-way or *ternary* relations among triplets of items.

Although the above analysis of memory in ASD is consistent with Halford's (1992) relational complexity account, it needs further confirmation by more systematic, hypothesis led investigations. Nevertheless, it is corroborated by evidence from other areas of psychological functioning in ASD. Andrews *et al.* (2003) report that the standard 'Sally-Anne' false belief task on which children with ASD are characteristically delayed (Baron-Cohen *et al.* 1985) correlates highly with performance on tasks of ternary relational processing, and Bowler *et al.* (2005) report similar levels of delay in children with ASD on a non-social task of complex reasoning and the Sally-Anne task. Both tasks are consistent with a ternary processing analysis, suggesting that it is the processing complexity and not the mental state nature of the Sally-Anne task that poses particular difficulty for the children with ASD.

Difficulty in processing three-way relations is also a theme that recurs in two of the major theoretical accounts of the development of ASD. Early in development, infants who fail to engage in joint attention behaviours are almost certainly on an autistic developmental trajectory. Joint attention, which involves children's co-ordinating attention between themselves, an object and another person involves what Bakeman and Adamson (1984) refer to as *triadic deployment of attention*. A similar conceptualisation of the child's relation between self, other and objects of shared attention is put forward by Hobson (1993), who argues that the core of autism is a difficulty with the patterning of affectively charged interactions with other people. Earlier on we saw how difficulties with emotion spill over into the memory performance of individuals with ASD. But Hobson's characterisation of the structure of interpersonal relatedness and its role in the development of symbolic understanding also invokes the child's developing awareness of themselves in relation to another person and to objects to which both themselves and that person also stand in relation (see Hobson, 1993, pp. 140–153 and Chapter 8 of this volume). In a similar vein, albeit from a radically different theoretical perspective, Leslie's (1987) analysis of children's understanding of pretence and mental state representation emphasises the importance of the child's developing awareness of *action-centred representations*, metarepresentations or M-representations (Leslie and Roth, 1993). This development marks an enlargement of the child's conception of objects from one which considers their true identity (e.g. a banana as a piece of fruit) to one where they can also be defined in terms of the pretend actions of an agent (e.g. Mummy pretends that the banana is a telephone). This last development involves the child's being able to coordinate its own relation to the object with that of another person's relation to it in the context of a playful interpersonal exchange. Both Leslie and Hobson see autism as resulting from a breakdown in their respective systems, and the position advocated here is that the two systems may be different manifestations of a wider difficulty with processing ternary relations, which also has repercussions in the domain of memory.

A further advantage of adopting Halford's relational complexity account is that it elaborates on a position first advocated by Minshew and her colleagues (Minshew *et al.* 2001) who argue that autism is a disorder of complex information processing. This position makes intuitive sense when the pattern of performance across memory tasks identified by Minshew and colleagues is considered, but runs the risk of circularity by defining any task that poses difficulty for people with ASD as being 'complex', without establishing any *a priori* criteria for what constitutes complexity. Relational complexity allows predictions to be made in advance about which tasks should be easy and which difficult for individuals with ASD. In addition, its resonance with other behavioural characteristics of ASD suggests that difficulties with ternary relations may be a pervasive cause of a range of psychological atypicalities in this population.

Finally, readers of this section may be tempted to draw parallels between our account of relational processing difficulties and the Weak Central Coherence (WCC) theory put forward by Frith and Happé (Happé and Frith, 2006 – see Chapter 7 in this volume). However, the two approaches differ in a number of respects. For example, the way they envision how elements are processed both singly and in combination has knock-on effects for the kinds of predictions the two accounts make. Our account emphasises the processes that enable an individual to constitute complex representations, often on the basis of limited exposure. This process-oriented view has the potential to provide a developmental description of how people with ASD build representations of their experience in the world and formulates testable hypotheses about the kinds of complexity that people with ASD might find difficult. WCC theory by contrast locates complexity or 'wholeness' in the stimulus and characterises individuals with ASD as being intrinsically more detail-focused and consequently less aware of wholes. This leads WCC theory, for example, to predict that individuals with ASD would be less susceptible to memory illusions because of their tendency to focus on the detail of individual words to the detriment of global relations among them. Our theory of diminished relational processing, by contrast, predicts that it is only when the relational complexity of the inter-item relations crosses the threshold from binary to ternary relations that individuals with ASD experience memory difficulties. Relations below that threshold (as is the case with memory illusions) tend not to pose problems.

10.4 Memory and the brain

An important development in the typical memory literature in recent years has been an increasing refinement of our understanding of how the brain mediates our capacity to remember the past. In combination with our growing knowledge of memory in ASD, this development can help to enhance our understanding of functional and structural brain atypicalities in that population. The literature on structural brain atypicalities in ASD is converging on four broad themes. First, studies of brain size indicate that the brains of infants with ASD are often larger than normal and that the developmental trajectory of brain size is atypical (Akshoomoff *et al.* 2002; Aylward *et al.* 2002; Courchesne *et al.* 2001). Second, neurological abnormalities at the cellular level have been reported for the cerebellum, the frontal cortex and certain medial temporal lobe (MTL) structures such as the hippocampus and the amygdala (see Bachevalier, 2000; Bauman and Kemper, 2005; Casanova *et al.* 2002; DiCicco-Bloom *et al.* 2006; Palmen *et al.* 2004 for relevant reviews). Third, functional imaging studies indicate abnormalities in these same regions, particularly MTL structures and the frontal lobes (e.g. Bachevalier and Loveland, 2006). Finally, behavioural and neuroscientific evidence is starting to converge on the idea that MTL structures and the frontal lobes are characterised by abnormalities in their functional connectivity with one another and with other areas of the brain (e.g. Bachevalier and Loveland, 2006; Gaigg and Bowler, 2007; Just *et al.* 2007; Rippon *et al.* 2007). It is perhaps no coincidence that two of the three brain regions that manifest greatest structural abnormalities in ASD are also those that are implicated in memory, especially those aspects of memory that appear to operate atypically in this population. Although we should be careful about seeing 'memory' as residing in one or more specific areas of the brain (see Graham *et al.* (2008) for discussion), there is now a broad consensus that declarative memory is mediated by frontal and MTL structures (see Brown and Aggleton, 2001 for review).

Support for some frontal involvement in memory in ASD is evidenced by the greater need of these individuals for task support in memory. The need for task support is also a characteristic of memory in typically ageing individuals, especially those in whom there is a suspicion of frontal lobe dysfunction evidenced by diminished performance on executive function tasks (Craik and Anderson, 1999; Craik *et al.* 1990). Similarly, patients with acquired frontal lobe damage also show a pattern of performance across memory tasks that is not dissimilar to that seen in people with ASD (Schacter, 1987). More specifically, such frontal lobe patients exhibit difficulties with minimally cued recall and episodic memory tasks while their performance on tests of recognition memory is undiminished. Together with the literature on executive dysfunction in ASD (see Hill (2004a; 2004b) for reviews), this parallel between ASD, typically aging and frontal lobe patients provides converging evidence for frontal dysfunction as a component of memory difficulty in ASD.

Although the arguments for frontal contributions to memory in ASD are strong, there is increasing evidence pointing to the involvement of other brain areas. In typically developed individuals, the most severe memory disorders result from damage to the medial temporal lobes, especially the hippocampus and associated structures of the ento- and perirhinal cortices and the amygdala (see Mayes and Boucher, 2008 for review). It was this observation that led Boucher and colleagues (Boucher, 1981; Boucher and Warrington, 1976) to suggest that autism might be a variant of the amnesic syndrome and as such would involve medial temporal structures. In the period since this earlier work, which was carried out mostly in children with severe and low-functioning ASD, this view has been less and less advocated (see, for example, Bowler *et al.* 1997). The reason for this change is partly because it is evident that individuals with ASD are not amnesic in the same way as individuals with severe temporal lobe damage are, but also because our conception of 'autism' has enlarged to a spectrum view that encompasses subtler forms of the condition and includes individuals of normal cognitive and language ability and who therefore present subtler forms of memory difficulty. Nevertheless, the most recent empirical findings are prompting a return to a consideration of medial temporal lobe structures as contributing to atypical memory in ASD.

The capacity to recollect context implies that the disparate elements that constitute an episode have to be bound together in memory in a way that enables subsequent retrieval. There is now considerable evidence that this relational binding is mediated by the hippocampus (Brown and Aggleton, 2001), while related medial temporal lobe structures such as the perirhinal and entorhinal cortices mediate the processing of individual elements. As noted in the previous section, the patterning of memory in ASD suggests that such individuals experience difficulties in processing relations among elements of experiences in memory while their processing of the individual elements seems preserved. Recall, for instance, the observation of diminished recognition of episodically defined combinations of elements in the presence of undiminished recognition of the individual elements themselves (Bowler *et al.*, unpublished data) or of diminished influence of item-context relatedness on recall but not on recognition of context (Bower *et al.* 2008b), or the finding that individuals with ASD experience relatively specific difficulties in drawing on relations amongst words to facilitate recall while their use of information specific to individual words is undiminished (Gaigg *et al.* 2008). All of these findings, together with the general difficulties in episodic memory characterising ASD, strongly suggest compromised hippocampal and spared perirhinal and entorhinal functioning in this population. In addition, this framework is compatible with the analysis of complexity by Halford (1992) and thus provides a useful starting point for investigating the importance of relational information in other cognitive domains such as 'Theory of Mind' and logical reasoning. Many theorists argue that an important function of the hippocampus is the ability to encode objects, events and relations among them rapidly and in a way that allows the adaptive use of encoded information in different settings (Eichenbaum, 2000). This ability is evidenced by tasks such as *Transitive Inference* (TI) in which an individual can infer that A > C having been told that A > B and B > C. TI performance is reflected in hippocampal activation (Greene *et al.* 2006), is sensitive to hippocampal damage and is impaired in people with amnesia (Smith and Squire, 2005). On the basis of the arguments presented here on diminished relational processing in ASD, we would predict diminished TI performance in this population and, moreover, would predict that TI performance would correlate both with those aspects of semantic organisation of material – clustering and the use of categories to aid recall – that pose difficulty for people with ASD, and with measures of binding and memory as well as measures of episodic remembering.

In an earlier section, we noted that an important characteristic of episodic memory is an awareness of self in time. Although the evidence from the domain of memory does not suggest that abnormalities in the experience of such temporally extended self-awareness are solely responsible for the episodic memory difficulties evident in ASD, abnormalities in this domain may nevertheless contribute to it. Given the close relation between self-awareness and episodic remembering, it is therefore possible, and perhaps even likely, that neural correlates of self-awareness are compromised in ASD. There is currently considerable debate about the neural correlates of self-awareness (see Feinberg and Keenan, 2005; Keenan *et al.* 2005; LeDoux, 2002; Morin, 2005) and although some recent studies suggest abnormalities in this domain in ASD (Chiu *et al.* 2008) more work is clearly needed before one can draw any conclusions.

Although the patterning of memory functioning in ASD is consistent with the idea that it stems from hippocampal dysfunction, albeit with some frontal involvement, it does not follow that such atypical function results from hippocampal damage *per se*. The hippocampus receives rich sensory information from a range of cortical and sub-cortical areas of the brain via the entorhinal cortex, which in turn relays information from the hippocampus back to a host of cortical areas (e.g. Squire, 1992). This arrangement is ideal for its function in relation to episodic memory and relational processing as it is in a position (literally) to integrate information processed in various different parts of the cortex and also modulate the processing of information in those cortical areas accordingly. It also means, however, that the patterning of memory functioning in ASD is not necessarily a reflection of hippocampal dysfunction *per se* but could also be the result of atypical connectivity between the hippocampus and functionally associated areas. Or the information flowing along those pathways could be abnormal. Both the empirical and theoretical literature offer some support for these possibilities. As mentioned above, a considerable amount of evidence suggests that disparate brain areas are abnormally connected in ASD (e.g. Rippon *et al.* 2007) suggesting that the hippocampus may receive inadequate input, or may have difficulty in adequately transmitting outputs. The finding that emotional arousal atypically modulates forgetting in ASD (Gaigg and Bowler, 2008) is particularly relevant in this context, since such modulation is widely thought to be mediated by interactions between the amygdala and the hippocampus (e.g. Hamann, 2001). It is also possible that the information from primary sensory areas that is marked for bound representation by the hippocampus is atypical because of compromised functioning in those areas. This account has resonances with the *Enhanced Perceptual Functioning* model of ASD advocated by Mottron and colleagues (Mottron *et al.* 2006). Their argument is that the processing of information by people with ASD is characterised by the retention of lower-level perceptual features that remain available even when higher-level, conceptual processing has taken place. This has consequences in situations where typical individuals process in a predominantly global or conceptual manner. In such situations, individuals with ASD may tend to process perceptually rather than conceptually, even when both options are available, often producing atypical performance patterns. There is some evidence that this happens in memory. Bowler *et al.* (2008a) found that adults with ASD showed less inter-individual convergence of subjective organisation of unrelated words than did typical individuals, suggesting that whereas the latter group organised words along semantic/associative lines, the ASD group may, in addition to this strategy, have organised the words along more perceptual features such as phonology or number of syllables. What is needed to confirm this account is a series of demonstrations of enhanced perceptual influence on psychological processes other than memory.

The argument just outlined leaves open the possibility that atypical hippocampal function may be the result of structural or functional problems elsewhere in the brain, which modify information fed to the hippocampus. But it ignores one fundamental aspect of ASD, namely that it is fundamentally a *developmental* problem, that is to say it affects the trajectory of development of the individual in a way that yields an atypical endpoint. We can reasonably expect this atypical developmental trajectory to be as evident in brain structures as in adaptive behaviour. So, for example, it may be the case that enhanced perceptual functioning may feed information to the hippocampus in a manner that influences the bindings it makes, and that these different bindings in turn affect the way in which the hippocampus develops and influences processing in other brain areas. There is some evidence from the neuroimaging literature that is consistent with this position. Schumann *et al.* (2004) report atypical development of the hippocampus in children and adolescents across the autism spectrum. They also report atypicalities in the development of the amygdala in these groups. As we have seen, the amygdala plays an important role in emotional memory. In view of the connectivity between the hippocampus and the amygdala (Smith *et al.* 2006), it can be argued that diminished emotional modulation of memory in ASD is a specific aspect of more general difficulties with binding in memory.

10.5 Conclusions

It is now well established that ASD is characterised by a particular pattern of spared and impaired performance across different memory tasks. This pattern points to difficulties in the processing of information in ways that require binding of those elements of experience that uniquely define episodes, in the flexible relations among features that can be organised hierarchically, and in the emotional modulation of memory. Processing of individual items by contrast is relatively spared. All these types of processing implicate different structures of the medial temporal lobe of the brain, most particularly the hippocampus, the amygdala and the entorhinal and perirhinal cortices, as well as modulation of the functioning of these areas by the frontal lobes. Although these implications have yet to be systematically tested, they are consistent with the current state of knowledge of the development of these structures in the autistic brain. What also needs to be established is the extent to which atypical developmental trajectories in these structures are the outcome of abnormal input resulting from atypical processing in other brain areas or from some initial damage to the structures themselves. As well as providing a framework within which to test neural underpinnings of psychological underpinnings in ASD, the behavioural findings in memory also provide a window into the inner experience of these individuals by showing that they have diminished self-involvement in their memories for past experience and that the quality of these experiences, the connections that the individual makes between experiences and the here-and-now consequences of a particular memory can at times be radically different from those of a typical individual.

10.6 Acknowledgements

The authors would like to acknowledge the financial support of the Medical Research Council (UK) and Autism Speaks during the preparation of this chapter.

10.7 References

Akshoomoff, N., Pierce, K., Courchesne, E. (2002). The neurobiological basis of autism from a developmental perspective. *Development and Psychopathology*, **14**: 613–634.

Ameli, R., Courchesne, E., Lincoln, A., Kaufman, A.S., Grillon, C. (1988). Visual memory processes in high-functioning individuals with autism. *Journal of Autism and Developmental Disorders*, **18**: 601–615.

Anderson, J.R., Bower, G.H. (1972). Recognition and retrieval processes in free-recall. *Psychological Review*, **79**: 97–123.

Andrews, G., Halford, G.S., Bunch, K.M., Bowden, D., Jones, T. (2003). Theory of mind and relational complexity. *Child Development*, **74**: 1476–1499.

Aylward, E.H., Minshew, J.J., Field, K., Sparks, B.F., Singh, N. (2002). Effects of age on brain volume and head circumference in autism. *Neurology*, **59**: 175–183.

Bachevalier, J. (2000). The amygdala, social behaviour, and autism. In *The Amygdala*, 2nd edn. Oxford: Oxford University Press, pp. 509–543.

Bachevalier, J., Loveland, K.A. (2006). The orbito-frontal-amygdala circuit and self-regulation of social-emotional behaviour in autism. *Neuroscience and Biobehavioural Reviews*, **30**: 97–117.

Baddeley, A.D. (1986). *Working Memory*. Oxford: Clarendon Press.

Baddeley, A.D., Hitch, G. (1974). Working memory. In *The Psychology of Learning and Motivation*, Volume 8. New York: Academic Press, pp. 47–90.

Bakeman, R., Adamson, L. (1984). Co-ordinating attention to people and objects in mother-infant and peer-infant interaction. *Child Development*, **55**: 1278–1289.

Baron-Cohen, S., Leslie, A., Frith, U. (1985). Does the autistic child have a 'theory of mind'? *Cognition*, **21**: 37–46.

Barth, C., Fein, D., Waterhouse, L. (1995). Delayed match-to-sample performance in autistic children. *Developmental Neuropsychology*, **11**: 53–69.

Bauman, M.L., Kemper, T.L. (2005). Neuroanatomic observations of the brain in autism: a review and future directions. *International Journal of Developmental Neuroscience*, **23**: 183–187.

Ben Shalom, D., Mostofsky, S.H., Hazlett, R.L. *et al.* (2006). Normal physiological emotions but differences in expression of conscious feelings in children with high-functioning autism. *Journal of Autism and Developmental Disorders*, **36**: 395–400.

Bennetto, L., Pennington, B.F., Rogers, S.J. (1996). Intact and impaired memory function in autism. *Child Development*, **67**: 1816–1835.

Beversdorf, D.Q., Anderson, J.M., Manning, S.E., *et al.* (1998). The effect of semantic and emotional context on written recall for verbal language in high-functioning adults with autism spectrum disorder. *Journal of Neurology, Neurosurgery, and Psychiatry*, **65**: 685–692.

Beversdorf, D.Q., Smith, B.W., Crucian, G.P., *et al.* (2000). Increased discrimination of 'false memories' in autism spectrum disorder. *Proceedings of the National Academy of Sciences USA*, **97**: 8734–8737.

Bjork, R.A., Whitten, W.B. (1974). Recency-sensitive retrieval processes in long-term free recall. *Cognitive Psychology*, **6**: 173–189.

Boucher, J. (1978). Echoic memory capacity in autistic children. *Journal of Child Psychology and Psychiatry*, **19**: 161–166.

Boucher, J. (1981). Immediate free recall in early childhood autism: Another point of behavioural similarity with the amnesic syndrome. *British Journal of Psychology*, **72**: 211–215.

Boucher, J. (2001). Lost in a sea of time. In *Time and Memory: Issues in Philosophy and Psychology*. Oxford: Oxford University Press, pp 111–135.

Boucher, J., Lewis, V. (1989). Memory impairments and communication in relatively able autistic children. *Journal of Child Psychology and Psychiatry*, **30**: 99–122.

Boucher, J., Warrington, E.K. (1976). Memory deficits in early infantile autism: some similarities to the amnesic syndrome. *British Journal of Psychology*, **67**: 73–87.

Boucher, J., Pons, F., Lind, S., Williams, D. (2007). Temporal cognition in children with autistic spectrum disorders: Tests of diachronic perspective taking. *Journal of Autism and Developmental Disorders*, **37**: 1413–1429.

Bousfield, W.A. (1953). The occurrence of clustering in the recall of randomly arranged associates. *The Journal of General Psychology*, **49**: 229–240.

Bowler, D.M. (2007). *Autism Spectrum Disorders: Psychological Theory and Research*. Chichester: Wiley.

Bowler, D.M., Matthews, N.J., Gardiner, J.M. (1997). Asperger's syndrome and memory: Similarity to autism but not amnesia. *Neuropsychologia*, **35**: 65–70.

Bowler, D.M., Gardiner, J.M., Grice, S. (2000a). Episodic memory and remembering in adults with Asperger's syndrome. *Journal of Autism and Developmental Disorders*, **30**: 305–316.

Bowler, D.M., Gardiner, J.M., Grice, S., Saavalainen, P. (2000b). Memory illusions: false recall and recognition in high functioning adults with autism. *Journal of Abnormal Psychology*, **109**: 663–672.

Bowler, D.M., Gardiner, J.M., Berthollier, N. (2004). Source memory in Asperger's syndrome. *Journal of Autism and Developmental Disorders*, **34**: 533–542.

Bowler, D.M., Briskman, J.A., Gurvidi, N., Fornells-Ambrojo, M. (2005). Autistic and non-autistic children's performance on a non-social analogue of the false belief task. *Journal of Cognition and Development*, **6**: 259–283.

Bowler, D.M., Gardiner, J.M., Gaigg, S.B. (2007). Factors affecting conscious awareness in the recollective experience of adults with Asperger's syndrome. *Consciousness and Cognition*, **16**: 124–143.

Bowler, D.M., Gaigg, S.B., Gardiner, J.M. (2008a). Subjective organisation in the free recall of adults with Asperger's syndrome. *Journal of Autism and Developmental Disorders*, **38**: 104–113.

Bowler, D.M., Gaigg, S.B., Gardiner, J.M. (2008b). Effects of related and unrelated context on recall and recognition by adults with high-functioning autism spectrum disorder. *Neuropsychologia*, **46**: 993–999.

Bowler, D.M., Limoges, E., Mottron, L. (2009). Different verbal learning strategies in high-functioning autism: evidence from the Rey Auditory Verbal Learning Test. *Journal of Autism and Developmental Disorders*, **39**: 910–915.

Bowler, D.M., Gaigg, S.B., Gardiner, J.M. (2010). Multiple list learning in adults with autism spectrum disorder: parallels with frontal lobe damage or further evidence of diminished relational processing? *Journal of Autism and Developmental Disorders*, **40**: 179–187.

Bray, N.W., Fletcher, K.L., Turner, L.A. (1997). Cognitive competencies and strategy use in individuals with mental retardation. In *Ellis' Handbook of Mental Deficiency, Psychological Theory and Research*, 3rd edn. Mahwah, NJ: Erlbaum, pp 197–217.

Brown, G.D.A., Neath, I., Chater, N. (2007). A temporal ratio model of memory. *Psychological Review*, **114**: 539–576.

Brown, M.W., Aggleton, J.P. (2001). Recognition memory: what are the roles of the perirhinal cortex and hippocampus? *Nature Reviews: Neurosciences*, **2**: 51–61.

Casanova, M.F., Buxhoeveden, D.P., Switala, A.E., Roy, E. (2002). Minicolumnar pathology in autism. *Neurology*, **58**: 428–432.

Chalfonte, B.L., Johnson, M.K. (1996). Feature memory and binding in young and older adults. *Memory and Cognition*, **24**: 403–416.

Chiu, P.H., Kayali, M.A., Kishida, K.T., *et al.* (2008). Self responses along cingulated cortex reveal quantitative neural phenotype for high-functioning autism. *Neuron*, **57**: 463–473.

Colle, L., Baron-Cohen, S., Wheelwright, S., Van Der Lely, H. (2008). Narrative discourse in adults with high-functioning autism or Asperger syndrome. *Journal of Autism and Developmental Disorders*, **38**: 28–40.

Conway, M.A., Pleydell-Pearce, C.W. (2000). The construction of autobiographical memories in the self-memory system. *Psychological Review*, **107**: 261–288.

Courchesne, E., Karns, C.M., Davis, H.R., *et al.* (2001). Unusual brain growth patterns in early life in patients with autistic disorder: an MRI study. *Neurology*, **57**: 245–254.

Craik, F.I.M., Anderson, N.D. (1999). Applying cognitive research to the problems of ageing. *Attention and Performance*, **17**: 583–615.

Craik, F.I.M., Lockhart, R.S. (1972). Levels of processing: a framework for memory research. *Journal of Verbal Learning and Verbal Behavior*, **11**: 671–674.

Craik, F.I.M., Morris, L.W., Morris, R.G., Loewen, E.R. (1990). Relations between source amnesia and frontal lobe functioning in older adults. *Psychology and Aging*, **5**: 148–151.

Crane, L., Goddard, L. (2008). Episodic and semantic autobiographical memory in adults with autism spectrum disorder. *Journal of Autism and Developmental Disorders*, **38**: 498–506.

Crowder, R.G. (1976). *Principles of Learning and Memory*. Hillsdale, NJ: Erlbaum.

Deruelle, C., Hubert, B., Santos, A., Wicker, B. (2008). Negative emotion does not enhance recall skills in adults with autistic spectrum disorders. *Autism Research*, **1**: 1–96.

Deese, J. (1959). On the prediction of occurrence of particular verbal intrusions in immediate recall. *Journal of Experimental Psychology*, **58**: 17–22.

DiCicco-Bloom, E., Lord, C., Zwaigenbaum, L., *et al.* (2006). The developmental neurobiology of autism spectrum disorder. *The Journal of Neuroscience*, **26**: 6897–6906.

Eichenbaum, H. (1999). Conscious memory, awareness and the hippocampus. *Nature Neuroscience*, **2**: 775–776.

Eichenbaum, H. (2000). A cortical-hippocampal system for declarative memory. *Nature Reviews: Neuroscience*, **1**: 41–50.

Farrant, A., Blades, M., Boucher, J. (1998). Source monitoring in children with autism. *Journal of Autism and Developmental Disorders*, **28**: 43–50.

Feinberg, T.E., Keenan, J.P. (2005). Where in the brain is the self? *Consciousness and Cognition*, **14**: 661–678.

Ferrari, M., Matthews, W.S. (1983). Self-recognition deficits in autism: syndrome-specific or general developmental delay? *Journal of Autism and Developmental Disorders*, **13**: 317–324.

Gaigg, S.B., Bowler, D.M. (2007). Differential fear conditioning in Asperger's syndrome: Implications for an amygdala theory of autism. *Neuropsychologia*, **45**: 2125–2134.

Gaigg, S.B., Bowler, D.M. (2008). Free recall and forgetting of emotionally arousing words in autism spectrum disorder. *Neuropsychologica*, **46**: 2336–2343.

Gaigg, S.B., Bowler, D.M. (2009). Illusory memories for emotionally charged words in autism spectrum disorder: Further evidence for atypical emotional processing outside the social domain. *Journal of Autism and Developmental Disorders*, **39**: 1031–1038.

Gaigg, S.B., Gardiner, J.M., Bowler, D.M. (2008). Free recall in autism spectrum disorder: the role of relational and item-specific encoding. *Neuropsychologia*, **46**: 983–992.

Gardiner, J.M. (2008). Concepts and theories of memory. In *Memory in Autism: Theory and Evidence*. Cambridge: Cambridge University Press, pp. 3–20.

Gardiner, J.M., Bowler, D.M., Grice, S. (2003). Perceptual and conceptual priming in autism: An extension and replication. *Journal of Autism and Developmental Disorders*, **33**: 259–269.

Graham, K.S., Lee, A.C.H., Barense, M.D. (2008). Impairments in visual discrimination in amnesia: implications for theories of the role of medial temporal lobe regions in human memory. *European Journal of Cognitive Psychology*, **20**: 655–696.

Greene, A.J., Gross, W.L, Elsinger, C.L., Rao, S.M. (2006). An fMRI analysis of the human hippocampus: inference, context and task awareness. *Journal of Cognitive Neuroscience*, **18**: 1156–1173.

Halford, G.S. (1992). *Children's Understanding: the Development of Mental Models*. Hillsdale, NJ: Erlbaum.

Hamann, S. (2001). Cognitive and neural mechanisms of emotional memory. *Trends in Cognitive Sciences*, **5**: 394–400.

Happé, F., Frith, U. (2006). The weak coherence account: detail-focused cognitive style in autism spectrum disorders. *Journal of Autism and Developmental Disorders*, **36**: 5–25.

Henderson, H.A., Zahka, N.E., Kojkowski, N.M., *et al.* (2009). Self-referenced memory, social cognition, and symptom presentation in autism. *Journal of Child Psychology and Psychiatry*, **50**: 853–861.

Hermelin, B., O'Connor, N. (1967). Remembering of words by psychotic and subnormal children. *British Journal of Psychology*, **58**: 213–218.

Hermelin, B., O'Connor, N. (1970). *Psychological Experiments with Autistic Children*. Oxford: Pergamon Press.

Hill, E.L. (2004a). Executive dysfunction in autism. *Trends in Cognitive Sciences*, **8**: 26–32.

Hill, E.L. (2004b). Evaluating the theory of executive dysfunction in autism. *Developmental Review*, **24**: 189–233.

Hill, E., Berthoz, S., Frith, U. (2004). Brief report: cognitive processing of own emotions in individuals with autistic spectrum disorder and in their relatives. *Journal of Autism and Developmental Disorders*, **34**: 229–235.

Hillier, A., Campbell, H., Kiellor, J., Phillips, N., Beversdorf, D.Q. (2007). Decreased false memory for visually presented shapes and symbols among adults on the autism spectrum. *Journal of Clinical and Experimental Neuropsychology*, **29**: 610–616.

Hobson, R.P. (1993). *Autism and the Development of Mind*. Hove: Psychology Press.

Howe, M.L., Courage, M.L. (1993). On resolving the enigma of infantile amnesia. *Psychological Bulletin*, **113**: 305–326.

Hunt, R.R., Seta, C.E. (1984). Category size effects in recall: The roles of relational and individual item information. *Journal of Experimental Psychology: Learning, Memory and Cognition*, **10**: 454–464.

Jacoby, L.L. (1991). A process dissociation framework: Separating automatic from intentional uses of memory. *Journal of Memory and Language*, **30**: 513–541.

Johnson, S.A., Filliter, J.A, Murphy, R.R. (2009). Discrepancies between self- and parent-perceptions of autistic traits and empathy in high functioning children and adolescents on the autism spectrum. *Journal of Autism and Developmental Disorders*, Epub. Jul 21, doi: 10.1007/s10803-009-0809-1.

Just, M.A., Cherkassky, V.L., Keller, T.A., Kana, R.K., Minshew, N.J. (2007). Functional and anatomical cortical underconnectivity in autism: Evidence from an fMRI study of an executive function task and corpus callosum morphometry. *Cerebral Cortex*, **17**: 951–961.

Keenan, J.P., Rubio, J., Racioppi, C., Johnson, A., Barnacz, A. (2005). The right hemisphere and the dark side of consciousness. *Cortex*, **41**: 695–704.

LeDoux, J. (2002). *The Synaptic Self: How our Brains Become Who We Are*. New York: Viking.

Lee, A., Hobson, R.P. (1998). On developing self-concepts: A controlled study of children and adolescents with autism. *Journal of Child Psychology and Psychiatry*, **39**: 1131–1144.

Leekam, S., Lopez, B. (2003). Do children with autism fail to process information in context? *Journal of Child Psychology and Psychiatry*, **44**: 285–300.

Leslie, A.M. (1987). Pretense and representation: the origins of 'theory of mind'. *Psychological Review*, **94**: 412–426.

Leslie, A., Roth, D. (1993). What autism teaches us about metarepresentation. In *Understanding Other Minds: Perspectives from Autism*, Oxford: Oxford Medical Publications, pp. 83–111.

Lind, S.E. (2010). Memory and the self in autism: A review and theoretical framework. *Autism* Advanced online publication. doi:10.1177/1362361309358700.

Lind, S.E., Bowler, D.M. (2009). Delayed self-recognition in autism spectrum disorder. *Journal of Autism and Developmental Disorders*, **39**: 643–650.

Lombardo, M.V., Barnes, J.L., Wheelwright, S.J., Baron-Cohen, S. (2007). Self-referential cognition and empathy in autism. *Plos One*, **2**: e883.

Losh, M., Capps, L. (2003). Narrative ability in high-functioning children with autism or Asperger's syndrome. *Journal of Autism and Developmental Disorders*, **33**: 239–251.

Martin, J.S., Poirier, M., Bowler, D.M., Gaigg, S.B. (2006). *Short-term serial Recall in Individuals with Asperger's Syndrome*. Poster presented at the International Meeting for Autism Research, Montreal.

Mayes, A., Boucher, J. (2008). Acquired memory disorders in adults: implications for autism. In *Memory in Autism: Theory and Evidence*. Cambridge: Cambridge University Press, pp. 43–62.

Minshew, N.J., Goldstein, G. (1993). Is autism an amnesic disorder? Evidence from the California Verbal Learning Test. *Neuropsychology*, **7**: 209–216.

Minshew, N.J., Goldstein, G. (2001). The pattern of intact and impaired memory functions in autism. *Journal of Child Psychology and Psychiatry*, **42**: 1095–1101.

Minshew, N.J., Johnson C., Luna, B. (2001). The cognitive and neural basis of autism: a disorder of complex information processing and dysfunction of neocortical systems. *International Review of Research in Mental Retardation*, **23**: 111–138.

Mitchell, P., Ropar, D. (2004). Visuo-spatial abilities in autism: a review. *Infant and Child Development*, **13**: 185–198.

Morin, A. (2005). Self-awareness and the left hemisphere: the dark side of selectively reviewing the literature. *Cortex*, **43**: 1068–1073.

Mostofsky, S.H., Goldberg, M.C., Landa, R.J., Denckla, M.B. (2000). Evidence for a deficit in procedural learning in children and adolescents with autism: implications for a cerebellar contribution. *Journal of the International Neuropsychological Society*, **6**: 752–759.

Mottron, L., Morasse, K., Belleville, S. (2001). A study of memory functioning in individuals with autism. *Journal of Child Psychology and Psychiatry*, **42**: 253–260.

Mottron, L., Dawson, M., Soulières, I., Hubert, B., Burack, J. (2006). Enhanced perceptual functioning in autism: an update and eight principles of autistic perception. *Journal of Autism and Developmental Disorders*, **36**: 27–43

Murdock, B.B. (1962). The serial position effect of free recall. *Journal of Experimental Psychology*, **64**: 482–488.

O'Connor, N., Hermelin, B. (1967). Auditory and visual memory in autistic and normal children. *Journal of Mental Deficiency Research*, **11**: 126–131.

O'Connor, N., Hermelin, B. (1978). *Seeing and Hearing and Space and Time*. London: Academic Press.

Palmen, S.J.M.C., van Engeland, H., Hof, P.R., Schmitz, C. (2004). Neuropathological findings in autism. *Brain*, **127**: 1–12.

Perner, J. (1991). *Understanding the Representational Mind*. Cambridge, MA: MIT Press.

Perner, J. (2001). Episodic memory: essential distinctions and developmental implications. In *The Self in Time: Developmental Issues*. Hillsdale, NJ: Erlbaum, pp. 181–202.

Pesta, B.J., Murphy, M.D., Sanders, R.E. (2001). Are emotionally charged lures immune to false memory? *Journal of Experimental Psychology: Learning, Memory, and Cognition*, **27**: 328–338.

Poirier, M., Martin, J. (2008). Working memory and immediate memory in autism spectrum disorders. In *Memory in Autism: Theory and Evidence*. Cambridge: Cambridge University Press, pp. 231–248.

Reisberg, D., Hertel, P. (2004). *Memory and Emotion*. Oxford: Oxford University Press.

Renner, P., Klinger, L.G., Klinger, M. (2000). Implicit and explicit memory in autism: Is autism an amnesic disorder? *Journal of Autism and Developmental Disorders*, **30**: 3–14.

Rippon, G., Brock, J., Brown, C., Boucher, J. (2007). Disordered connectivity in the autistic brain: Challenges for the 'new psychophysiology'. *International Journal of Psychophysiology*, **63**: 164–172.

Roediger, H., McDermott, K. (1993). Implicit memory in normal human subjects. In *Handbook of Neuropsychology*, Volume 8. Amsterdam: Elsevier, pp. 63–131.

Roediger, H.L., McDermott, K.B. (1995). Creating false memories: remembering words not presented in lists. *Journal of Experimental Psychology: Learning, Memory and Cognition*, **21**: 803–814.

Schacter, D.L. (1987). Memory, amnesia, and frontal lobe dysfunction. *Psychobiology*, **15**: 21–36.

Schacter, D.L., Tulving, E. (1994). What are the memory systems of 1994? In *Memory Systems, 1994*. Cambridge, MA: MIT Press, pp. 1–38.

Schumann, C.M., Hamstra, J., Goodlin-Jones, B.L., *et al.* (2004). The amygdala is enlarged in children but not adolescents with autism; the hippocampus is enlarged at all ages. *The Journal of Neuroscience*, **24**: 6392–6401.

Smith, A.P.R., Stephan, K.E., Rugg, M.D., Dolan, M.D. (2006). Task and content modulate amygdala-hippocampal connectivity in emotional retrieval. *Neuron*, **49**: 631–638.

Smith, B.J., Gardiner, J.M., Bowler, D.M. (2007). Deficits in free recall persist in Asperger's syndrome despite training in the use of list-appropriate learning strategies. *Journal of Autism and Developmental Disorders*, **37**: 445–454.

Smith, C., Squire, L.R. (2005). Declarative memory, awareness and transitive inference. *The Journal of Neuroscience*, **25**: 10138–10146.

South, M., Ozonoff, S., Suchy, Y., *et al.* (2008). Intact emotion facilitation for non-social stimuli in autism: Is amygdala impairment in autism specific for social information? *Journal of the International Neuropsychological Society*, **14**: 42–54.

Squire, L.R. (1992). Memory and the hippocampus: A synthesis from findings with rats, monkeys, and humans. *Psychological Review*, **99**: 195–231.

Summers, J.A., Craik, F.I.M. (1994). The effects of subject-performed tasks on the memory performance of verbal autistic children. *Journal of Autism and Developmental Disorders*, **24**: 773–783.

Tager-Flusberg, H. (1991). Semantic processing in the free recall of autistic children: Further evidence of a cognitive deficit. In *Autism: Nature, Diagnosis, and Treatment*. New York: Guilford Press, pp. 92–109.

Toichi, M., Kamio Y. (2002). Long-term memory and levels-of-processing in autism. *Neuropsychologia*, **40**: 964–969.

Toichi, M. (2008). Episodic memory, semantic memory and self-awareness in high-functioning autism. In *Memory in Autism: Theory and Evidence*. Cambridge: Cambridge University Press, pp. 143–165.

Tulving, E. (1962). Subjective organisation in the free recall of 'unrelated' words. *Psychological Review*, **69**: 344–354.

Tulving, E. (1985). Memory and consciousness. *Canadian Psychologist*, **26**: 1–12.

Tulving, E. (2001). Episodic memory and common sense: how far apart? *Philosophical Transactions of the Royal Society, Part B*, **356**: 1505–1515.

Uttl, B., Ohta, N., Siegenthaler, A.L. (2006). *Memory and Emotion: Interdisciplinary Perspectives*. Oxford: Blackwell Publishing Ltd.

Wheeler, M.A., Stuss, D.T. (2003). Remembering and knowing in patients with frontal lobe injuries. *Cortex*, **39**: 827–846.

Williams, D., Happé, F. (2009). Pre-conceptual aspects of self-awareness in autism spectrum disorder: The case of action monitoring. *Journal of Autism and Developmental Disorders*, **39**: 251–259.

Williams, D.L., Goldstein, G., Minshew, N.J. (2006). The profile of memory function in children with autism. *Neuropsychology*, **20**: 21–29.

Wyatt, B.S., Conners, F.A. (1998). Implicit and explicit memory in individuals with mental retardation. *American Journal on Mental Retardation*, **102**: 511–526.

11

Measuring executive function in children with high-functioning autism spectrum disorders: what is ecologically valid?

AYLA HUMPHREY, OFER GOLAN, BARBARA A. WILSON
AND SARA SOPENA

Clinical experience and anecdotal written accounts suggest that school-age children with high-functioning autism spectrum disorders (ASD) have difficulties which can be described as 'executive dysfunction'. Problems with organisation, planning and task completion impede academic achievement and cause disruption in daily routine. The authors review research of executive function in this population and conclude that clinicians will find little in the scientific literature to guide them in neuropsychological assessment and remediation. They describe their study of 23 clinic-referred children (18 boys, 5 girls; mean age of 9) illustrating the challenges facing clinicians who would measure executive function. Tests of executive function (including the NEPSY and the BADS-C) were administered. Parent and Teacher questionnaires (DEX-C, BRIEF and VABS) were completed. Scores on tests of executive function and other areas of cognition were found to be in the average or above average range. In contrast, responses on both teacher and parent questionnaires indicated significant executive dysfunction. Parents' responses on the BRIEF and on the DEX-C were not correlated with teacher responses on the BRIEF. The authors consider the importance of a "halo effect" on questionnaire responses and challenge the notion that questionnaire measures have more ecological validity than laboratory measures. Suggestions for future research include observation, interviews and graded modification of the testing environment.

Researching the Autism Spectrum: Contemporary Perspectives, ed. I. Roth and P. Rezaie. Published by Cambridge University Press.

11.1 Introduction

Not enough attention is given to identifying individual neuropsychological deficits of children with ASD in the clinical setting with the aim of remediation despite being recommended by the National Autism Plan for Children (2003). This is partly because child mental health services and educational psychology services do not usually undertake detailed neuropsychological assessments and often cannot agree on who should take responsibility for this work (Humphrey, 2006). Even if existing services were to routinely offer such assessment, the question of which measures to use is open.

The study we are describing in this chapter was undertaken with the wish to identify measures which would enable the identification of executive dysfunction in the clinical setting for children with high-functioning ASD (HFA). Our results have, surprisingly, suggested to us that there is no 'best' measure, and that the evaluation of executive dysfunction and possibly all neuropsychological function in this group of children should be approached as a synthesis of information from several different sources. Our work has also shown the importance of considering and studying how the expectations of parents and teachers of children with ASD influence their view and reporting of a child's abilities and disabilities.

School age children with HFA are routinely observed to have difficulty organising, planning and completing tasks such as school activities, homework and dressing. These difficulties can lead to time spent out of class, detentions and exclusions. They often require additional educational support. There are numerous anecdotal accounts of such difficulties:

> Transitional periods may be the hardest part of the day . . . just give Justin a few minutes to organise his materials before and after instruction. (Betts *et al.*, 2007)

> [They] have difficulty with organization, with knowing, remembering, and attending to what is important. (Jacobsen, 2005)

> . . . [We] are often unable to shift our attention away from the point at which we have become stuck, or generate new strategies . . . Organization abilities . . . were also affected. At secondary school, I adopted the strategy of carrying everything I might conceivably need at any point in the week . . . out of fear I might be caught without something I needed. (Sainsbury, 2000)

The difficulties described above can be classified as executive dysfunction. Executive function has been characterised as including: (1) inhibition: the ability to inhibit a pre-potent response; (2) intention: the ability to formulate appropriate goal-directed plans and follow complex behavioural sequences to a satisfactory conclusion; and (3) executive/working memory: the mental representation of tasks and goals. These abilities are scaffolded by a host of skills such as flexibility and set-shifting, self-monitoring, sustaining attention and utilising feedback (Burgess *et al.* 1998; Emslie *et al.* 2003) as well as fluency and estimation (Baron, 2004). Eslinger (1996) offers a discussion of the various definitions of 'executive function'. Executive function is considered a higher order cognitive function integrating more basic functions. Baron (2004) helpfully describes executive function as: *'Metacognitive capacities that allow an individual to perceive stimuli . . . respond adaptively, flexibly change direction, anticipate future goals, consider consequences, and respond in an integrated or common-sense way, utilizing all these capacities to serve a common purposive goal'.*

While the anecdotal accounts clearly point to executive dysfunction, laboratory studies of executive function in children with HFA have been equivocal in their findings. In general, meta-analyses suggest that there are inconclusive results with a lack of replication, that the deficits that are measured are mild and circumscribed, and that the evidence that executive dysfunction is characteristic of HFA is mixed (Hill and Bird, 2006; Kleinhans *et al.* 2005; Pennington and Ozonoff, 1996; Sergeant *et al.* 2002).

There are several possible explanations for the lack of consistent findings described above. Sampling differences in studies of children with ASD is, of course, one hindrance to replication. Historically, it has been difficult to recruit large samples of children with a single reliable diagnosis and samples will include children who fall into the diagnostic hinterlands between Asperger Disorder, High-Functioning Autism and Pervasive Developmental Disorder Not Otherwise Specified. A perusal of the literature on adults and children with ASD does suggest that deficits are less apparent in individuals without global learning disability (Baron-Cohen *et al.* 1999; Bogte *et al.* 2009; Hill, 2004).

Another threat to the validity of laboratory studies of executive function is the unavoidable fact that strict examination conditions differ from most conditions in the real world (Burgess *et al.* 1998). Several authors have identified an over-reliance on laboratory measures and the structured nature of the test setting (Gilotty *et al.* 2002; Liss *et al.* 2001). The need to use ecologically valid tests of executive function has been widely documented (Kenworthy *et al.* 2005; Lezak, 1995; Shallice and Burgess, 1991) as executive dysfunction is better captured when the cognitive demands required to do a particular task/s resemble real life.

Hill (2004) and Baron (2004) address the difficulty partitioning components of executive tasks. For example, the Wisconsin Card Sorting Test requires flexibility, working memory, inhibition and monitoring as well as set-shifting. The complexity of our measures challenges their discriminant validity; what are we really measuring? Anderson carried out a review of the most commonly used tests of executive function for children and indicated several methodological limitations such as no standardised administration or valid developmental norms as well as lack of specificity of what the tests are supposed to measure (Anderson, 1998).

Clinicians working with children diagnosed with an ASD who have an IQ above 70 and are attending mainstream schools will, therefore, find little in the scientific literature to guide them in targeting and remediating areas of cognitive deficit that may be contributing to a child's maladaptive behaviours or academic difficulties. However, while there may not be agreement on a pathognomonic profile of executive dysfunction or function in individuals with ASD, there is no reason that clinicians cannot choose from a range of well normed tests measuring executive function when working with individual children. Despite a lack of concordance in our scientific findings, clinically, it is of paramount importance to determine the strengths and weaknesses of students with ASD in order to facilitate learning, especially within a mainstream school environment where tailored educational approaches may depend on a comprehensive test report.

We wanted to measure and further characterise the difficulties with planning and organisation in daily life that the children we assessed and treated in our Tier 3 Child and Adolescent Mental Health Asperger Service were experiencing. We undertook a small study in a clinic-referred sample of children with ASD who had an IQ above 70 and were attending mainstream school. Rather than attempting to identify core and causal deficits in ASD, we wanted to identify an evidence-based assessment protocol that could guide intervention. We hypothesised that children in this sample would have executive function impairments as measured by neuropsychological and behavioural measures and that scores on laboratory and ecologically valid measures of executive function would be positively correlated.

11.2 Participants

Twenty-three children (18 boys and 5 girls) attending mainstream schools, with a diagnosis of ASD (Asperger Disorder, 65%; High Functioning Autism, 13%; or Pervasive Developmental Disorder Not Otherwise Specified, 22%) between the ages of 7 and 12 years (mean = 9.4, SD = 1.6) and with an IQ above 70 (mean = 104.5, SD = 10.8), participated in this study. This age group was chosen because our clinical observation suggested that children with ASD had increasing difficulty with executive function in the latter part of primary school and during the transition into secondary school. The sample was recruited by contacting all cases open to the Asperger Outreach Service (Cambridge and Peterborough Mental Health Partnership NHS Trust). A total of 65 families were contacted to participate in the study. All children whose parents consented to the study were included. Two children who took part in the study had a co-morbid diagnosis, one of ADHD, the other of partial epilepsy, for which they were medicated. Since many of their task scores differed from the group's average by more than one standard deviation, they were excluded from the sample. Families who declined to participate in the study cited several reasons such as their children already had psychological testing, they didn't want their child to feel different, they were on holiday or they felt it was going to take too long.

11.3 Materials

We chose tests normed for our age group with acceptable psychometric properties. Most executive function measures are designed to assess individual executive function components. We wanted to use test batteries and questionnaires which were inclusive and tapped into a range of executive function properties rather than choosing many separate tests. In addition, we wanted to use a battery which would also assess other cognitive functions including verbal and non-verbal ability. This narrowed our choice of measures significantly.

11.3.1 *Neuropsychological assessment*

NEPSY (A Developmental Neuropsychological Assessment) (Korkman *et al.* 1998). The NEPSY is normed for children from age 3 to 12 years and contains five domains: language, attention and executive function, memory, visuospatial ability and sensorimotor ability. The core sub-tests for children from 5 to 12 years of age were administered. The sub-tests included in the Attention/Executive Function domain, together with the areas of function tested, are shown below:

1. Tower: planning, monitoring, self-regulation and problem solving. Move three balls to target positions on three pegs in a prescribed number of moves.
2. Auditory Attention and Response Set: continuous performance task, vigilance, selective auditory attention, shift set, maintain complex mental set. Place a red square in a box when hearing the word 'red' in Part A. Place a blue square when hearing the word 'red' in Part B.
3. Visual Attention: speed and accuracy scanning an array and locating target. Scan an array of pictures and mark targets quickly and accurately.

The normative mean scores for all domains is 100 with a standard deviation of 15. Normative mean scores for individual sub-tests is 10 with a standard deviation of 3. The core domains exhibit moderately high reliability scores for internal consistency (0.88 to 0.91 for 3–4-year-olds, and 0.79 to 0.87 for 5–12-year-olds). Inter-rater reliability has a coefficient of 0.99 (Nash, 1995).

Behavioural Assessment of Dysexecutive Syndrome in Children (BADS-C) (Emslie *et al.* 2003). The BADS-C is normed for children between the ages of 7 and 16 years and measures planning, flexibility, impulse inhibition and novel problem solving. The tasks included in the BADS-C are shown below:

1. Playing Cards: change established pattern of response. Part 1, say 'yes' to red card, 'no' to black. Part 2, say 'yes' to card that is same colour as card before and 'no' to card that is a different colour.
2. Water Test: develop a plan of action to solve a problem. Get a cork out of a tube using any of the objects placed out without touching beaker lid, stand, beaker and tube.
3. Key Search: plan an efficient, systematic, feasible plan of action, self-monitor, take into account unstated factors. Draw a line from a dot showing how they would search a field to find their keys.
4. Zoo Map: planning. Ability to plan a route in order to visit 6/12 possible locations in the zoo when there are restrictions on the number of times certain paths can be used. Zoo Map 1 is a demanding open-ended task with little structure provided. Zoo Map 2 is a low demand, rule governed task.
5. Six Part Test: planning, task scheduling and performance monitoring. Three different coloured coded tasks to do (arithmetic, naming, sorting). Each task includes two parts. Children need to schedule their time to attempt something from all 6 parts over 5 minutes with restrictions on the order in which the parts can be completed.

The mean score on the BADS is 100, SD is 15. The inter-rater reliability for the BADS-C is high, ranging between 0.53 and 1.00. Test–retest reliability correlation ranged from 0.289 to 0.814.

11.3.2 *Behavioural assessments*

Dysexecutive Questionnaire for Children (DEX-C) (Emslie *et al.* 2003). This is a 20 item Likert scale questionnaire that asks about executive difficulties in everyday life. Table 11.1 details the executive functions covered by the questionnaire. The DEX-C was completed by parents of children taking part in the study. The mean score is 15, SD is 13.

Behaviour Rating Inventory of Executive Function (BRIEF) (Gioia *et al.* 2002). This inventory of executive function provides a parent and a teacher rating form, each with 86 items yielding a Global Executive Composite score. The mean score

Table 11.1 *Child characteristics measured by the Dysexecutive Syndrome Questionnaire for Children (DEX-C)*

Abstract thinking problems
Impulsivity
Confabulation
Planning problems
Euphoria

Temporal sequencing problems
Lack of insight and social awareness
Apathy
Loss of decision-making ability
Disinhibition
Disturbed impulse control
Aggression
Perseveration
Lack of concern

Restlessness
Inability to inhibit
Distractibility
Unconcern for social rules

Example questions and response choices
'Gets events mixed up with each other, and gets confused about the correct order of events'
'Acts without thinking, doing the first thing that comes to mind'
Never; Occasionally; Sometimes; Fairly Often; Very Often

is 50, SD is 10. In addition, the BRIEF includes two broad indexes (Behavioural Regulation and Metacognition) and eight scales. These are:

1. Behaviour Regulation Index:
   - Inhibit: resist
   - Shift: move freely, change focus
   - Emotional Control: moderate emotional responses
2. Metacognition Index:
   - Initiate
   - Working Memory
   - Plan/Organise
   - Organise Materials
   - Monitor: work checking habits

Internal consistency for both parent and teacher forms (Cronbach's alpha) was high, ranging from 0.80 to 0.98. Mean test–retest correlations across clinical scales were 0.81 (range = 0.76–0.85). Construct correlations with ADHD rating scale were good (DuPaul *et al.* 1998).

Vineland Adaptive Behaviour Scales – Survey Form (VABS-S) (Sparrow *et al.* 1984). The VABS is a measure of adaptive behaviour in the areas of communication (receptive, expressive and written), daily living (personal, domestic, community), socialisation (interpersonal relationships, play and leisure time, coping skills) and motor skills. The mean score for each domain is 100, with a standard deviation of 15. The Vineland provides age norms for the general population, as well as scores for various clinical groups. Internal consistency for both parent and teacher forms (Cronbach's alpha) was high, ranging from 0.80 to 0.98. Mean test–retest correlations across clinical scales were 0.81 (range = 0.76–0.85). In the current study, the scales were completed by interviewing one parent of each child.

Normative data were obtained from all the instruments' standard scores. A clinical comparison group would have been preferable. However, resource and time limitations prevented this. In addition, the central aims of the study related to how this sample of children would compare to their same age peers and whether neuropsychological and behavioural measures of executive function would be positively correlated. Both these questions can be answered by using the measures' own population norms.

11.4 Procedure

Families were asked to attend our clinic for the administration of all measures which took approximately three hours (including measures given to the child and interview and questionnaires administered to the parent). All measures were administered by a research assistant. Parents were asked to give their child's teacher the BRIEF and requested to send it back using a pre-paid envelope. All parents and all but one of the teachers completed and returned the questionnaires.

11.5 Results

First, normality of the different scores was tested, using one-sample Kolmogorov-Smirnov tests. Distribution of none of the scores significantly differed from a normal distribution. Next, in order to test for possible differences between diagnoses, Kruskal-Wallis non-parametric tests were conducted on the different task scores. No significant differences were found. In order to test whether scores of our sample differed significantly from the tasks' normative averages one sample t-tests were conducted for the different scores, using Bonferroni correction for multiple comparisons. Contrary to our hypothesis, the sample's average score on the attention/executive function domain of the NEPSY (mean (M) = 102.9,

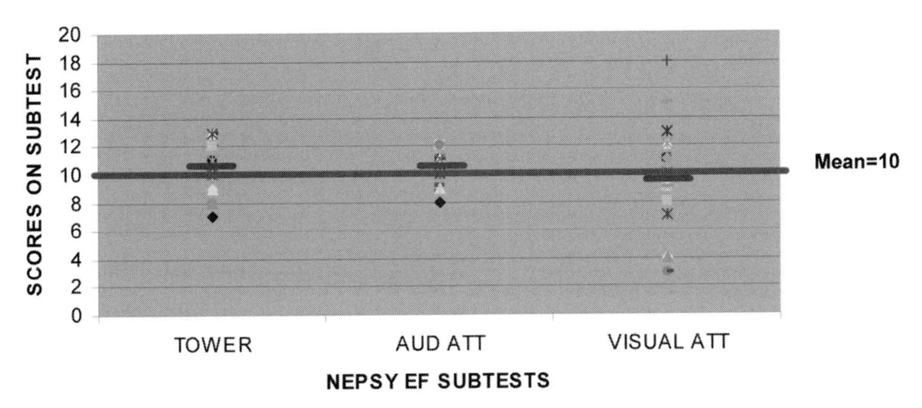

Figure 11.1 Individual scores on NEPSY Attention/Executive Function Domain sub-tests. See plate section for colour version.

SD = 12.2) did not significantly differ from the norm (t(22) = 1.13, NS) and 69.6% of the sample scored within ±1 SD of the scale's average score. All of the participants were within 2 SDs of the domain average. Furthermore, individual scores clustered around the population mean for the Tower and Auditory Attention sub-tests.

However, scores on the Visual Attention sub-tests were more diverse: three participants scored more than 1 SD above average (one of them scoring more than 2 SDs above average) and four participants scored more than 1 SD below average (two of them scoring more than 2 SDs below average). The group mean was, however, in the middle of the average range (M = 9.6, SD = 3.6). Figure 11.1 illustrates the distribution of participants' scores around the sub-test means.

The sample's average score on the language (M = 101.6, SD = 16.2) and memory (M = 102.7, SD = 13.4) scales did not differ from the normative average (t(22) = 0.48 for language, and 0.98 for memory, NS). However, the sample scored significantly higher than the norm on the visuospatial scale of the NEPSY (M = 113.0, SD = 13.0; t(22) = 4.77, $P < 0.001$), with 47.8% of the participants scoring more than one standard deviation above the normative average. In addition, the sample's average on the sensorimotor scale of the NEPSY (M = 95.5, SD = 10.3) was lower than the normative average, although after correction for multiple comparisons, this difference did not reach significance (t(22) = 2.11, P = 0.047).

Contrary to our hypothesis, the sample's average did not differ from the normative average on the BADS overall score (M = 97.8, SD = 24.9; t(22) = 0.42, NS). Sixty percent of the participants scored within ±1 SD of the BADS average score, and 73.9% scored within ±2 SD of the average. As with the NEPSY Attention/Executive Function sub-tests, the sample's average scores on all sub-tests of the BADS were in the average range. However, the standard deviation for each sub-test was relatively large (SD for the sub-tests ranged between 3.7 and 4.7). Figure 11.2

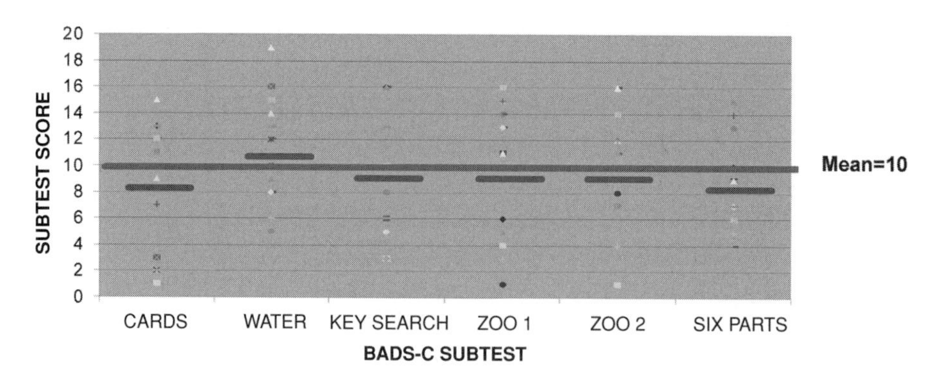

Figure 11.2 Individual Bads-C sub-test scores. See plate section for colour version.

illustrates the distribution of participants' scores around the BADS sub-test means.

Our hypothesis was, however, supported by parent and teacher ratings which were significantly higher for our sample, compared to the normative measures on the DEX-C (M = 42.9, SD = 10.9; t(22) = 12.25, $P < 0.001$), on the parent version of the BRIEF (M = 73.3, SD = 6.1, t(22) = 18.38, $P < 0.001$) and on the teacher version of the BRIEF (M = 70.2, SD = 11.9; t(21) = 7.99, $P < 0.001$). Higher scores indicate greater impairment on these measures. Ratings parents gave their children on the more general measure of adaptive behaviour, the VABS-S, were also lower than the average for their age (VABS-S overall score: M = 69.7, SD = 15.9; t(22) = 9.18, $P < 0.001$) indicating greater impairment in the sample under study. Parent ratings on the DEX and the BRIEF were significantly correlated with each other (r = 0.66, $P < 0.01$). None of the parents' measures correlated with the teachers' ratings on the BRIEF.

In order to test whether NEPSY scores can predict the behavioural measures scores, three hierarchical regression analyses were conducted for the DEX, parent BRIEF and teacher BRIEF. In each of the analyses, the first block included the demographic variables: age, gender and IQ, followed by a second block which included all NEPSY sub-tests. A stepwise method was used to enter variables into the regression in each block.

The analysis conducted for the teacher BRIEF yielded four significant predictors: sex ($\beta = 0.59$, $P < 0.005$), NEPSY visual attention, from the Attention/Executive Function domain of the battery ($\beta = -0.43$, $P < 0.05$) and two sub-tests from the NEPSY sensorimotor domain: imitating hand positions ($\beta = -0.36$, $P < 0.05$) and finger tapping ($\beta = -0.34$, $P < 0.02$). Together these four variables explained 68.6% of the variance in the dependent variable (Adj. $R^2 = 0.686$). Table 11.2 shows the steps included in this regression.

Table 11.2 *Steps included in the NEPSY hierarchical regression for the teacher BRIEF*

Step	Predicting variables	β	t	Adj R^2
1	Sex (1 = male, 2 = female)	0.59	3.25***	0.313***
2	Sex	0.60	3.77***	0.478*
	NEPSY visual attention	−0.43	−2.71*	
3	Sex	0.59	4.18***	0.578*
	NEPSY visual attention	−0.56	−3.67**	
	NEPSY imitating hand positions	−0.36	−2.35*	
4	Sex	0.57	4.62***	0.686*
	NEPSY visual attention	−0.66	−4.81***	
	NEPSY imitating hand positions	−0.39	−2.96**	
	NEPSY finger tapping	−0.34	−2.68*	

***$P < 0.005$ **$P < 0.01$ *$P < 0.05$.

In the regression analysis for the parent BRIEF only one significant predictor was included: NEPSY auditory attention ($\beta = -0.46$, $P < 0.03$), with only 17.7% explained variance. The regression analysis for the DEX revealed no significant predictors.

Three regression analyses, similar to those described above, were conducted with the BADS sub-test in the second block instead of the NEPSY sub-tests. Results revealed no significant predictors for the DEX or the parent BRIEF. The teacher BRIEF was predicted by two variables: sex ($\beta = 0.59$, $P < 0.005$) and the BADS cards sub-test ($\beta = -0.39$, $P < 0.05$), which together explained 43.6% of the variance of the teacher BRIEF.

In order to understand the sex effect on the teacher BRIEF scores, a t-test for independent groups was conducted, comparing teacher BRIEF scores of boys and girls (see Figure 11.3). The test was found to be significant ($t(20) = 3.3$, $P < 0.005$), suggesting girls (M = 82.8, SD = 7.0) were rated by teachers as having greater executive dysfunction than boys (M = 66.5, SD = 10.4). No such difference was found on parent BRIEF ($t(21) = 1.1$, NS) or the DEX ($t(21) = 1.2$, NS).

Lastly, in an attempt to predict more general adaptive scores on the VABS-S, a hierarchical regression with three blocks was conducted: the first block included the demographic variables and the second block included the NEPSY and BADS scores, as done in the regression analyses described above. The third block included the DEX-C and the parent and teacher BRIEF scores. The stepwise method was used for all three blocks. None of these variables had a significant contribution to the prediction of the VABS-S scores.

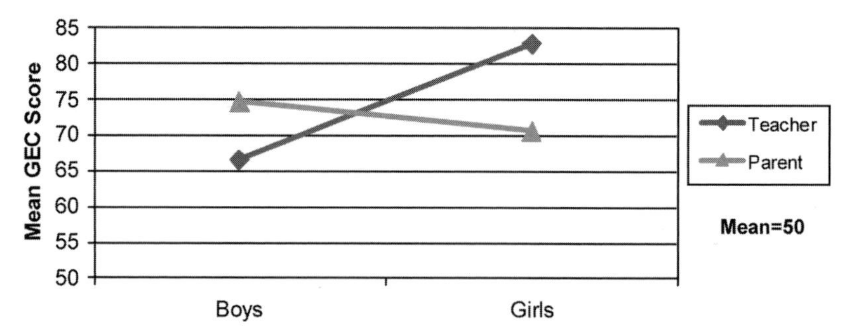

Figure 11.3 Mean Global Executive Composite Score for Parent and Teacher by sex of child.

11.6 Limitations of study

We initially hoped to recruit only children with an Asperger Disorder diagnosis but expanded our inclusion criteria when faced with restricting our sample size to very small numbers. Future research with larger samples will need to undertake analysis of executive function in discrete diagnostic groups. It is worth noting that functionally, the children included in our sample were not idiosyncratic and shared common strengths and difficulties. It may, therefore, be more useful to analyse the association between symptom severity across defining domains of ASD such as repetitive behaviours with executive function. We excluded children who had co-morbid psychiatric disorders. However, a separate analysis in a larger sample of children with HFA and, for example, attention deficit disorder, would be valuable in understanding core deficits and in planning interventions.

11.7 Discussion

The findings of this study confirm the anecdotal and clinical view that children with HFA have difficulty with executive function. This is evidenced in teacher and parent responses on ecologically valid questionnaire measures of executive function. However, evidence of executive dysfunction was not found using laboratory administered standardised measures of executive function. Indeed, the children in our sample performed in the average range as compared to same age peers on most of the laboratory measures employed.

Our sample demonstrated weakness on the Sensory-Motor domain of the NEPSY only and while the group mean for the sample was significantly lower than the population test norms, this was by five points only. The sample mean was, therefore, still in the average range. The other laboratory measure of executive function, the BADS-C, also yielded a mean score in the average range for the group. There was, however, a large standard deviation on all of the BADS-C sub-tests. It is possible, therefore, that in a larger sample the BADS-C score would have predicted scores on the questionnaire measures including on the DEX which was developed to complement the BADS-C and for which its authors have reported a high agreement with the BADS-C, especially for clinical groups.

Regression analysis found the only predictor of parent BRIEF to be the Auditory Attention sub-test of the NEPSY. It is important to remember that while some of the scores on the neuropsychological measures predicted variance on the ecological measures, these scores are not in themselves indicating impairment. We might expect children who have difficulty with auditory attention to have difficulty attending to parental instruction and subsequent difficulty organising their behaviour. In fact, the children in our sample were not having difficulty with auditory attention although parents' perception of auditory attention may have, perhaps, been influencing parental scoring of the BRIEF. Similarly, teachers appeared to be influenced by pupils' visual attention and sensorimotor ability as measured on the NEPSY and flexibility as measured by the BADS-C, although these scores were in the average range.

How can we explain what appears to be a heightened sensitivity by parents and teachers to particular aspects of the cognitive and motor ability of children with HFA? We would like to discuss several explanations and to suggest that some of these possible explanations deserve particular attention. One hypothesis is that there is something about the 'real-life' demands on executive function which we have not captured in our laboratory measures of executive function. One aspect of 'real-life' that we might consider are multiple task demands in contrast to the item-by-item approach in the laboratory setting. Studies of auditory processing in children with Asperger disorder have shown that they have significant difficulty attending to specific auditory stimuli in the context of ongoing background noise (Alcantara *et al.* 2004). Future research could create an approximation of a 'real-life' setting in which to administer standardised laboratory measures of executive function. If multiple demands contribute to the deterioration of executive function in this group of children, we would expect to see test scores indicating greater executive dysfunction and this would need to be significantly different when compared to a typically developing control group under the same conditions.

Another feature of 'real-life' executive function demands is the presence of social demands inherent in executive function tasks above and beyond one tester. In a study of novel problem-solving, Channon *et al.* (2001) showed videos of social 'predicaments' to adolescents with Asperger syndrome. An example of a scenario involved a story about a man who is not sleeping enough because of new neighbours who have a barking dog. The subjects were asked to offer a solution to this man's predicament. They found that compared to the control group, adolescents with Asperger disorder did not differ on Problem Apperception or Effectiveness of their solutions, but did differ significantly on the Social Appropriateness of their solutions. Because executive function demands in 'real-life' require not just application of the core attributes contained within the construct of executive function, but also require social judgement, parent and teacher ratings of executive function may, therefore, be indicating greater impairment than laboratory measures. While the children in our sample may have effectively implemented tasks requiring executive function, they may do so in a way which is not socially appropriate and, therefore, appears ineffective to parents and teachers, and may indeed prove to be ineffective in real-life settings.

The discrepancy we report here between laboratory and ecologically valid measures of executive function in children with HFA has been found by other researchers. Kenworthy and colleagues (2005) found in a sample of 72 children with high-functioning autism and Asperger disorder that parent ratings on the BRIEF, the Behaviour Assessment System for Children, and the VABS indicated significant impairment. However, the only laboratory test on which the same children scored significantly below the population mean was the reaction time on TOVA (Test of Variables of Attention) which was one standard deviation below population mean. Gilotty *et al.* (2002) also reported high scores on the Parent BRIEF and low scores on the VABS indicating executive dysfunction and deficits in adaptive behaviour in a comparable group of children. These authors conclude that their study illustrates the ecological validity of such standardised questionnaire measures of executive function and cognition with this group of children.

We would like to suggest that there may be a reporting bias on questionnaire measures of executive function for this group of children. The strong predictive power of sex in relation to the teacher BRIEF also points to this possibility. Perhaps, teachers are rating girls with ASD as having greater executive dysfunction than boys because they have expectations that girls will demonstrate better executive function than boys. While we assumed that all teachers completing the teacher BRIEF knew that the children had a diagnosis of an autism spectrum disorder, we did not directly ask this question. We are not, therefore, able to comment on whether teachers might have different expectations of girls compared to boys, or girls with ASD compared with boys with ASD.

There is strong evidence of a 'halo effect' in teachers' reporting of symptoms of Attention Deficit Hyperactivity Disorder (ADHD) and Oppositional Defiant Disorder (ODD) interacting with the sex of the child. Teachers scoring video-tapes of boys acting out 'pure' ADHD symptoms also rated ODD symptoms highly and rated ODD symptoms significantly higher than when the actor was a girl. However, when rating video-tapes of girls acting out 'pure' ODD symptoms they also rated ADHD symptoms highly and significantly more highly as compared to their rating of boy actors (Jackson and King, 2004). Other researchers have found that parent as opposed to teacher ratings of ADHD behaviors in 'real-life' settings differ less as a function of the child's sex (Achenbach *et al.* 1990; McGee *et al.* 1987). It has been suggested that these sex effects are a result of differing teacher expectations.

While parents' reports on the BRIEF and DEX were not influenced by the child's sex, the fact that ratings were partially predicted by auditory attention scores (despite the fact that these abilities were average) may also indicate that parental views about executive function are highly sensitive to neuropsychological function and that this sensitivity has a halo effect on assessment of executive function.

We suggest that the study of neuropsychological function in children with ASD would benefit from a less dichotomous view of the validity of laboratory versus ecological measures of executive function and, indeed, of other areas of cognitive function. Researchers and clinicians alike should consider employing qualitative and observational methods to understand the findings we describe here and to advance screening of cognitive function in ASD. For example, carefully constructed classroom observation may help us to understand teachers' views and expectations of children with ASD, as would interviews with teachers and children themselves. Graded modification of our laboratory test environments, for example altering the number of social demands or distractions, may help us to understand how we could develop more valid measures for use in the clinic. The additional benefit of these methodologies is that they provide us with valuable information with which to construct interventions and remedial strategies. If we can understand just how and when intact executive function deteriorates, we may be able to alter the conditions under which the children with ASD are asked to employ these functions.

11.8 References

Achenbach, T.M., Bird, H.R., Canino, G., *et al.* (1990). Epidemiological comparisons of Puerto Rican and U.S. mainland children: parent, teacher, and self-reports. *Journal of the American Academy of Child and Adolescent Psychiatry*, **29**: 84–93.

Alcantara, J.I., Weisblatt, E.J., Moore, B.C., Bolton, P.F. (2004). Speech-in-noise perception in high-functioning individuals with Autism or Asperger's Syndrome. *Journal of Child Psychology and Psychiatry*, **45**: 1107–1114.

Anderson, V. (1998). Assessment of executive function in children. *Neuropsychological Rehabilitation*, **8**: 319–349.

Baron I.S. (2004). *Neuropsychological Evaluation of the Child*. Oxford: Oxford University Press.

Baron-Cohen, S.B., Wheelwright, S., Stone, V., Rutherford, M. (1999). A mathematician, a physicist, and a computer scientist with Asperger Syndrome: performance on folk psychology and folk physics tests. *Neurocase*, **5**: 475–483.

Betts, S.W., Betts, D.E., Gerber-Eckard, L.N. (2007). *Asperger Syndrome in the Inclusive Classroom: Advice and Strategies for Teachers*. London: Jessica Kingsley.

Bogte, H., Flamma, B., Van Der Meere, J., Van Engeland, H. (2009). Divided attention capacity in adults with autism spectrum disorders and without intellectual disability. *Autism*, **13**: 229–243.

Burgess, P.W., Alderman, N., Evans, J., Emslie, H., Wilson, B.A. (1998). The ecological validity of tests of executive function. *Journal of the International Neuropsychological Society*, **4**: 547–558.

Channon, S., Charman, T., Heap, J., Crawford, S., Rios, P. (2001). Real-life-type problem-solving in Asperger's syndrome. *Journal of Autism and Developmental Disorders*, **31**: 461–469.

DuPaul, G., Power, T., Anastropoulos, A., Reid, R. (1998). *ADHD Rating Scale-IV: Checklist, Norms and Clinical Interpretation*. New York: Guilford Press.

Emslie, H., Wilson, C., Burden, V., Nimmo-Smith, I., Wilson, B. (2003). *Behavioral Assessment of Dysexecutive Syndrome for Children (BADS-C)*. Bury St. Edmunds, England: Thames Valley Test Company.

Eslinger, P.J. (1996). Conceptualizing, describing, and measuring components of executive function. In *Attention, Memory and Executive Function*. Baltimore, MD: Paul H. Brookes, pp. 367–395.

Gilotty, L., Kenworthy, L., Sirian, L., Black, D.O., Wagner, A.E. (2002). Adaptive skills and executive function in autism spectrum disorders. *Child Neuropsychology*, **8**: 241–248.

Gioia, G., Isquith, P., Guy, S., Kenworthy, L. (2002). *Behavior Rating Inventory of Executive Function (BRIEF)*. Odessa, Florida; Psychological Assessment Resources.

Hill, E.L. (2004). Executive dysfunction in autism. *Trends in Cognitive Sciences*, **8**: 26–32.

Hill, E.L., Bird, C.M. (2006). Executive processes in Asperger Syndrome: patterns of performance in a multiple case series. *Neuropsychologia*, **44**: 2822–2835.

Humphrey A. (2006). Children behaving badly – a case of misunderstanding? The development of a CAMHS based child neuropsychology service. *The Psychologist*, **19**: 494–495.

Jackson, D.A., King, A.R. (2004). Gender differences in the effects of oppositional behavior on teacher ratings of ADHD symptoms. *Journal of Abnormal Child Psychology*, **32**: 215–224.

Jacobsen, P. (2005). *Understanding How Asperger Children and Adolescents Think and Learn*. London: Jessica Kingsley.

Kenworthy, L.E., Black, D.O., Wallace, G.L., *et al.* (2005). Disorganization: the forgotten executive dysfunction in high-functioning autism (HFA) spectrum disorders. *Developmental Neuropsychology*, **28**: 809–827.

Kleinhans, N., Akshoomoff, N., Delis, D.C. (2005). Executive functions in Autism and Asperger's Disorder: flexibility, fluency, and inhibition. *Developmental Neuropsychology*, **27**: 379–401.

Korkman, M., Kirk, U., Kemp, S. (1998). *NEPSY: A Developmental Neuropsychological Assessment*. San Antonio, Texas: Psychological Corporation.

Lezak, M. (1995). *Neuropsychological Assessment*, 3rd edn. New York: Oxford University Press.

Liss, M., Fein, D., Allen, D., *et al.* (2001). Executive functioning in high-functioning children with autism. *Journal of Child Psychology and Psychiatry, and Allied Disciplines*, **42**: 261–270.

McGee, R., Williams, S., Silva, P.A. (1987). A comparison of girls and boys with teacher-identified problems of attention. *Journal of the American Academy of Child and Adolescent Psychiatry*, **26**: 711–717.

Nash, D.L. (1995). Interrater reliability of behavioural observations on NEPSY. Unpublished Master's Thesis, Trinity University, San Antonio, TX.

National Autism Plan for Children (NAPC). (2003). *National Initiative for Autism: Screening and Assessment (NAISA) Guidelines*. London: National Autistic Society.

Pennington, B.F., Ozonoff, S. (1996). Executive functions and developmental psychopathology. *Journal of Child Psychology and Psychiatry, and Allied Disciplines*, **37**: Jan, 51–87.

Sainsbury, C. (2000). *Martian in the Playground*. Bristol: Lucky Duck Publishing Ltd.

Sergeant, J.A., Geurts, H., Oosterlaan, J. (2002). How specific is a deficit of executive functioning for attention-deficit/hyperactivity disorder? *Behavioral Brain Research*, **130**: 3–28.

Shallice, T., Burgess, P. (1991). Higher order cognitive impairments and frontal lobe lesions in man. In *Frontal Lobe Function and Dysfunction*. New York: Oxford University Press.

Sparrow, S., Balla, D., Cicchetti, D. (1984). *Vineland Adaptive Behavior Scales – Survey Form*. Circle Pines, MN: American Guidance Service.

12

Autism spectrum disorders in current educational provision

RITA JORDAN

This chapter examines the research evidence for the learning style in autism spectrum disorders and ways in which this impacts on educational provision. It considers international evidence but has a focus on educational provision in England. The particular and dual role of education is considered and the effects of differences and difficulties in key areas of development (sensory, perceptual, conceptual, motivational, memory, language and social aspects). Key features of learning style and the implications for certain curriculum areas are analysed, including the need for homework support and the notion of a '24 hour curriculum'. The pervasive effects of anxiety and stress are discussed, and the factors that influence relationships with peers. The evidence of the value of different kinds of educational placement is also considered and the need for further research in this, and other, areas identified.

12.1 The role of education

Given that there is no medical 'treatment' for Autism Spectrum Disorders (ASD) and that even the idea of ASD as a medical disorder is problematic (Jordan, 2009), education has a special therapeutic role to play. Children and young people with ASD have the same entitlement as anyone else to acquisition of the culturally valued skills, knowledge and understanding that will enable full participation in their society, but, in addition, they need an education that will enable them to acquire the additional skills, knowledge and understanding that others acquire naturally and intuitively, without explicit instruction. In that sense, education has to take on the therapeutic role of compensating for the effects of ASD.

Researching the Autism Spectrum: Contemporary Perspectives, ed. I. Roth and P. Rezaie. Published by Cambridge University Press.

This dual role of education in ASD can be a source of conflict between parents and educational authorities. The latter will most commonly respond to what they see as their statutory obligation: to enable access to the same 'broad and relevant curriculum' as is provided for others. Parents may want this too, but, especially in the early years, may give a higher priority to the therapeutic aspects of education; they want an education that will help their children deal with or even overcome the difficulties that arise from their ASD. In an ideal world, the child should have access to both kinds of educational input, but first, both aspects have to be recognised.

This chapter will concentrate on the educational system. However, education continues throughout life and is not confined to the school years or to school hours. The relative failure to learn intuitively means that individuals with ASD need to be educated throughout their lives and in all aspects of their lives. It is also important that education prepares the individual to acquire life skills and social competence more naturally, to make education more self-sustaining, although this is unlikely to be entirely successful for everyone with ASD.

Above all, education needs to be individualised, to encompass the heterogeneity of the population, and to allow for different teaching goals at different times. Reviews of educational interventions that are adopting a therapeutic role, often in the early years, fail to support the use of any single intervention to meet all needs for all learners (e.g. Humphrey and Parkinson, 2006; Jones and Jordan, 2008; McConachie and Diggle, 2007; Perry and Condillac, 2003; Spreckley and Boyd, 2007). In all the comparative evaluations of educational interventions, it is always the case that some children do well in each intervention and others do not (e.g. Magiati *et al.* 2007; Remington *et al.* 2007). It is also true that children with ASD tend to learn what they are taught, and seldom go beyond it (e.g. Gulsrud *et al.* 2007; Howlin *et al.* 2007). Educators, therefore, need to take great care to select and monitor their teaching to ensure they are meeting the needs of each particular learner and that what is being taught is worthwhile and appropriate. Detailed case studies and single subject case designs often provide the most appropriate research for answering these questions. Randomised controlled trials (RCTs), even where these are possible and ethical, can only answer questions about the likely value of an intervention in general, and have little to say when it comes to individuals.

12.2 The particular challenges of the autism spectrum

As has been evidenced in the earlier chapters in this book, development in ASD is atypical. In ASD, without additional learning impairments, there will be some academic tasks that are easily mastered, at least if presented in an accessible way. Yet in other aspects of life, in common sense, social awareness, understanding of the world and how to behave in it, the child with ASD may be barely functioning at all. When such everyday tasks are mastered they are achieved at such high cost in terms of effort that the child may be exhausted, and the continual confrontation of such difficult situations may lead to ongoing anxiety and stress. All this will naturally affect that child's capacity to undertake academic tasks, in time, and so the ASD may come to have a general depressing effect on the child's overall functioning in education. If there are additional learning difficulties of any kind (language impairment, cognitive impairment, sensory impairment, dyslexia, dyspraxia, etc.) then these too will interact with the ASD to cause greater difficulties.

However, it is not just the complexity of needs that causes problems. When development follows a typical path, even if severely slowed, educators can appreciate the problems faced by the child and, with some effort, good will and training, can adapt to meet the child's needs. When development is atypical, this natural adjustment does not occur. It is as hard for the teacher to intuitively understand the mind of someone with an ASD as it is for children with ASD to understand their teacher. In other words they have a mutual failure in natural empathy. Just as the child with an ASD has to work cognitively to try to understand others so the educators of the child with an ASD (parents, teachers, therapists) have to adopt the same explicit cognitive ways of understanding the child, not being able to rely on typical natural intuition nor professional training. They will need education in understanding ASD, and time and resources to study each individual, to manage this successfully, and even then it will be exhausting. The extra cognitive load of teaching children with ASD needs to be researched, as do effective ways of managing this extra load. Peeters and Jordan (1999) draw on experience to characterise the qualities needed by an effective educator in ASD, but such assumptions need to be tested.

12.3 Core issues in learning in ASD

This section will examine some of the key differences and difficulties in ASD to explore their effect on education. The list is in no way comprehensive but demonstrates some of the core issues that need to be addressed.

12.3.1 *Sensory difficulties*

Difficulties in sensory processing are commonly attributed to people with ASD, and autobiographies of individuals with ASD often give them a key role in their disorder, especially hypersensitivities to sound and sharp contrasts in light (Grandin and Scariano, 1986; Lawson, 2003; Shore, 2003). Some professionals also support the notion of abnormal sensory responsiveness having a key role in ASD (Bogdashina, 2003). Yet the research evidence is not clear. Rogers and Ozonoff (2005) in a review found more evidence for hyposensitivity than hypersensitivity.

Hyposensitivity to pain (or at least an extreme delay in response to pain) is often reported in the literature but is not supported by well-conducted studies (Nader *et al.* 2004). This is at odds with the common experience that pain is not a deterrent in many children with ASD, who may return repeatedly to hold their hands in the steam from a kettle, in spite of what appears to be painful scalding, or will return to climbing a surface from which they have recently fallen with apparently painful outcomes (broken limbs) and yet with no apparent fear. Although most parents and teachers will seek to train children to avoid danger, there is inevitably some reliance on the fact that children will learn from their mistakes. Whatever the truth of responsivity to pain, it is clear that learning from it cannot be relied upon in ASD, so greater vigilance is needed to keep individuals with ASD safe.

Theories about attention distribution in ASD (Murray *et al.* 2005) may offer a partial explanation for inconsistent responses to pain. Other inconsistencies in sensory responsiveness may be due to individual variation; it has been suggested that responsiveness to sensory stimulation may vary across individuals, sense modalities and within an individual over time. If hypersensitivity is caused by a neurochemical imbalance then there is likely to be over adjustment in receptors and contrary responsiveness over time. Thus, for example, a young man detailed his extreme reaction to noise and light (describing sunlight as painful and the teacher's voice as like bullets hitting him) being replaced a few hours later by extreme under-responsiveness (the view appearing misty and faint and the teacher appearing to whisper indistinctly). There is research showing that individuals with ASD tend to cluster at the extremes of sensory responsiveness (Kientz and Dunn, 1997), which would make some 'sensory seekers' and others 'sensory avoiders'. This has led to programmes designed to assess individuals in terms of their responsiveness to different sensory modalities (seven senses usually being the number chosen – five 'outer' senses plus proprioception and vestibular senses), and then design a 'sensory diet' to meet their needs. There is a need to research the validity of such analyses and the efficacy of such programmes (American Association of Pediatrics, 2001).

Although the research base may be poor, there is sufficient concern about sensory issues in individuals with ASD themselves, and in educators, for attempts to have been made to adjust educational environments to reduce sensory effects. Whether there is a domain-independent sensory integration disorder is still an empirical question, and there is pressure to get such a disorder recognised in new formulations of the diagnostic manuals (Miller, 2008). Even if such a disorder were established, there would remain the issue of whether it was an integral part of ASD or a separate disorder that may or may not be co-morbid with ASD. Until more and better research provides answers to such questions, sensory issues should be considered:

1. as a possible explanation for some erratic or troubled behaviour which may be alleviated by eliminating or reducing the stressful stimuli, giving the child access to a way of blocking the stimuli, or giving access to less diffuse stimuli (e.g. a firm hold rather than a light one)
2. as a possible source of stress that may interact with cognitive or social demands calling for reduction of potentially disturbing stimuli in high demand situations or periods of respite from the stimulation
3. as a need (e.g. for deep pressure) that may have to be met before a child can concentrate on other tasks

The existence of a deficit in sensory integration has not yet been firmly established. The research gives inconclusive results (Reynolds and Lane, 2008) and undoubtedly more is needed, especially well conducted case studies on the use of sensory integration programmes to tease out variables that would warrant more systematic research. In the UK there is insufficient occupational therapy resource to make such programmes generally available, so it is vital to establish both the evidence base of effectiveness but also a model for their delivery. Are these programmes needed by all with ASD or only some, and what criteria should be used to decide on eligibility? How long and for what intensity should such programmes be given and do they need to be given by specialists such as occupational therapists or physiotherapists, or could such specialists provide management programmes for delivery by parents and professionals in daily contact? At the moment the situation is confused and needs a proper evidence base for treatment. If sensory integration is a significant problem then there are huge implications for the multi-sensory environments that exist in most schools (as elsewhere) so these issues need to be resolved.

What also remains unknown is how sensory reactivity relates to perceptual issues. There are two possibilities. If the sensory problem is core (whether it is one of hypersensitivity or of inability to integrate senses), as some believe, then it would help explain some of the problems in forming concepts and in idiosyncratic perceptions. However, it is possible, as many cognitive psychologists would hold, that the core problem is a perceptual one. This would mean the individual's primary difficulty would lie in 'chunking' environmental stimuli to make sense of the world around them. A failure to do this would leave the individual responding, like a baby, to the 'booming and buzzing' (James, 1892) confusion around, interpreted by self and others, perhaps as being hypersensitive to detailed stimulation simply because each detail would need to be responded to, rather than 'seen' as part of a more meaningful whole. It is not possible with current knowledge to choose between these 'chicken and egg' explanations. At a practical level it appears helpful, and certainly kinder, to work on both aspects: reducing stimulation to give individuals with ASD a better chance of interpreting their world; and helping individuals make sense of their environment and produce meaningful concepts to reduce the 'overwhelming' sensation from the environment and enable them to cope better with different kinds of stimulation.

12.3.2 *Perceptual understanding*

Regardless of the validity of the different theories about the underlying mechanisms in ASD, there is evidence of differences in making sense of the world. Perceptual understanding typically develops under social tutorage (Vygotsky, 1962) where mechanisms of joint attention, social referencing and social imitation give a framework for both understanding and acting on the world. What this means is that the child with ASD is literally on his/her own in making sense of the environment and thus is liable to develop very idiosyncratic perceptions. The child (like his/her parent or teacher) will be unaware of the idiosyncracy of those perceptions and, exacerbated by problems with communication, those differences may remain unrevealed. Educators need to use careful observation and investigation to try to uncover the child's perspective or initial confusion may be further compounded.

In particular, educators need to compensate for the lack of natural intuitive mechanisms such as joint attention by teaching meaning explicitly. Without this understanding, educators may continue to refer to items they are holding up or pointing to without checking that the child knows how (and when) to direct attention to the appropriate item. Words and phrases used by the child with an ASD may have a particular meaning tied to a particular context and this also needs to be investigated and the meaning expanded, where necessary. In the same way, the child may attach particular meaning to certain sequences of events in a 'superstitious' way so that the occurrence of one event comes to mean a particular outcome; there is then extreme distress if the expected outcome does not materialise or, even more likely, the child is unable to recreate the events she or he believes are necessary for the next event to occur. Gerland (1999), an adult with Asperger syndrome, describes such a situation when, as a child, an arrangement of objects on a table had coincided with the longed-for arrival home of her sister from school. Thereafter she had struggled to recreate that arrangement to bring about her sister's arrival and had experienced extreme distress when these efforts were thwarted. In a similar way a child with ASD, without social guidance, may not know which perceptual feature is the relevant one in any given situation and may easily attend to some irrelevant detail. In education systems social signals are used rapidly and continuously to direct and redirect attention to different aspects of events and, without the educator understanding the child's potential problems with this, and allowing for it by specific instruction and time for attention switching, the child with ASD may become confused and distressed or switch attention to something better understood (some repetitive action, perhaps).

Finally, there is the perception of novelty. There is some research (Plaisted *et al.* 1998) that shows that individuals with ASD have a particularly strong response to novelty and anecdotal evidence suggests that this can be experienced as aversive. The consequence is that almost all new situations (unless introduced with considerable preparation) are likely to give rise to a negative response at first, and that the child or young person will need time to adjust to new situations before they can be expected to learn in them. New experiences need to be introduced with knowledge (usually presented as a visual schedule) of how many of these experiences there will be, and when they will end. If the new experience is of a situation (such as a new school or class) that is not responsive to the individual's choice, or to a fixed number of occasions, then a somewhat different strategy is needed of helping the individual find the familiar within the new setting and making clear what aspects can be changed or adapted and what has to be endured (perhaps with additional support).

12.3.3 *Conceptual understanding*

It is often reported in the literature that individuals with ASD have problems with 'abstract' concepts, although it is not always clear what is meant by this and to what research evidence it refers. Certainly it would be difficult to defend this empirically as applying to all with an ASD, since subjects which many individuals with ASD excel in and enjoy utilise numerous abstract concepts: science, mathematics, music, for example. If it is only meant to apply to those with learning difficulties alongside their ASD, then it has little meaning, since it does not distinguish people with ASD from those with learning difficulties and, since learning difficulties are partly defined by difficulties in understanding and using abstract concepts, it becomes a tautology.

There is a problem in concept formation, however, in 'abstracting' (the verb, not the adjective) the 'essence' of experiences to give the 'prototypes' on which typical concept formation depends (Klinger and Dawson, 2001). Typical human perception is characterised by an ability to 'gloss over' insignificant differences when 'chunking' information into meaningful wholes, paying attention to what unites rather than divides members of a category. Thus, typically, human processing gives a fast 'good enough' categorisation of the world, and has to be trained to go beyond that perception to identify those differences that discriminate when necessary. Typical processing is speedy, enabling everyday efficient functioning. In ASD, the focus on detail makes it easier for individuals to detect difference rather than similarity and they find it hard to ignore what they see as pronounced differences, in order to group items into a single category or concept. One consequence of this is 'concepts' that consist of a single exemplar. De Clercq (2003) describes her son with Asperger syndrome as having three separate 'concepts' of a bicycle: 'wheels in the mud', 'keep your feet on the pedals' and 'off you go', respectively.

Grandin (1995a) (an intellectually able person with autism) recognised her own differences in concept formation, which in the beginning were also single exemplars, so that 'old' meant a particular old man she knew, 'cat' a particular cat, 'red' a particular red object. She recognised the restrictions on her thinking brought about by this method of conceptualisation, and also that other people's concepts were not tied to particular items or events in this way. Not having access to the typical process of concept formation, she claims to have devised her own, very closely related to methods used in artificial intelligence. She describes this as a process of constructing mental 'libraries' of common objects against which she would assess objects she came across, searching for a match. Thus, if what might be a chair was found not to be represented in her library she would decide it was not a chair unless told it was, whereupon she would add it to her library. This is clearly cognitively inefficient and time consuming and could only work in someone with her high level of intelligence and exceptional powers of memory.

Paradoxically, Grandin has no problems with the truly abstract concepts she encounters in her daily work as an animal scientist and designer, since scientific concepts are defined by criterial features in a way that everyday concepts are not. It might seem then, that educators could attack the problem with concept formation in ASD by giving explicit criterial features for all concepts, but in practice this is unlikely to succeed. Every-day concepts are referred to by psychologists as 'fuzzy' concepts, since they are characterised by their relationship to other things in a functional world, not by set definitional criteria. We only 'know' what a chair is because we have had experience of chairs and of treating them in the same functional way, not because anyone has defined a chair. Grandin's strategy would also have limited application, given the high cognitive load entailed. Using discrimination training to pick out concepts works with identifying particular items but does not address the problem of 'single exemplar' categories; in fact, it is likely to reinforce the idea that this one object is 'red', only to lead to confusion when other objects or hues of red are used. The answer lies in 'general case programming', more generally known in education as 'sorting'. This enables the child to gain practice in paying attention to the one feature (say, the colour 'red') that unites a large collection of items as against a similarly large collection of objects that lack this attribute. Computer programs have made such sorting activities more accessible to educators and should also make their effectiveness easier to evaluate. It is not clear how widespread this difficulty with concept formation is in ASD; interest levels and motivation appear to be key determinants of success, but this also needs more research.

The problem with 'fuzzy' concepts may also relate to the fact that people with ASD appear to have conceptual boundaries that are less amenable to modification. This also applies to action schema. Peterson (2002) proposes that there are difficulties in ASD with 'dialogical processing', which typically allows concepts in working memory to act together, influence one another and thus be flexible and amenable to context. Vermeulen (2001) has offered a similar account of 'context blindness' to account for many of the problems in ASD. At the current state of understanding, there are no simple solutions to this other than explicit strategies to draw attention to contextual features when concepts or schema are being activated. A cumbersome, but worthwhile, alternative for educators is to try to teach all possible contextual variations during the initial teaching of the schema, but this is far from easy or satisfactory.

12.3.4 Motivation

One of the hardest issues for educators to resolve in relation to children with ASD is whether failure to perform in acceptable ways is due to difficulties in cognition or conation (i.e. is it that they can't or won't?). Of course, 'willing' does not happen in a cognitive vacuum and undoubtedly what a person can or cannot do is hugely influenced by motivational factors; in practice, both aspects must be considered. Certainly, nearly all specialist techniques for educating children with ASD give a high profile to motivation. Applied Behaviour Analysis (ABA) claims to be able to override 'within child' factors by providing a suitably high level of external motivation, delivered in a highly contingent way for desired responses. In principle, if not always in practice, the reinforcers used to deliver such motivation move from materialistic towards social, as training progresses, although Tauber (1986) gives a useful warning of the dangers of using social reinforcement contingently in educational settings. 'Structured teaching', as developed under the Treatment and Education of Autistic and Related Communication Handicapped Children (TEACCH) programme (Mesibov and Howley, 2003), uses the Premack and Collier (1962) principle of more preferred activities rewarding less preferred ones in a motivational chain (often made explicit to the child in a visual schedule), and this has been shown to be adaptable to most educational settings. There is much talk about using the child's interests and strengths as motivators in education, and some systematic use of special talents is beginning to develop (Clark, 2005).

The need for predictability is so strong in ASD that that alone has been suggested as a way of developing motivation in the 'hard to motivate' child (Jordan, 2001). Many of the factors that motivate children in general also apply to those with ASD: active engagement, meaningfulness, time to complete activities, knowing what to do and when it is finished, and what will happen next (Peeters, 1997). The biggest difference is that individuals with ASD are likely to be less aware of how to please others and care less about doing so. They may also suffer from executive function difficulties that make it harder to postpone immediate gratification for long-term gain.

12.3.5 *Memory*

The issue of memory in ASD is complex (Boucher and Bowler, 2008; see Bowler *et al.* Chapter 10 of this volume), but it is clear that what is sometimes presented as a strength is in fact a reaction to a problem with memory. Children and young people with ASD often rely on single strategies for memorising, which work well for rote learning tasks but are less efficient and even unhelpful for other educational situations. Such strategies often entail exact repetition of experiences (even including the non-verbal soundtrack of memorised films, for example) with the inability to give the gist of the event or to select memories that have relevance to the current situation. The apparently impressive feat of remembering the full soundtrack of a movie is usually without meaning for the individual and is not available to recall unless prompted in some way. Educators can help the child with ASD make use of their memories by teaching cues to the key aspects at the time of encoding and rehearsing the 'gist' of the memory, using these cues. The reconstruction of memories from the gist and from general semantic knowledge, that typically takes place naturally, can be taught explicitly, using these same cues and prompts to access stored knowledge. More able individuals with ASD do seem to develop ways of recalling personal events, at least where there is emotional involvement, but may need training in how to relate the event as a narrative and when it is appropriate to do so. Children with ASD also need to be taught that memories relate to actual events rather than learning routines to respond to certain questions, such as 'what did you do at school today?' Visual cues can be helpful but have the danger of suggesting a memory, which may not be accurate.

12.3.6 *Language*

Although it is communication rather than language problems *per se* that characterise ASD, language development is important for the child expressively as an educational tool and receptively to help make sense of the educational world (see Chapter 9 in this volume for a discussion of the relationship between language deficits and ASD). The minority of children with ASD who do not develop any useful spoken language have a poorer prognosis, but suffer less from being misunderstood and being the subject of unhelpful pressure at school. Faced with a child who is not speaking, all staff will have a natural response of slowing down their own speech and speaking in shorter sentences – both helpful strategies in enabling the child with ASD to process the language. Educators are also less likely to assume that a failure to speak is willful and will appreciate, if not fully understand, that the child is likely to have cognitive and linguistic problems. Sometimes this can lead to unnecessarily low expectations of the child, but usually it leads to helpful support, often extending to the use of visual forms of communication.

For the child with an ASD who has speech, but otherwise has very similar difficulties to non-verbal children with ASD, the response of educators and peers can be very different. It is harder for educators to recognise that the speaking child may be unable to communicate, deficiencies are often thought to be wilful and the child said to be suffering from a behavioural disorder. Problems in processing language are similarly often unrecognised, with the educator failing to slow down to the rate the child needs in order to understand. Nor do educators realise that the language the child has may not be available as language for thought, and that visual modes of thinking are still likely to dominate (Grandin, 1995b). The child's capacity to 'hold the floor' (and, even more tellingly, reluctance to 'yield the floor') is seldom recognised as a strategy to avoid the difficult task of participating in conversation or relating to the topics raised by others. Being able to talk about one's own interests is very different from being able to adjust to the interests of others. The child also will need specific training in pragmatics and conversational skills and peers will need to be shown how to support the individual in interactions in which both parties have an interest.

'Educational' language can also prove a particular barrier to understanding in children and young people with ASD. It is a particular genre of language based on the assumption that children will already know about how language is used for everyday communication, and introducing particular forms geared to particular educational purposes. This is particularly puzzling for the child with an ASD, who may be trying to learn about communication for the first time in the educational setting and be thus trying to use and understand this special genre as a means of everyday communication. As was discussed above, educators will often assume early communication skills such as the capacity to follow a point or realise that the object of attention is that held in the teacher's hand, but the child may have no, or a completely wrong, idea of what is being discussed if he or she is absorbed by something else. Educators will often introduce topics by asking questions, usually ones to which they already know the answer, but the child who copies this strategy is bewildered to be told that 'I'm not answering that; you know the answer to that'. Given the role of theory of mind difficulties in ASD, children on the spectrum are unlikely to realise that others may know things they do not and so are only likely to ask questions (like the teacher) to get the desired response. There are many other aspects of educational language that need explicit translation for the child with an ASD, but, for this to happen, educators have to be aware of the genre they are using and the problems this may pose for those with ASD.

On the positive side, having speech makes it possible for the child to learn ways of thinking in language, which may not be the best mode for the child but will help with generalisation; visual modes of thinking are very particular and context bound so language can be useful in freeing events from that context and in drawing attention to commonalities across settings. It can also be used in training the child to 'self prompt' to deal with anxiety or to problem solve in ways that are easier to generalise than image-based formats. Written language can provide an ideal compromise, being available to the child in a preferred visual mode but having the language properties that aid generalisation.

12.3.7 *Social aspects*

Education is both socially and linguistically mediated, at least in its traditional forms. The problems with linguistic mediation were raised above, but social mediation is also often overlooked as an issue, in spite of the recognition of social difficulties lying at the heart of ASD (Hobson, 1993; see also Chapter 8 of this volume). Evidence presented in earlier chapters suggests that individuals with ASD do not respond to (or even notice) social signals as a priority and are only able to understand social stimuli by working them out cognitively (Frith and Happé, 1994). These social difficulties have certain key consequences in relation to education. Children will need to be taught to recognise and respond to social signals (such as their name being called) as a way of gaining their attention. Once this is achieved, the same recognition will have to be developed for all other such attention-getting signals such as 'Everybody!', 'Class x!', 'All the boys!', an imperious hand clap, a whistle or whatever form these signals take in that particular environment. However, educators have then to remember to use these taught phrases or actions as signals, and not bury them in the middle or at the end of an instruction. Individuals with ASD are not particularly non-compliant (Golding, 1997), as long as they understand the instruction and that it is addressed to them.

Having to process social information through general cognitive routes has further implications for the social context of education. If individuals with ASD are required to learn something new, then they are least able to do so when having to cope with social demands at the same time; unfamiliar tasks need to be introduced asocially (by organising the material as in a structured teaching setting, or using computer assisted learning, for example) or, if appropriate, in one to one instruction with a single adult. The corollary of this is that if the child or young person is required to engage socially, or even just take part in a group, then she or he is best able to do this if the task set is a familiar one, so all the cognitive effort can be directed to the social domain. Just as for most people, it will be easier to interact with and understand someone familiar than a stranger.

Children with ASD vary significantly in the extent they wish to engage socially with others; what they have in common is difficulty in doing so. Wing and Gould (1979) and Wing (1996) found different sub-types in the degree of sociability in children with ASD; these were categorised as 'withdrawn', 'passive', 'active but odd' and 'eccentric'. They pointed out that children might change sub-category with time and training and it has been shown that stress and mental illness can also cause individuals with ASD to move from a more sociable category to a more withdrawn one, at least temporarily. It is also likely that degree of familiarity of the persons and the environment will affect degree of sociability. Given the effect of social engagement on cognitive capacity in individuals with ASD, it is surprising that degree of sociability is seldom considered when deciding on a teaching approach. Based on analysis and experience, rather than research, I suggest the following guide:

1. a 'withdrawn' child requires both didactic one to one teaching to engage interest but also desensitisation to enable him/her to work with others
2. a 'passive' child needs intensely interactive high stimulation techniques with structure to encourage engagement
3. an 'active but odd' child needs to know the social rules (through Social Stories (Gray, 1994) perhaps) and then support to carry them out as in 'Buddy' schemes or Circles of Friends (Whitaker *et al.* 1998)
4. an 'eccentric' child may just need help in analysing situations, managing his/her own reactions and good models to imitate or to act as guides

12.4 Features of learning style

The extreme heterogeneity of those with ASD means that there will always be exceptions to most generalisations about learning style. However, research has established certain features of learning style that are more likely to be true across the spectrum.

12.4.1 Visual rather than verbal mediation

As suggested above, many children and young people have problems processing language and are more able to use visual forms of instruction, whether this is written or in diagrammatic form. Grandin (1995b) gives a good analysis of her own very visual learning style and programmes such as TEACCH (Mesibov and Howley, 2003; Peeters, 1997) use visual structure for time and work schedules and to enable the individual to literally see what has to be done, where, with whom, how, when it will be finished and what happens next. TEACCH can be adapted for those with visual impairments (Howley and Preece, 2003; Jordan, 2004) although even for the visually impaired with ASD, augmented vision may remain a preferred mode, where possible. Jordan (2003a) shows how a visual flow chart can be used with young people with Asperger syndrome to help them understand where they have choices in situations and to take responsibility for the consequences of their own behaviour.

12.4.2 *'Bottom-up' processing*

Part of typical development is to move from perception and cognition being led by the details of the stimulation experienced, to a learning style that perceives and processes the world through imposed structures and expectations (Piaget, 1929). Although there is evidence that individuals with ASD do develop conceptual thinking, it also appears that the 'bottom-up' processing of early childhood persists into adulthood as a preferred mode, at least in many situations (Behrmann *et al.* 2006). The situation is complex because stress and anxiety can also lead to switching from 'top-down' to 'bottom-up' processing styles (Smock, 1955), which we are all more likely to use in new and confusing situations where we have not yet established expectations or routines. It may be that it is the effects of stress or lack of understanding that lead to the long term maintenance of this learning style in ASD, rather than a cognitive bias. However, evidence from biology of more local processing in certain brain regions and fewer connections between areas (Belmonte *et al.* 2004) would suggest that a bottom-up processing style, less influenced by existing knowledge and structures, has a biological substrate.

In the classroom, there is a clear necessity to reduce stress and anxiety to promote more advanced learning styles and to allow time for processing so that existing concepts and schema can be brought into play. There will also be a need to teach about alternative learning styles and to encourage the adoption of strategies to overcome some of the limitations of a very detailed focused learning style, without losing some of its benefits (a 'fresher' and unique vision in the arts resulting in valuable skills in poetry and painting in some, the attention to detail which will be an important asset in some professions, and the fine discriminations that not only enable careers but also provide much appreciated leisure pursuits such as astronomy, playing a musical instrument by ear and bird watching).

One debilitating problem that often remains is understanding how details are grouped together and which details to include or exclude when building cognitive structures. It will be obvious to most children when the teacher switches from explaining some aspect of history or mathematics, to reprimanding a child for misbehaving, for example, but that may not be the case in children with ASD. Educators need to develop habits of giving 'advance organisers' (Ausubel *et al.* 1978) to signal the content of the lesson (or part of the lesson) to come, reducing the guess work for the child with ASD, and benefiting many others who also struggle to be prepared to take in information. At the same time, the child with ASD needs to be helped to recognise the cues that indicate when educators change topic or addressee and to react accordingly.

12.5 Access to the curriculum

Having an ASD carries no automatic entailments about which curriculum subjects will prove easy or difficult to access. There are some predispositions that arise from ASD, but these are overridden by the child's characteristics of intelligence, interest, particular relevant abilities and experience as well as factors such as the teaching style and mode of presentation of the teacher, the teaching environment and so on. Thus, no general assumptions should be made about which subjects should be taught to individuals with ASD. They have the same entitlement to a 'broad and relevant' curriculum as any other child and having a particular marketable skill may do as much for their future adjustment as an adult as participation in social skills classes (Howlin *et al.* 2004). Decisions need to be made on an individual basis, taking account of both current and likely future needs, in planning a suitable curriculum. Within each subject domain, however, there are some common issues related to certain curriculum subjects and some of these are discussed below.

12.5.1 English

Many children with ASD learn to read through their interest in computer games, just as they may start to speak through copying what is said (in an exact mimicry of the accent and intonation) in favourite television programmes. There are teaching programmes that harness such natural learning processes in, for example, teaching children to read through animated interactive computer programs (Heimann *et al.* 1995). Some children with ASD may find it easier to learn to read (in a mechanical sense) than to speak and so the child can be taught to communicate through written language before (or sometimes, but rarely, instead of) doing so through speech. This can be helped by the child learning to type on a computer but this must be taught as an independent skill and not by leaving the child to be 'assisted' in typing as in Facilitated Communication (Konstantareas and Gravelle, 1998). Later on in development, learning to use a word processor for essays and other school work not only helps overcome some of the dyspraxic problems that may accompany ASD and interfere with handwriting, but may also help anxious 'perfectionist' children overcome their fear of getting things wrong in general. By emphasising the role of 'drafting' in eventually reaching a 'perfect' copy the child can accept the modifications that may be needed to an early draft as simply part of the process, rather than feeling judged and too anxious to try again.

Children with ASD have some specific problems with narrative forms (Bruner and Feldman, 1993; Jordan, 2008; Losh and Capps, 2003). Some of these problems may arise from early missed experiences and many children will be helped by learning to act out everyday events and so 'tell a story' through drama (Sherratt and Peter, 2002). Learning specific story structures by, for example, analysing the key elements of a newspaper story and reporting on events in class 'newspapers' can also help. However, as Jordan (2008) found, failing to understand human emotion and intention is the biggest barrier to understanding stories, as it is to understanding life events, so teaching children on the spectrum to analyse frequently watched television 'soap' programmes for these aspects underlying people's words and actions can be a valuable tool. Soap characters are chosen because motivations and intentions are often both exaggerated and stylised and thus form a more advanced version of Thomas the Tank Engine stories, part of whose attraction for children with ASD lies in the characters' unvarying motivation and clear intentions. Learning from video is becoming a useful tool in the education of children with ASD (Sturmey, 2003) in many ways, allowing the necessary repetition and focus.

12.5.2 *History*

Aspects of the history curriculum that depend on memorising lists of dates of battles or kings and queens have particular appeal to children with ASD. They have more difficulty when they are expected to use their imaginations and show empathy for people living in past times far from their own experiences (Jordan and Guldberg, 2002). This can be tackled by omitting those aspects of teaching for the child with an ASD who can be given an alternative task, perhaps to do with fact-finding and recording events; sometimes this will be the best course of action to take. However, aspects of subjects and lessons that cause problems for children with ASD often do so because they focus on key barriers to learning. This means that they also represent key opportunities to help the children with ASD overcome these barriers. Thus, empathising with a Roman soldier allows the opportunity to investigate what empathy means and how one would go about exploring the thoughts and feelings of another person who has a very different experience to one's own. This kind of lesson will be valuable for all children, but particularly so for those with ASD because it makes explicit what is usually hidden and assumed.

12.5.3 *Mathematics*

Mathematics is often an area of strength in ASD, but not invariably so, Sometimes individuals do very well in some aspects, but find others a stumbling block. It has been suggested that algebra presents a particular problem in this respect and so Jordan and Hewett are currently undertaking trials of a visual tool for use in algebra to see if this will help.

12.5.4 *Science*

A typical early understanding of the physical world is through an anthropomorphised view (Carey, 1985), which can persist at a deep level into adulthood and present problems when counterposed with alternative physical explanations. It is likely, although not yet adequately researched, that individuals with ASD do not share this developmental pathway and use 'folk physics' in preference to 'folk psychology' (Baron-Cohen, 2004) from the beginning. This should mean they do not have to overcome earlier modes of thinking when tackling science and should find scientific thinking more comfortable. This appears to be the case. However, there are aspects of science that are likely to be more problematic in ASD. Science proceeds through a 'democratic' process of empirical work, testing and verification of hypotheses rather than a set of rules laid down by authorities. Even the most venerable laws in science may be subject to modification or even refutation over time and what is 'true' is always a temporary state of affairs until disproved. This level of uncertainty about what is the case and the fact that hypotheses may be proved or disproved, can be difficult for people with ASD to accept, adding to the confusion of a very confusing world. One way round, that experience suggests may be helpful, is to introduce statistics. The young person who is very disturbed to learn that the results of an experiment are uncertain in advance may take comfort in being able to put a number to that level of uncertainty and also when given numbers to show the degree of certainty in a 'fact'. This has sometimes led to a lifetime's fascination with, and a career in, statistics.

12.5.5 *Modern foreign languages*

When looking for subjects that may be regarded as less 'suitable' for children and young people with ASD (perhaps to replace them with social skills classes) it is common for educators to select modern foreign languages. Since all such decisions should be made on an individual basis, there are cases where this is appropriate, but the benefits of modern foreign language teaching in ASD are often overlooked. In a mainstream curriculum, this is often the only time when children are taught everyday social skills, how to use common facilities, how to conduct conversations and how to leave them. The fact that all this is being taught in a foreign language is in reality a minor point compared with the explicit learning opportunities provided. In addition the fact that it is a foreign language means that idioms, metaphors, sarcasm are all explained and the child gains some meta-awareness of how language is used. Many children with ASD enjoy this opportunity to have clarified what has been puzzling before, and again may pursue languages as further study or even as a career. If they have access to dead languages such as Latin, they often enjoy that even more, because the structure remains unchanged, but there are few opportunities to learn (or use) Latin in the UK now.

12.6 Parental support, homework and the '24 hour' curriculum

Since so much that has to be learnt concerns understanding of people, relationships and daily living, the involvement of parents as educators is an important contributor to educational success in ASD. At the lowest level of involvement, parents will be needed to support and extend the teaching begun at school and will inevitably become involved over issues such as homework. Parents may have to explain to teachers the necessity for clear (preferably written) instructions for all homework, and for extra support in lessons to draw the attention of the child with ASD to relevant aspects that will form part of his/her homework. Parents may also need to advocate on behalf of the child who is becoming over-stressed at school (usually through excess social demands or perhaps bullying), even if the effects of the stress build-up are not apparent until the child 'relaxes' at home. Just as the education of a child with an ASD cannot be confined to school hours or premises, nor can the stress. Whenever there are problems they are likely to reflect factors at home and school and so a common approach needs to be adopted. The child who explodes in a rage each night on returning from school is unlikely to be reacting solely to something at home, but may be responding to unreleased tensions that have built up during the day. By working together, schools and parents can identify times or occasions when the child needs a respite break to calm down or escape a difficult situation before re-entering the situation as she/he has been taught to do. This may avoid episodes where the child loses control and enable the child (and peers) to be taught better ways of coping with stress.

As the child with ASD gets older, and sometimes even for younger children, parents find it increasingly difficult to manage this 24 hour curriculum at the same time as providing a reasonable quality of life for the rest of the family. Families need a break, as does the child with ASD, both at crisis points and also regularly, as a planned strategy for meeting needs. Preece and Jordan (2007) reinforce the need to relieve stress in families but also demonstrate the inadequacy of provision, even in a well resourced county in the UK that has a long history of specialist provision for children with ASD. The problem seems to lie in the view of social service planning that short breaks services are by their nature a 'last resort', to prevent crises in families and to be given only when all else has failed. In fact, well trained staff and well resourced provision should be part of a planned service to meet the child's 24 hour educational needs, apart from the side benefits that may accrue from relief of care for families. Failure to get this right may result in residential schooling being sought and/or in family breakdown (Randall and Parker, 1999).

12.7 Anxiety and stress

In respect of schooling, it is important to recognise the debilitating effects of stress and anxiety on the child's capacity to learn and so reducing stress needs to be a top curriculum aim. Sources of stress will be very individual but are likely to include the following:

1. Endogenous stress arising with hormone changes at the onset of puberty. Exercise, both aerobic and anaerobic, can help reduce this stress (Campbell, 2007; Campbell and Jordan, unpublished data) as can specific relaxation techniques and periods of quiet enjoyable activity.
2. Sensory overload in the environment, particularly noise, seems to cause the most stress. Local solutions might include putting pads on the bottom of chair legs on a vinyl floor, or the child may be given a proximal block such as earphones.
3. Frustration from not understanding or not being able to communicate needs. Educators should watch for the signs of communicative need so it can be addressed before frustration sets in, and the child or young person needs to be taught a system of communication.
4. Anger or panic at having routines disrupted, especially when these routines are themselves indicators of a high level of stress. Staff and peers may need to be taught to respect routines once they have started. Equally, the child or young person with ASD needs to learn to identify early signs of their own stress and to learn to engage in safe activities that reduce stress, rather than resorting to open-ended routines that may fail to resolve the underlying anxiety. It is important that the child is taught to act on early signs of stress as just drawing attention to them may exacerbate the anxiety in a transactional way.
5. Having to leave tasks incomplete or being unable to put items back in what the child regards as a 'proper' relation to one another (e.g. the chair exactly parallel to the table, the pencils all facing the same way in parallel rows, etc.) often leads to extreme stress. It may be that the child needs a programme so that in the longer term he/she can learn to tolerate slight deviations from the 'ideal' situation with less stress. In the meantime it is best to reduce the size of tasks to allow completion, and to allow the child extra time for packing up, to allow for the exact arranging of materials.

6. Not understanding one's own emotional states and so being unable to control them leads to further stress. Children need to become aware of their own emotions if they are to understand what they are, to recognise them in themselves and in others, and then learn to manage them. Greig and MacKay (2005) have recently developed a programme for children and young people with Asperger syndrome, based on the idea of 'little men in the head' – 'homunculi'. Children are taught to name these 'men' as mental states in a representation of their own heads and to manipulate them in ways that help control their activities. This is 'Cognitive Behavioural Therapy' but in a form that is accessible to young children and does not require clinical psychologists to administer.

12.8 Relationships with peers

One of the key benefits in attending school, rather than being educated at home or in a clinic based setting, is that it allows opportunities to engage with and learn with and from peers. Research shows that when individuals with ASD interact in positive ways with peers, all benefit in terms of development and social maturity (Roeyers, 1995; Yang *et al.* 2003). If children with ASD can interact happily with others all three aspects of impaired or atypical development are likely to be affected: the child will engage more socially, communicate more and become more flexible as others' thoughts, feelings and intentions 'interfere' with one's own. One feature of the Young Autism Project (Lovaas, 1987) was that children were taught 'entry' skills to their local nursery and the most successful children were those who engaged in the group from an early age. There have also been successful programmes targeting the development of peer interaction through pivotal response training (Odom and Strain, 1986) or other proactive techniques (Strain and Hayson, 2000). Peers can also be part of support teams for the child through Buddy schemes or Circles of Friends. A recent suggested remodelling of the diagnostic criteria for ASD (van Lang *et al.* 2006) has play as a key aspect of the definition of the disorder, in acceptance of its key role in development. Jordan (2003b) has analysed the benefits of teaching both cognitive and social aspects of play to children with ASD, to bring them into successful relationship with their peers, so this too should form a vital part of the educational curriculum.

12.9 Information and communication technologies (ICT)

Engagement with computers has a vital role to play in the education of children and young people with ASD, and in their quality of life thereafter

(Jordan, 2007a; 2007b; Murray, 1997; Murray and Aspinall, 2006). Computer assisted learning can help take the place of social or linguistic mediation of learning, allowing the child or young person to work at their own pace and work to their strengths. Information technology can also provide tools to teach aspects of learning that are otherwise difficult to attempt, such as the use of virtual reality to teach about thinking and imagination (Herrera *et al.* 2008). Use of laptops with interactive white boards allows teachers to individualise class teaching and monitor the child with ASD, who is working at his/her own pace, at the same time as giving class instruction. The increased use of such 'laboratory' classrooms will help make schools considerably more 'autism friendly'. It is also clear that at least some people with ASD do like to engage socially with others and share ideas and views when they can do so at their own pace in a 'safe' environment, and for many, computer social network sites provide such an opportunity (Biever, 2007).

12.10 Kinds of placement

Alongside growing understanding of ASD and specialist educational approaches to meet their needs has come a worldwide movement for inclusion, where many argue that inclusion should be the default position (as a right) and that it is exclusion or segregation that has to be justified by evidence of a 'greater good' (UNESCO, 1994). There is no evidence (and little research) on which kind of educational provision is 'best' for children with ASD and little agreement on the criteria for 'best' practice. The Department for Education and Skills, UK (2002) has produced consensual (rather than research-based) recommendations for good practice in ASD, but this is based on policies and processes rather than types of provision. Nevertheless, a recent research review in England (Jones *et al.* 2008) has identified some positive examples of good inclusive practice, while also identifying the common view of all stakeholders that the main barrier to effective inclusion was the lack of understanding among school staff. A new initiative on inclusive practice in ASD (National Strategies Schools Development Programme, 2009) that provides an interactive resource for mainstream schools, may help to remedy this.

The role of research in evaluating broader kinds of educational entitlement is almost invisible. It is rare for the outcome measures of educational placement to be specified, let alone monitored. Thus, there is some evidential base to the policy of inclusion in education in that large international surveys found that segregated schooling made social inclusion as an adult more difficult (Hegarty, 1993). However, given the very atypical experiences of children with ASD in supposedly 'inclusive' settings (e.g. Jordan and Powell, 1994) it is not clear that this is also true for them (Chamberlain *et al.* 2007; Simpson *et al.* 2003). Children with ASD in mainstream schools, when there is no or inadequate specialist support, often

Table 12.1 *Comparative benefits of single curricula versus eclectic curricula for pupils with ASD*

Single curriculum	Eclectic curriculum
Enables staff expertise	Can match to goal
Better monitoring & easier evaluation	All needs can be addressed
Builds staff & parent confidence	Needs compatibility checks & child perspective
Enables positive views	Takes strengths from each approach

feel isolated rather than included, are frequently bullied and are more likely than most other groups to be excluded (Barnard *et al.* 2000; Batten *et al.* 2006). There is anecdotal evidence of a high use of home tutoring among children with ASD (especially at secondary transfer) and it is suggested that this is a response to lack of better options rather than a real choice.

All too often there is conflict between the educational placement that will best meet the child's therapeutic needs and one that will provide the best access to a broad curriculum and to typically developing peers.

The areas where research evidence would be helpful include:

1. whether being fully included in a mainstream school leads to more social inclusion in society as an adult
2. whether attending specialist provision leads to greater skills, independence and a better quality of life as an adult than either supported mainstream provision or a generic special school
3. whether children with ASD attending mainstream schools have more or fewer positive social contacts with peers than those attending special or specialist schools

Even in specialist provision there is a division between those schools which follow eclectic curricula and those which adopt a single form of intervention, although even in such 'single approach' schools there is usually a degree of eclecticism, as other approaches are incorporated. Since, as was shown above, there is no evidence for the value of a single kind of educational intervention to meet all needs, there is equally no evidence for the superiority or otherwise of single approach schools. There are likely to be pros and cons, as illustrated in Table 12.1.

Resource bases appear to provide more flexible provision for children and young people than separate classes or units (Hesmondhalgh and Breakey, 2001). The difference is that in resource bases the child 'belongs' to his or her peer group class and the class teacher works with the resource base specialist to plan the child's individual educational plan and to work out effective programmes for integrated lessons and for support. This means the child can attend mainstream classes when ready but, if extra stress or particular circumstances mean the child cannot cope on a particular occasion, the resource base is always there to provide a safe working environment. The resource teacher also has a role in advocating for the children with ASD and in arranging training and support for colleagues in the main part of the school and for the children's peers. Specialist schools may still be needed for some children whose needs or circumstances are extreme, but they should become true centres of excellence, developing innovatory practice, conducting research for evidence-based practice, and supporting mainstream and generic special schools.

Children and young people with ASD who have additional severe (or even profound) learning difficulties also need to have their autism addressed since they are always going to need support and supervision in their daily life. However, specialist teaching is about the understanding and expertise available, not about location. There is no reason why a generic special school for children with moderate or severe learning difficulties could not be an appropriate placement, as long as the conditions for specialist teaching were in place, the school was organised to be 'autism friendly' and the peer group was a suitable one for the child with the ASD (Jordan *et al.* 1999). Just as in mainstream settings, specialist teaching might be available to individuals supported in the ordinary classes in the special school, or there might be a specialist ASD class or a resource base in the school.

Reports from parent surveys, and other research (English and Essex, 2001), show that periods of transition are particularly difficult for children with ASD and their families, and lead to the greatest problems with respect to placement. There are crucial times of transition:

1. from diagnosis to intervention
2. from home and/or pre-school intervention to school
3. from primary to secondary provision
4. from school to adult life/post-school provision

Parents will have a key role at these times but they and students with ASD also need support and guidance to develop transition programmes to ease progress across these boundaries (Emis and Manns, 2004).

12.11 Concluding remarks

In spite of its crucial role in enhancing life opportunities for people on the autism spectrum, education remains poorly researched. This chapter has used data from other areas of research to draw out the educational implications for students with ASD, as well as reviewing some of the few studies on educational provision itself. As other research in ASD illustrates, individual factors remain key and few specific generalisations can be made. Many areas that would benefit from further research have been identified, while recognising that the research question for the educationalist (whether parent or professional) concerns the needs of an individual, rather than making general statements on the value of particular interventions.

12.12 References

American Association of Pediatrics. (2001). Technical Report: The Pediatrician's Role in the Diagnosis and Management of Autistic Spectrum Disorder in Children. *Pediatrics*, **107**: 85–103.

Ausubel, D.P., Novak, J.D., Hanesian, H. (1978). *Educational Psychology: A Cognitive View.* New York: Holt, Rinehart and Winston.

Barnard, J., Prior, A., Potter, D. (2000). *Inclusion and Autism: Is it Working?* London: National Autistic Society.

Baron-Cohen, S. (2004). *The Essential Difference: The Truth About the Male and Female Brain.* London: Penguin Books.

Batten, A., Corbett, M., Withers, L., Yule, R. (2006). *Make School Make Sense*. London: National Autistic Society.

Behrmann, M., Thomas, C., Humphreys, K. (2006). Seeing it differently: visual processing in autism. *Trends in Cognitive Science*, **10**: 258–264.

Belmonte, M.K., Allen, G., Bechel-Mitchener, A., *et al.* (2004). Autism and abnormal development of brain connectivity. *The Journal of Neuroscience*, **24**: 9228–9231.

Biever, C. (2007). Let's meet tomorrow in Second Life. *New Scientist*, **194**: 26–27.

Bogdashina, O. (2003). *Sensory Perceptual Issues in Autism: Different Sensory Perception, Different Perceptual Worlds.* London: Jessica Kingsley.

Boucher, J., Bowler, D. (2008). *Memory in Autism: Theory and Evidence*. Cambridge: Cambridge University Press.

Bruner, J., Feldman, C. (1993). Theories of mind and the problem of autism. In Baron-Cohen, S., Tager-Flusberg, H., Cohen, D.J. (eds.) *Understanding Other Minds: Perspectives from Autism*. Oxford: Oxford University Press, pp. 267–291.

Campbell, C. (2007) An investigation into the effects of exercise on children with autism within the Daily Life Therapy intervention. Msc Thesis, School of Education, University of Birmingham, UK.

Carey, S. (1985). *Conceptual Change in Childhood*. Cambridge, MA: Bradford Books, MIT Press.

Chamberlain, B., Kasari, C., Rotheram-Fuller, E. (2007). Involvement or isolation. The social networks of children with autism in regular classrooms. *Journal of Autism and Developmental Disorders*, **37**: 230–242.

Clark, T. (2005). Autistic savants: educational strategies for the functional application of savant and splinter skills in children with autism and Asperger's disorder. Paper presented at the Australian Autism Research Symposium, 23–24 July 2005, Sydney, Australia: Autism Spectrum.

De Clercq, H. (2003). *Mum, Is That a Human Being or an Animal?* Bristol: Lucky Duck Publishers.

Department for Education and Skills. (2002). *Autistic Spectrum Disorders: Good Practice Guidance*. Nottingham: Department for Education and Skills.

Emis, D., Manns, C. (2004). *Breaking Down Barriers: Practical Strategies for Achieving Successful Transition for Students with Autism and Asperger Syndrome*. Surrey Children's Services.

English, A., Essex, J. (2001). *Carers' Views*. Birmingham: West Midlands Regional Special Educational Needs Partnership.

Frith, U. Happé, F. (1994). Autism: Beyond 'Theory of Mind'. *Cognition*, **50**: 115–132.

Greig, A., MacKay, T. (2005). Asperger's syndrome and cognitive behaviour therapy: new applications for educational psychologists. *Educational and Child Psychology*, **22**: 4–15.

Hepburn, H. (2008). From Beano to bravado, with the help of the little men. *Times Educational Supplement Scotland*, 29 August.

Gerland, G. (1999). *A Real Person*. London: Souvenir Press.

Golding, M.M. (1997). Beyond compliance: the importance of group work in the education of children and young people with autism. In *Autism and Learning: A Guide to Good Practice*. London: David Fulton, pp. 46–60.

Grandin, T. (1995a). How people with autism think. In *Learning and Cognition in Autism*. New York: Plenum Press.

Grandin, T. (1995b). *Thinking in Pictures and Other Reports from my Life with Autism*. New York: Doubleday.

Grandin, T., Scariano, M. (1986). *Emergence, Labelled Autistic*. California: Nevato Press.

Gray, C.A. (1994). *The Social Stories Book*. Arlington, TX: Future Horizons.

Gulsrud, A., Kasari, C., Freeman, S., Paparella, T. (2007). Children with autism's response to novel stimuli while participating in interventions targeting joint attention or symbolic play skills. *Autism: The International Journal of Research and Practice*, **11**: 535–546.

Hegarty, S. (1993). Reviewing the literature on integration. *European Journal of Special Needs Education*, **8**: 194–200.

Heimann, M., Nelson, K.E., Tjus, T., Gilberg, C. (1995). Increasing reading and communication skills in children with autism through an interactive multimedia computer program. *Journal of Autism and Developmental Disorders*, **25**: 459–480.

Herrera, G., Alcantua, F., Jordan, R., *et al.* (2008). Development of symbolic play through the use of virtual reality tools in children with autistic spectrum disorders: two case studies. *Autism: The International Journal of Research and Practice*, **12**: 143–157.

Hesmondhalgh, M., Breakey, C. (2001). *Access and Inclusion for Children with Autistic Spectrum Disorders: Let me in*. London: Jessica Kingsley.

Hobson, P. (1993). *Autism and the Development of Mind*. London: Erlbaum.

Howley, M., Preece, D. (2003). Structured teaching for individuals with visual impairments. *British Journal of Visual Impairment*, **21**: 78–83.

Howlin, P., Goode, S., Hutton, J., Rutter, M. (2004). Adult outcome for children with autism. *Journal of Child Psychology and Psychiatry*, **45**: 212–229.

Howlin, P., Gordon, R.K., Pasco, G., Wade, A., Charman, T. (2007). The effectiveness of Picture Exchange Communication System (PECS) training for teachers of children with autism: a pragmatic group randomized controlled trial. *Journal of Child Psychology and Psychiatry*, **48**: 473–481.

Humphrey, N., Parkinson, G. (2006). Research on interventions for children and young people on the autistic spectrum: a critical perspective. *Journal of Research in Special Educational Needs*, **6**: 76–86.

James, W. (1892). Psychology (Briefer Course). University of Notre Dame Press [Reprinted in 2001 by Dover Publications, New York].

Jones, G., Jordan, R. (2008). Research base for interventions in Autism Spectrum Disorders. In *An Integrated View of Autism*. Oxford: Oxford University Press, pp. 281–302.

Jordan, R. (2001). *Autism with Severe Learning Difficulties*. London: Souvenir Press.

Jordan, R. (2003a). School-based interventions for children with specific learning difficulties. In *Learning and Behavior Problems in Asperger Syndrome*. New York: The Guilford Press, pp. 212–243.

Jordan, R. (2003b). Social Play and autistic spectrum disorders: a perspective on theory, implications and educational approaches. *Autism: The International Journal of Research and Practice*, **7**: 347–360.

Jordan, R. (2004). Educational implications of autism and visual impairment. In *Autism and Blindness: Research and Reflections*. Oxford: Oxford University Press, pp. 142–157.

Jordan, R. (2007a). Using computer assisted learning to aid communication in individuals with autism spectrum disorders [Italian translation]. *Autism Today*, **10**: 13–17.

Jordan, R. (2007b). Computer assisted learning and ASD. *Autism News: Orange County and the Rest of the World*, **4**: 10–13.

Jordan, R. (2008). Narrative ability in children with autism tested through the Karmiloff-Smith (1985) stories. Poster presented at International Meeting for Autism Research, London, 15–17 May.

Jordan, R.R. (2009). Medicalisation of autism spectrum disorders: implications for services? *British Journal of Hospital Medicine*, **70**: 128–129.

Jordan, R., Guldberg, K. (2002). Web wise: new training opportunities in autistic spectrum disorders. *Special Children*, **147**: 3–5.

Jordan, R.R., Powell, S.D. (1994). Whose curriculum? Critical notes on integration and entitlement. *European Journal of Special Needs Education*, **9**: 27–39.

Jordan, R., Macleod, C., Brunton, L. (1999). Making special schools 'specialist': a case study of the provision for pupils with autism in a school for pupils with severe learning difficulties. In *GAP: Good Autism Practice. Occasional Papers 2*. Birmingham: University of Birmingham School of Education, pp. 27–44.

Kientz, M.A., Dunn, W. (1997). Comparison of the performance of children with and without autism on the sensory profile. *American Journal of Occupational Therapy*, **51**: 530–537.

Klinger, L.G., Dawson, G. (2001). Prototype formation in autism. *Development and Psychopathology*, **13**: 111–124.

Konstantareas, M.M., Gravelle, G. (1998). Facilitated communication: the contribution of physical, emotional and mental support. *Autism: The International Journal of Research and Practice*, **2**: 389–414.

Lawson, W. (2003). *Sensory Perceptual Issues in Autism: Different Sensory Perception, Different Perceptual Worlds*. London: Jessica Kingsley.

Losh, M., Capps, L. (2003). Narrative ability in high functioning children with autism or Asperger syndrome. *Journal of Autism and Developmental Disabilities*, **33**: 239–251.

Lovaas, I.O. (1987). Behavioural treatment and normal educational and intellectual functioning in young autistic children. *Journal of Consulting and Clinical Psychology*, **55**: 3–9.

Magiati, I., Charman, T., Howlin, P. (2007). A two year prospective follow-up study of community based early intensive behavioural intervention and specialist nursery provision for children with autism spectrum disorders. *Journal of Child Psychology and Psychiatry*, **48**: 803–812.

McConachie, H., Diggle, T. (2007). Parent implemented early intervention for young children with autism spectrum disorder: a systematic review. *Journal of Evaluation in Clinical Practice*, **13**: 120–129.

Mesibov, G., Howley, M. (2003). *Accessing the Curriculum for Pupils with Autistic Spectrum Disorders*. London: David Fulton.

Miller, L.J. (2008). *Sensational Kids: Hope and Help for Children with Sensory Processing Disorder (SPD)*. Knowledge in Development Foundation. New York: Perigee Books.

Murray, D. (1997). Autism and information technology: therapy with computers. In Powell, S., Jordan, R. (eds.) *Autism and Learning: A Guide to Good Practice*. London: David Fulton, pp. 100–117.

Murray, D., Aspinall, A. (2006). *Using Information Technology to Empower People with Communication Difficulties*. London: David Fulton.

Murray, D., Lesser, M., Lawson, W. (2005). Attention, monotropism and the diagnostic criteria for autism. *Autism: The International Journal of Research and Practice*, **9**: 139–156.

Nader, R., Oberlander, T.F., Chambers, C.T., Craig, K.D. (2004). Expression of pain in children with autism. *The Clinical Journal of Pain*, **20**: 88–97.

National Strategies Schools Development Programme (2009). *Primary and Secondary: Supporting Pupils on the Autism Spectrum – An Interactive Resource*. London, Department of Children, Schools and Families. Available at: www.standards.dcsf.gov.uk/nationalstrategies/inclusion/sen/idp (accessed May 2010).

Odom, S.L., Strain, P.S. (1986). A comparison of peer-initiation and teacher-antecedent interventions for promoting reciprocal social interaction of autistic preschoolers. *Journal of Applied Behaviour Analysis*, **19**: 59–72.

Peeters, T. (1997). *Autism: From Theoretical Understanding to Educational Practice*. London: Whurr.

Peeters, T., Jordan, R. (1999). What makes a good practitioner in the field of autism? In *GAP: Good Autism Practice*. Birmingham: University of Birmingham School of Education.

Perry, A., Condillac, R. (2003). *Evidence-based Practices for Children and Adolescents with ASD: Review of the Literature and Practice Guide*. Toronto: Children's Mental Health Report.

Peterson, D.M. (2002). Mental simulation, dialogical processing and the syndrome of autism. In *Simulation and Knowledge of Action*. Amsterdam: John Benjamins, pp. 185–197.

Piaget, J. (1929). *The Child's Conception of the World*. New York: Harcourt Brace.

Plaisted, K., O'Riordan, M., Baron-Cohen, S. (1998). Enhanced discrimination of novel, highly similar stimuli by adults with autism during a perceptual learning task. *Journal of Child Psychology and Psychiatry*, **39**: 765–775.

Preece, D., Jordan, R. (2007). Short breaks services for children with autistic spectrum disorders: factors associated with service use and non-use. *Journal of Autism and Developmental Disorders*, **37**: 374–385.

Premack, D., Collier, G.H. (1962). Analysis of non-reinforcement variables affecting response probability. *Psychological Monographs*, **76**: 1–20.

Randall, P., Parker, J. (1999). *Supporting Families of Children with Autism*. Chichester: Wiley and Sons.

Remington, B., Hastings, R.P., Kovshoff, K., *et al.* (2007). Early intensive behavioral intervention: outcomes for children with autism and their parents after two years. *American Journal of Mental Retardation*, **112**: 418–438.

Reynolds, S., Lane, J. (2008). Diagnostic validity of sensory over-responsivity: a review of the literature and case reports. *Journal of Autism and Developmental Disorders*, **38**: 516–529.

Roeyers, S.H. (1995). A peer-mediated proximity intervention to facilitate the social interactions of children with a pervasive developmental disorder. *British Journal of Special Education*, **22**: 161–164.

Rogers, S.J., Ozonoff, S. (2005). Annotation: What do we know about sensory dysfunction in autism? A critical review of the empirical evidence. *Journal of Child Psychology and Psychiatry*, **46**: 1255–1268.

Sherratt, D., Peter, M. (2002). *Developing Play and Drama in Children with Autistic Spectrum Disorders*. London: David Fulton.

Shore, S. (2003). *Beyond the Wall: Personal Experiences with Autism and Asperger Syndrome*, 2nd edn. New York: Autism Asperger Publications.

Simpson, R.L., Boer-Ott, S.R., Smith-Myles, B. (2003). Inclusion of learners with autism spectrum disorders in general education settings. *Topics in Language Disorders*, **23**: 116–133.

Smock, C. (1955). The influence of stress on the perception of incongruity. *Journal of Abnormal and Social Psychology*, **50**: 354–356.

Spreckley, M., Boyd, R. (2007). Efficacy of applied behavioural intervention for pre-school children with autism on cognitive, behavioural and language outcomes: a systematic review and meta analysis. Melbourne, Australia: NHS Reviews.

Strain, P.S., Hayson, M. (2000). The need for longitudinal intensive social skill intervention: LEAP follow-up outcomes for children with autism. *Topics in Early Childhood Special Education*, **20**: 116–122.

Sturmey, P. (2003). Video technology and persons with autism and other developmental disabilities: an emerging technology for PBS. *Journal of Positive Behavior Interventions*, **5**: 3–4.

Tauber, R. (1986). The negative side of praise and the positive side of negative reinforcement. *Durham and Newcastle Research Review*, **10**: 299–302.

United Nations Educational Scientific and Cultural Organization (UNESCO). (1994). *The Salamanca Statement and Framework for Action on Special Needs Education World Conference on Special Needs Education: Access and Equality*. Salamanca, Spain: UNESCO.

Van Lang, N.D.J., Boomsma, A., Sytema, S., *et al.* (2006). Structural equation analysis of a hypothesized symptom model in the autism spectrum. *Journal of Child Psychology and Psychiatry*, **47**: 37–44.

Vermeulen, P. (2001). *Autistic Thinking: This is the Title*. London: Jessica Kingsley.

Vygotsky, L.S. (1962). *Thought and Language*. New York: MIT Press.

Whitaker, P., Barratt, P., Joy, H., Potter, M., Thomas, G. (1998). Children with autism and peer group support: using 'Circles of Friends'. *British Journal of Special Education*, **25**: 60–64.

Wing, L. (1996). *The Autistic Spectrum: A Guide for Parents and Professionals*. London: Constable.

Wing, L., Gould, J. (1979). Severe impairments of social interaction and associated abnormalities in children: epidemiology and classification. *Journal of Autism and Developmental Disorders*, **9**: 11–29.

Yang, T-R., Wolfberg, P.J., Wu, S-CH., Hwu, P-Y. (2003). Supporting children on the autism spectrum in peer play at home and in school: piloting the integrated peer groups model in Taiwan. *Autism: The International Journal of Research and Practice*, **7**: 437–454.

Index

Note: The following abbreviations are used: ADHD for attention deficit hyperactivity disorder; ASD for Autism Spectrum Disorders; ASD-LI for autistic spectrum disorders with language impairment; CNVs for copy number variations; EEG for Electro-encephalography; fMRI for functional magnetic resonance imaging; HFA for high-functioning autism; MEG for magnetoencephalography; MRI for magnetic resonance imaging.